Thyroid FNA Cytology
Differential Diagnoses & Pitfalls

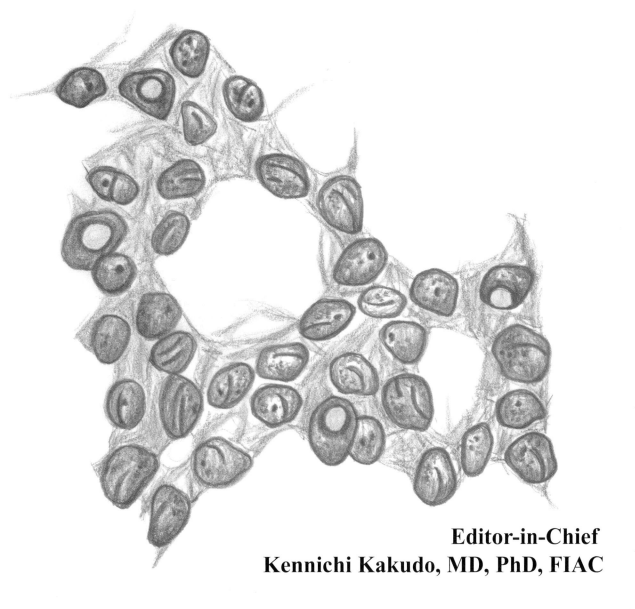

Editor-in-Chief
Kennichi Kakudo, MD, PhD, FIAC

Associate Editor
Zhiyan Liu, MD, PhD

Associate Editor
Mitsuyoshi Hirokawa, MD, PhD, FIAC

Two illustrations in the front book cover and back are artworks by Emiko Taniguchi, CT, CTIAC.

Thyroid FNA Cytology: Differential Diagnoses and Pitfalls

Editor-in-Chief:

Kennichi Kakudo, MD, PhD, FIAC

Professor
Department of Pathology, Nara Hospital
Kindai University Faculty of Medicine
Nara, Japan
kakudo@thyroid.jp

Associate Editor:

Zhiyan Liu, MD, PhD

Associate Professor
Department of Pathology
Shandong University School of Medicine
Shandong, China
zhiyanliu@sdu.edu.cn

Associate Editor:

Mitsuyoshi Hirokawa, MD, PhD, FIAC

Department of Diagnostic Pathology and Cytology
Kuma Hospital
Kobe, Japan
mhirokawa@kuma-h.or.jp

Printed by ONO KOUSOKU INSATSU CO.,LTD.
Published by Kakudo Medical Education
Copyright©2016 Kakudo Medical Education
Distributed by BookWay GLOBAL (https://bookway-global.com/)

Contents

Preface to Print Edition
  Thyroid FNA Cytology: Differential Diagnoses and Pitfalls
  Kennichi Kakudo, Zhiyan Liu and Mitsuyoshi Hirakawa 8

Book review   N. Paul Ohori 11

List of Frequently Used Abbreviations in This Book.. 12

Chapter 1: Factors Impacting Thyroid Fine Needle Aspiration Cytology and the Algorithm for Cytological Diagnosis
Kennichi Kakudo.. 14

Chapter 2: Comparison of Diagnostic Systems: The American, British, Italian, and Japanese Reporting Systems of Thyroid FNA Cytology
Kennichi Kakudo, Zhiyan Liu and Kaori Kameyama........................ 23

Chapter 3: Pitfalls in the Diagnosis of Papillary Thyroid Carcinoma
Xin Jing and Claire W. Michael 30

Chapter 4: Risk Stratification of Cases with Papillary Thyroid Carcinoma Type Nuclear Features into Low-risk, High-risk, and Malignancy Categories.
Zhiyan Liu and Kennichi Kakudo 39

Chapter 5: Diagnostic Criteria of AUS/FLUS in the Bethesda Reporting System and the Low-risk Indeterminate Category
Yubo Ren, Zhiyan Liu and Kennichi Kakudo 47

Chapter 6: The New Tumor Entity "NIFTP (Non-invasive Follicular Thyroid Neoplasm with Papillary-like Nuclear Features)" and the Conventional Papillary Carcinoma
Zhiyan Liu, Shinya Satoh and Kennichi Kakudo 61

Chapter 7: Cyst or Cystic Papillary Carcinoma
Kayoko Higuchi 69

Chapter 8: Tall Cell Variant of Papillary Thyroid Carcinoma vs. Conventional Papillary Thyroid Carcinoma
Miyoko Higuchi 78

Chapter 9: Cribriform Variant of Papillary Thyroid Carcinoma
Ayana Suzuki 83

Chapter 10: Papillary Carcinoma, Columnar Cell Variant - Diagnostic Pitfalls and Differential Diagnoses
Chiung-Ru Lai... 93

Chapter 11:	**Subacute Thyroiditis or Papillary Carcinoma** Tiesheng Wang 99	
Chapter 12:	**Hyalinizing Trabecular Tumor vs. Papillary Thyroid Carcinoma** Mitsuyoshi Hirokawa and Ayana Suzuki...................... 107	
Chapter 13:	**Hashimoto's Thyroiditis or Papillary Carcinoma** Yun Zhu and Tiesheng Wang 115	
Chapter 14:	**MALT Lymphoma vs. Hashimoto Thyroiditis** Mitsuyoshi Hirokawa and Ayana Suzuki...................... 125	
Chapter 15:	**Medullary (C Cell) Thyroid Carcinoma or Oxyphilic Follicular Neoplasms** Yun Zhu and Tiesheng Wang 132	
Chapter 16:	**Medullary (C Cell) Carcinoma or Metastatic Carcinoma to Thyroid** Junko Maruta 142	
Chapter 17:	**Intrathyroid Epithelial Thymoma/Carcinoma Showing Thymus-like Differentiation vs. Poorly Differentiated Carcinoma** Mitsuyoshi Hirokawa and Ayana Suzuki...................... 151	
Chapter 18:	**Parathyroid Adenoma and Its Differential Diagnoses** Kayoko Higuchi and Nami Takada 158	
Chapter 19:	**Risk-Classification of Follicular Pattern Lesions in Thyroid FNA Cytology (Part 1: Benign Follicular Pattern Lesions or Follicular Neoplasms)** Kennichi Kakudo, Emiko Taniguchi, Shinya Satoh and Kaori Kameyama 168	
Chapter 20:	**Risk-Classification of Follicular Pattern Lesions in Thyroid FNA Cytology (Part 2: Follicular Adenoma or Follicular Carcinoma)** Kennichi Kakudo, Kaori Kameyama, Keiko Inomata and Shinya Satoh 175	
Chapter 21:	**Poorly Differentiated Carcinoma vs. Well Differentiated Carcinoma** Mitsuyoshi Hirokawa and Ayana Suzuki...................... 185	
Chapter 22:	**Metastatic Renal Cell Carcinoma vs. Follicular Neoplasm** Ayana Suzuki 192	
Chapter 23:	**Biochemical Tests of Fine-needle Aspirate as an Adjunct to Cytologic Diagnosis for Patients with Thyroid Cancer or Primary Hyperparathyroidism** Shinya Satoh, Hiroyuki Yamashita and Kennichi Kakudo 198	
Chapter 24:	**Infectious Thyroiditis** Claire W. Michael and Xin Jing 207	

Chapter 25:	Necrotic Background in Thyroid FNA Cytology: Anaplastic Transformation or Infarction in Papillary Carcinoma Kennichi Kakudo, Shinya Satoh, Yusuke Mori, Hiroyuki Yamashita 213
Chapter 26:	Complications of Fine Needle Aspiration Biopsy Yasuhiro Ito and Mitsuyoshi Hirokawa 220
Chapter 27:	Cytological Features of Papillary Carcinoma on LBC Preparation, Comparison with Conventional Preparation Ayana Suzuki 225
Chapter 28:	Pitfalls in Immunocytochemical Study Using Fine Needle Aspiration Samples. Junko Maruta 232
Chapter 29:	Pitfalls in Molecular-based Diagnosis Using Thyroid Aspirates Toru Takano 237
Chapter 30:	Techniques of Thyroid Fine-Needle Aspiration Hongxun Wu 243
Chapter 31:	Standard and Rapid Stains in Fine-Needle Aspiration Cytology and Rapid On-Site Evaluation Takashi Koshikawa 251
Chapter 32:	Case Study and Mini-Tests (Multiple choice questions and differential diagnosis) Kennichi Kakudo, Masahiko Ura, Keiko Inomata, Ayana Suzuki, Yun Zhu, Zhiyan Liu, Yubo Ren, Xin Jing, and Shinya Satoh 255

Suppemental Chapter 1
   The Italian Reporting System for Thyroid Cytology
   Guido Fadda 276

Suppemental Chapter 2
   How to Follow Fine-needle Aspiration Biopsy-Proven Benign Thyroid Nodules, Active Surveillance *vs.* Diagnostic Lobectomy for Indeterminate Nodules and Individualized Treatments for Low-risk Thyroid Carcinomas
   Kennichi Kakudo 283

Suppemental Chapter 3
   Cyst Fluid Only (CFO)
   Nami Takada 293

Suppemental Chapter 4
   Thyroglossal Duct Cyst and Other Ectopic Thyroid Tissue in the Neck
   Andrey Bychkov 297

Suppemental Chapter 5
 Diagnostic Clues for Thyroid Fine Needle Aspiration Cytology
 Aki Ito and Ayana Suzuki 309

Contributors
(Alphabetical List)

Andrey Bychkov, MD PhD
Department of Pathology, Faculty of
Medicine, Chulalongkorn University,
Bangkok, Thailand
dr_bychkov@mail.com

Guida Fadda, MD, MIAC
Division of Anatomic Pathology and
Histology,
Catholic University,
Foundation "Agostino Gemelli"
University Hospital,
Rome, Italy
guido.fadda@unicatt.it

Kayoko Higuchi, MD, PhD, FIAC
Section of Anatomic Pathology
Aizawa Hospital
Matsumoto, Japan
byori-dr@ai-hosp.or.jp

Miyoko Higuchi, CT, IAC
Department of Laboratory Science
Kuma Hospital
Kobe, Japan
higuchi01@kuma-h.or.jp

Mitsuyoshi Hirokawa, MD, FIAC
Department of Diagnostic Pathology and
Cytology, Kuma Hospital
Kobe, Japan
mhirokawa@kuma-h.or.jp

Keiko Inomata, PhD
Department of Laboratory Medicine
Yamashita Thyroid and Parathyroid Clinic
Fukuoka, Japan
kinomata@kojosen.com

Aki Ito, CT
Department of Laboratory Science,
Kuma Hospital, Kobe, Japan
akiito@kuma-h.or.jp

Yasuhiro Ito, MD, PhD
Department of Surgery
Kuma Hospital
Kobe, Japan
ito01@kuma-h.or.jp

Xin Jing, MD
Department of Pathology
University of Michigan
Ann Arbor, Michigan, USA
xinjing@med.umich.edu

Kennichi Kakudo, MD, PhD, FIAC
Department of Pathology, Nara Hospital
Kindai University Faculty of Medicine
Nara, Japan
kakudo@thyroid.jp

Kaori Kameyama, MD, PhD
Division of Diagnostic Pathology
Keio University School of Medicine
Tokyo, Japan
kameyama@a5.keio.jp

Takashi Koshikawa, MD, PhD, FIAC
Department of Pathology
Shubun University Faculty of Nursing
Aichi, Japan
koshikawa.t@shubun.ac.jp

Chiung-Ru Lai, MD, FIAC
Department of Pathology
Taipei Veterans General Hospital
Taipei, Taiwan
crlai@vghtpe.gov.tw

Zhiyan Liu, MD, PhD
Department of Pathology
Shandong University School of Medicine
Shandong, China
zhiyanliu@sdu.edu.cn

Junko Maruta, CT, PhD
Noguchi Thyroid Clinic and Hospital Foundation
Oita, Japan
junko@noguchi-med.or.jp

Claire W. Michael, MD
Department of Pathology
University Hospitals Case Medical Center
Case Western Reserve University
Cleveland, OH, USA
claire.michael@uhhospitals.org

Yusuke Mori, MD, PhD
Department of Endocrine Surgery
Yamashita Thyroid and Parathyroid Clinic
Fukuoka, Japan
mori@kojosen.com

Yubo Ren, MD
Department of Pathology
Liaocheng People's Hospital,
Shandong, China
renli676312@163.com

Shinya Satoh, MD, PhD
Department of Endocrine Surgery
Yamashita Thyroid and Parathyroid Clinic
Fukuoka, Japan
shinya.satoh.48128@gmail.com

Ayana Suzuki, CT, CTIAC
Department of Laboratory Science
Kuma Hospital
Kobe, Japan
suzuki01@kuma-h.or.jp

Nami Takada, CT
Department of Laboratory Science
Kuma Hospital
Kobe, Japan
takada01@kuma-h.or.jp

Toru Takano, MD, PhD
Department of Metabolic Medicine
Osaka University
Graduate School of Medicine
Osaka, Japan
ttakano@labo.med.osaka-u.ac.jp

Emiko Taniguchi, CT, CTIAC
Formerly Chief Cytotechnologist (retired)
Department of Human Pathology
Wakayama Medical University
Wakayama, Japan
emi5106@yahoo.co.jp

Masahiko Ura, CT, CTIAC
Department of Pathology
Nara Hospital
Kindai University Faculty of Medicine
Nara, Japan
kensa@nara.med.kindai.ac.jp

Tiesheng Wang, MD
Department of Pathology
Jiangsu Institute of Nuclear Medicine
Wuxi, China.
1246513715@qq.com

Hongxun Wu, MD
Department of Ultrasound
Jiangsu Institute of Nuclear Medicine
Wuxi, China
wuhongxun@jsinm.org

Hiroyuki Yamashita, MD, PhD
Department of Endocrine Surgery
Yamashita Thyroid and Parathyroid Clinic
Fukuoka, Japan
yamaftc@kojosen.com

Yun Zhu, MD
Department of Pathology
Jiangsu Institute of Nuclear Medicine
Wuxi, China.
zhuyun@jsinm.org

Preface to Print Edition
Thyroid FNA Cytology: Differential Diagnoses and Pitfalls

We are happy to provide you a print edition of, "Thyroid FNA Cytology: Differential Diagnoses and Pitfalls". As there is a file size limit in the eBook edition, some important illustrations were deleted and all illustrations in the eBook edition were reduced in quality. To circumvent these conditions, the print edition was published. In this print edition, we provide you with all of the original illustrations in high quality and have incorporated some more illustrations which were deleted from the eBook edition.

The editors proudly announce that this is the first and only textbook for thyroid FNA cytology that incorporates borderline tumor categories in thyroid tumor classification, which are hyalinizing trabecular adenoma identified by Carney et al.(1), UMP (well differentiated tumor of uncertain malignant potential and follicular tumor of uncertain malignant potential) proposed by Williams (2), the recent reclassification of some indolent tumors currently classified as carcinoma into the borderline tumor category proposed by Kakudo et al. (3-7) and NIFTP (non-invasive follicular thyroid neoplasm with papillary-like nuclear features), a nomenclature revision of non-invasive encapsulated follicular variant papillary thyroid carcinoma proposed by Nikiforov et al. (8-15).

The E-Book edition was the first English-language textbook of thyroid FNA cytology textbook published in Asia. In the print edition, we invited some more authors, and we would like to highlight the new supplementary chapters only available in this print edition. Finally, this print edition is a more comprehensive and international textbook than our eBook edition, "Thyroid FNA Cytology: Differential Diagnoses and Pitfalls". The editors of the print edition, "Thyroid FNA Cytology: Differential Diagnoses and Pitfalls" thank all authors sincerely and appreciate their great efforts and contributions to this book.

The eBook version (reduced size version) is also available from the S&S Publications and distributed by Smashwords (https://www.smashwords.com/books/view/655745).

Chief Editor: Kennichi Kakudo, MD, PhD, FIAC
Department of Pathology, Nara Hospital
Kindai University Faculty of Medicine
Professor Emeritus, Wakayama Medical University, Japan

Associate Editor: Zhiyan Liu, MD, PhD
Department of Pathology and Pathophysiology
Shandong University School of Medicine, China

Associate Editor: Mitsuyoshi Hirokawa, MD, PhD, FIAC
Department of Pathology
Kuma Hospital, Kobe, Japan

References:

1. Carney JA, Hirokawa M, Lloyd RV, et al. Hyalinizing trabecular tumors of the thyroid gland are almost all benign. Am J Surg Pathol 2008; 32:1877-89.
2. Williams ED. Guest editorial: Two proposals regarding the terminology of thyroid tumors. Int J Surg Pathol 2000; 8:181-183.
3. Kakudo K, Bai Y, Katayama S et al: Classification of follicular cell trumors of thyroid gland: Analysis involving Japanese patients from one institute. Patholo Int 2009; 59:359-357.
4. Liu Z, Zhou G, Nakamura M, et al. Encapsulated follicular thyroid tumor with equivocal nuclear changes, so-called well-differentiated tumor of uncertain malignant potential: a morphological, immunohistochemical, and molecular appraisal. Cancer Sci 2011; 102:288-294.
5. Kakudo K, Bai Y, Liu Z et al: Classification of thyroid follicular cell tumors: with special reference to borderline lesions. Endocrine J 2012; 59:1-12.
6. Kakudo K, Bai Y, Liu Z, et al. Encapsulated papillary thyroid carcinoma, follicular variant: A misnomer. Pathol Int 2012; 62:155-60.
7. Nishigami K, Liu Z, Taniguchi E, et al. Cytological features of well-differentiated tumors of uncertain malignant potential: Indeterminate cytology and WDT-UMP. Endocrine J 2012; 59:483-7.
8. Liu J, Singh B, Tallini G, et al. Follicular variant of papillary carcinoma. A clinicopathologic study of a problematic entity. Cancer 2006; 107:1255-64.
9. Rivera M, Ricarte-Filho J, Knauf J, et al. Encapsulated papillary thyroid carcinoma: A clinic-pathologic study of 106 cases with emphasis on its morphologic subtypes (histologic growth pattern). Mod Pathol 2010; 23:1191-200.
10. Ganly I, Wang L, Tuttle RM, et al. Invasion rather than nuclear features correlates with outcome in encapsulated follicular tumors: further evidence for the reclassification of the encapsulated papillary thyroid carcinoma follicular variant. Hum Pathol 2015; 46:657-64.
11. Nikiforov Y, Seethala RR, Tallini G, et al. Nomenclature revision for encapsulated follicular variant of papillary thyroid carcinoma: A paradigm shift to reduce overtreatment of indolent tumors. JAMA Oncol, 2016, doi: 10.1001/jamaoncol.2016.0386 [Epub ahead of print].
12. Strickland KC, Howitt BE, Marquesee E, et al. The impact of non-invasive follicular variant of papillary thyroid carcinoma on rates of malignancy for fine-needle aspiration diagnostic categories. Thyroid 2015; 25:987-92.
13. Liu X, Medici M, Kwong N, et al. Bethesda categorization of thyroid nodule cytology and prediction of thyroid cancer type and prognosis. Thyroid 2015; [Epub ahead of print]
14. Faquin WC, Wong LQ, Afrogheh AH, et al. Impact of reclassifying noninvasive follicular variant of papillary thyroid carcinoma on the risk of malignancy in the Bethesda system for reporting thyroid cytopathology. Cancer Cytopathol 2015 Oct 12. doi: 10.1002/cncy.21631. [Epub ahead of print]
15. Maletta F, Massa F, Torregrossa L et al. Cytological features of "noninvasive follicular thyroid neoplasm with papillary-like nuclear features" and their correlation with tumor histology. Hum Pathol 2016, doi: 10.1016/j.humpath.2016.03.014. [Epub ahead of print]

Preface to eBook Edition
Thyroid FNA Cytology: Differential Diagnoses and Pitfalls

Thyroid fine needle aspiration (FNA) cytology is the most widely used clinical test for patients with thyroid nodules. This can be attributed to its accuracy and reliability in identifying high-risk patients who should undergo surgical treatments. It has been nearly 10 years since the National Cancer Institute of the United States of America proposed a reporting system for thyroid FNA cytology (1). Following this recommendation, Italy, England, and Japan developed their own reporting systems comparable with the American (Bethesda) system (2-4). These diagnostic systems have contributed to significantly better performance in thyroid cytology and improved communication among the different cytology practices. All four diagnostic systems focus on the standardization of 1) diagnostic terminologies, 2) clinical management, and 3) risk of malignancy. However, there remain a few of pitfalls that are important to address for cytopathologists to achieve a good performance in their practice. This E-Book, "Thyroid FNA Cytology: Differential Diagnoses and Pitfalls", focuses on how to avoid such pitfalls in thyroid FNA cytology. Good performance in your practice can only be achieved when you become familiar with these pitfalls and differential diagnoses in detail. The thyroid experts included in this E-Book demonstrate how to bypass these pitfalls using beautiful case presentations and detailed differential diagnoses based on their rich experiences and evidences from the literature. We believe this approach is essential for establishing high level performance in thyroid FNA cytology, regardless of the diagnostic system used.

This E-Book is the first English textbook of thyroid FNA cytology published in Asia, and all authors are of Asian background. The editors thank all authors sincerely and appreciate their great efforts on and contribution to this E-Book.

Chief Editor: Kennichi Kakudo, MD, PhD, FIAC

Associate Editor: Zhiyan Liu, MD, PhD

Associate Editor: Mitsuyoshi Hirokawa, MD, PhD, FIAC

References

1. Ali SZ and Cibas ES (ed). The Bethesda system for reporting thyroid cytopathology. Definitions, criteria and explanatory notes. 2010, Springer, New York, USA.
2. Fadda G, Basolo F, Bondi A, et al. Cytological classification of thyroid nodules. Proposal of the SIAPEC-IAP Italian consensus working group. Pathologica 2010; 102:405-6.
3. Lobo C, McQueen A, Beale T, et al. The UK Royal College of Pathologists thyroid fine-needle aspiration diagnostic classification is a robust tool for the clinical management of abnormal thyroid nodules. Acta Cytol 2011; 55:499-506.
4. Kakudo K, Kameyama K, Miyauchi A, et al. Introducing the reporting system for thyroid fine-needle aspiration cytology according to the new guidelines of the Japan Thyroid Association. Endocr J 2014; 61:539-52.

Book review

This book takes an unconventional but pragmatic approach of addressing many key issues in thyroid cytopathology through the use of case studies in many chapters. I believe this format is effective in engaging the reader to understand the subspecialty practice of thyroid cytopathology. The text is authored by many well-known thyroid cytologists and pathologists, mostly from Asia. The first few chapters discuss some key principles regarding thyroid cytopathology. The differences in the approaches to thyroid FNA cytology in various countries such as the USA, UK, Italy, and Japan are detailed nicely and are very insightful; they raise questions as to whether the differences are cultural or responses to external factors (e.g. medical-legal environment in the USA). While the expectation of having everyone practice in exactly the same manner globally may be too idealistic, better understanding of our similarities and differences bring us closer together.

The chapters based on case studies are organized systematically into sections on clinical summary, radiologic findings (with ultrasound images), cytologic findings, differential diagnosis, gross and histopathologic diagnosis, discussion, and references. The images are effective in addressing the main points of the authors. Sample chapter headings include *Diagnostic Criteria of AUS/FLUS, NIFTP (Non-invasive Follicular Thyroid Neoplasm with Papillary-like Nuclear Features) and Conventional Papillary Carcinoma, Hyalinizing Trabecular Tumor vs. Papillary Thyroid Carcinoma, Parathyroid Adenoma and Its Differential Diagnosis, and Poorly Differentiated Carcinoma vs. Well Differentiated Carcinoma.* In some chapters, the differential diagnoses are based on the cytologic findings, whereas in other chapters, they are based on the histologic findings of the resected lesion. In either case, pitfalls are discussed thoroughly.

The last chapters of this book cover the technical aspects of thyroid cytology. These include procedural complications, liquid-based cytology, immunocytochemistry, molecular diagnosis, FNA techniques, and staining procedures. As for the case study chapters, the images illustrate the authors' points very effectively. For some chapters, the technical procedures may be based primarily on the author's experience. Inquisitive readers are encouraged to broaden their scope by surveying the up-to-date references provided by the authors.

In summary, I recommend this book for residents and fellows in pathology training as well as those practicing thyroid cytopathology. The selection of chapter titles is excellent and addresses many common dilemmas in daily practice. Case examples are well illustrated and the thyroid cytology practitioners should find this book to be a valuable reference. While the reader may have to adjust to the writing style of some authors, the text is relatively easy to follow. Since some topics (e.g. diagnosis of AUS/FLUS) are controversial with many differing opinions, readers may want to use the text as a foundation and use the up-to-date references to build on their own understanding of the topics.

N. Paul Ohori, M.D.
Department of Pathology
University of Pittsburgh Medical Center
Pittsburgh, Pennsylvania, USA

List of Frequently Used Abbreviations in This Book

ATA:	The American Thyroid Association
ATC:	Anaplastic Thyroid Carcinoma (Undifferentiated Carcinoma)
AUS:	Atypia of Undetermined Significance
BRAF:	B-Raf Proto-oncogene, Serine/Threonine Kinase
CEA:	Carcinoembryonic Antigen
CNB:	Core Needle Biopsy (Core Biopsy)
CFO:	Cyst Flued Only
CT:	Computed Tomography
CV-PTC:	Cribriform Variant of Papillary Thyroid Carcinoma
FA:	Follicular Adenoma
FLUS:	Follicular Lesion of Undetermined Significance
FNA:	Fine Needle Aspiration
FNAC:	Fine-Needle Aspiration Cytology
FN/HCN:	Follicular Neoplasm/Hurthle Cell Neoplasm
FN/SFN:	Follicular Neoplasm/Suspicious Follicular Neoplasm
FT-UMP:	Follicular Tumor of Uncertain Malignant Potential
fT3:	free T3
fT4:	free T4
FTC:	Follicular Thyroid Carcinoma
FVPTC:	Follicular Variant Papillary Thyroid Carcinoma
HCN:	Hurthle Cell Neoplasm
HE:	Hematoxylin and Eosin
HT:	Hashimoto's Thyroiditis
IHC:	Immunohistochemical Stain
IL:	Indeterminate Lesion
ITET/CASTLE:	Intrathyroid Epithelial Thymoma/Carcinoma Showing Thymus-like Differentiation
LBC:	Liquid-Based Cytology
LT:	Lymphocytic Thyroiditis
MGG:	May Gruenwalds Giewsa
ML:	Malignant Lymphoma
MTC:	Medullary Thyroid Cancer or C Cell Carcinoma
N/C:	Nuclear/Cytoplasmic
NCI:	Nuclear Cytoplasmic Inclusions (Pseudoinclusions), Intranuclear Cytoplasmic Inclusions (Pseudoinclusions)
ND:	Non Diagnostic
NIFTP:	Non-Invasive Follicular Thyroid Neoplasm with Papillary-like Nuclear Features
PAP:	Papanicolaou
PAX8:	Paired Box Gene 8
PDC:	Poorly Differentiated Carcinoma
PHPT:	Primary Hyperparathyroidism
PMC:	Papillary Microcarcinoma
PTC:	Papillary Thyroid Carcinoma
PTC-N:	Papillary Thyroid Carcinoma Type Nuclear Features (Changes)
PTH:	Parathyroid Hormone
PTMC:	Papillary Thyroid Microcarcinoma

RAI:	Radioactive Iodine
ROM:	Risk of Malignancy
ROSE	Rapid On-site Evaluation
SM:	Suspicious for Malignancy
TBSRTC:	The Bethesda System for Reporting Thyroid Cytopathology
TG:	Thyroglobulin
TGD:	Thyroglossal Duct
TPO:	Thyroid Peroxidase
TSH:	Thyroid Stimulating Hormone or Thyrotropin
TTF1:	Thyroid Transcription Factor 1
UC:	Undifferentiated Carcinoma (Anaplastic Thyroid Carcinoma)
US:	Ultrasonography
WHAFFT:	Worrisome Histologic Alterations Following Fine needle aspiration of the Thyroid
WDT-UB:	Well Differentiated Tumor of Uncertain Behavior
WDT-UMP:	Well Differentiated Tumor of Uncertain Malignant Potential
WHO:	World Health Organization

Chapter 1

Factors Impacting Thyroid Fine Needle Aspiration Cytology and the Algorithm for Cytological Diagnosis

Kennichi Kakudo

1. **The American Thyroid Association (ATA) Management Guidelines and Thyroid Fine Needle Aspiration (FNA) Cytology**

   The ATA guidelines for thyroid nodules and differentiated thyroid carcinomas are the most well-known and established guidelines, with a new edition published recently (1). Recommendations (R7 to R24) regarding FNA cytology are also included in the 2015 ATA guidelines (1). Recommendation 8 suggests performing FNA cytology if the thyroid nodule is larger than 1 cm and with intermediate or highly suspicious pattern on sonography. Diagnostic FNA cytology is not recommended for thyroid nodules that are either purely cystic or smaller than 1 cm (please refer to Supplemental Chapter 3). Thus, papillary microcarcinomas smaller than 1 cm in diameter are clinically followed without cytological confirmation of malignancy. According to the 2015 ATA guidelines, a higher risk of malignancy should be suspected in cystic FNA samples from the USA than those from other countries. This is because according to the ATA guidelines, cystic FNA samples are often taken from the solid portion (high-risk for cystic papillary thyroid carcinoma [PTC]) of the cystic nodule, and purely cystic nodules should be excluded from FNA examination. The author of this textbook wishes cytopathologists, particularly those practicing in other geographic areas, to bear in mind that the risk of malignancy of cystic FNA samples from the American system may be different from the reader's samples, in which a significant number of samples are from purely cystic lesions (extremely low risk of malignancy).

   Furthermore, important improvements in the clinical management of AUS/FLUS (low-risk indeterminate) and FN/SFN (high-risk indeterminate) nodules have been included in the 2015 ATA guidelines. Although diagnostic surgery is the traditional and established standard for FN/SFN nodules in all clinical guidelines from Western countries, additional preoperative risk stratification is recommended for SN/SFN nodules in the 2015 ATA guidelines. According to Recommendation 16, the weak recommendation with moderate-quality evidence in FN/SFN cytology suggests molecular testing for supplementation of malignancy risk assessment data in lieu of proceeding directly with surgery, after consideration of clinical and sonographic features. Therefore, a diagnosis of FN/SFN on thyroid FNA cytology is no longer a compulsory order of immediate diagnostic surgery from cytopathologists to clinical doctors. In Recommendation 15, molecular testing was added as a supplement in risk assessment for AUS/FLUS nodules, in addition to the use of repeat FNA cytology and assessment of clinical and sonographic features. This triage of patients with AUS/FLUS or FN/SFN nodules is already a standard practice in Asian countries, and more than half of these patients with benign clinical tests are followed without surgical intervention. Higher risks of malignancy in surgically treated patients with AUS/FLUS or FN/SFN nodules have been reported in Korea (2, 3), China (4), and Japan (5-9), where risk stratification using cytological sub-classification, clinical tests, sonographic risk-stratification, and molecular analyses are usually performed for patients with indeterminate nodules. The increased role of conservative management using molecular testing and clinical/radiologic risk stratification are emphasized in the 2015 ATA clinical guidelines (1).

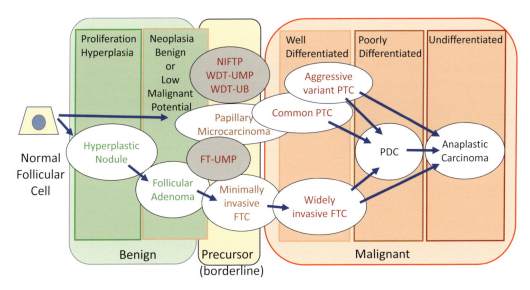

Figure 1. Progression and dedifferentiation of follicular cell neoplasia and precursor tumors in the multistep carcinogenesis theory. FTC: follicular thyroid carcinoma; FT-UMP: follicular tumor of uncertain malignant potential; NIFTP: non-invasive follicular thyroid neoplasm with papillary-like nuclear features; PTC: papillary thyroid carcinoma; PDC: poorly differentiated carcinoma; WDT-UB: well-differentiated tumor of uncertain behavior; WDT-UMP: well-differentiated tumor of uncertain malignant potential.

2. The New Classification of Thyroid Tumors in the 4th Edition (2017) of the WHO Classification of Endocrine Organs

The WHO classification of tumors serves as an international standard for histopathologic diagnosis and clinical practice for neoplastic diseases in all organ systems. The 3rd edition of endocrine tumor classification is under revision, and the 4th edition WHO classification of endocrine organs will be published in 2017. The thyroid tumors included in the contents of the 4th edition (Table 1) are essentially the same as those of the 3rd edition, but with one significant change. The 4th edition introduces a precursor tumor category in the classification schema of follicular cell neoplasia to better adhere to the multistep carcinogenesis theory (Figure 1). This category is the non-invasive follicular thyroid neoplasm with papillary-like nuclear features (NIFTP), introduced by Nikiforov et al. in 2016, and was formerly named the well-differentiated tumor of uncertain malignant potential (WDT-UMP) by Williams in 2000, or the well-differentiated tumor with uncertain behavior (WDT-UB) by Liu *et al.* in 2011 (10-12). All 109 cases of NIFTP in a patient series by Nikiforov *et al.* showed a benign course, with average follow-up of more than 14 years after surgery alone (without RAI treatments) (10). NIFTP is an encapsulated, follicular pattern tumor characterized by the worrisome nuclear features of papillary carcinoma, and with no invasion. This type of tumor shows significant observer disagreement among pathologists (13-15), and is usually classified as a malignant tumor (encapsulated follicular variant PTC without invasion) in Western practice, resulting in it being the most popular (10-30%) variant of PTC. While the so-called encapsulated follicular variant PTC without invasion is a rare malignancy (<1%) in Asian practice, the majority of NIFTPs are classified as benign hyperplastic nodules or follicular adenomas when evidence of invasion is not discernible (12). The use of a lower cut-off threshold in judging PTC type nuclear features (PTC-N) by Western cytopathologists compared with Asian cytopathologists may be the cause for such an increased number of malignant diagnoses (encapsulated follicular variant PTC), both histological and cytological, in Western practice. This was further demonstrated in recent publications from the USA, in which a significant number of malignancies in the indeterminate categories were shown to be NIFTP, and if NIFTP was no longer categorized as a malignant tumor, significant drops in the rates of malignancy were observed in the AUS/FLUS and suspicious for malignancy categories (16-18). Thus, there is a different diagnostic attitude regarding the diagnosis of PTC between Western and Eastern pathologists, contributing to significant inter-observer variation (11-15). Cytopathologists in Western countries must refine their cytological diagnostic criteria for PTC-N and adjust to the new WHO classification schema of PTC and precursor tumors (NIFTP).

Table 1. Classification of Thyroid Tumors in the 4th Edition

1	Follicular Adenoma
2	Hyalinizing Trabecular Adenoma/Tumor
2A	Other Encapsulated Follicular Patterned Thyroid Tumors
3	Papillary Carcinoma
4	Follicular Carcinoma
4A	Hurthle Cell Tumors
5	Poorly Differentiated Carcinoma
6	Undifferentiated Carcinoma
7	Squamous Cell Carcinoma
8	Medullary Carcinoma
9	Mixed Medullary and Follicular Cell Carcinomas
10	Mucoepidermoid Carcinoma
11	Sclerosing Mucoepidermoid Carcinoma with Eosinophilia
12	Mucinous Carcinoma
13	Ectopic Thymoma
14	Spindle Epithelial Tumor with Thymus-like Differentiation
15	Carcinoma showing Thymus-like Differentiation
16A	Paraganglioma
16B	Peripheral Nerve Sheath Tumors (including Schwannoma)
16C	Benign Vascular Tumors
16D	Angiosarcoma
16E	Smooth Muscle Tumors (including leiomyoma and leiomyosarcoma)
16F	Solitary Fibrous Tumor
17A	Langerhans Cell Histiocytosis
17B	Rosai-Dorfman Disease
17C	Follicular Dendritic Cell Tumor
17D	Primary Thyroid Lymphoma
18	Germ Cell Tumors
19	Secondary Tumors

3. Diagnostic Criteria and Observer Disagreement

Differences in the rates of thyroid tumor malignancy, proportions of histological types, and biological characteristics may exist among different geographic areas or patient populations. However, the author of this chapter emphasizes the importance of applying the diagnostic criteria of malignant thyroid tumors consistently throughout the world. From previous observer variation studies on the diagnostic criteria of PTC-N, possibly irreconcilable issues between the two types (Western and Eastern) of practice have been identified (13-15). These differences may also be observed not only in PTC type malignancies, but also in follicular adenoma (FA)/follicular thyroid carcinoma (FTC) tumors. Recently, Cipriani *et al.* from the USA reported that in a review of 66 FTC cases diagnosed over the past 50 years, 71% of the FTC diagnoses required reclassification, resulting in 36% of cases diagnosed as PTC, 8% as poorly differentiated carcinoma, and 27% as benign FA (19). The authors emphasized the importance of strict diagnostic criteria for thyroid tumors (19). In this chapter, issues that cause significant observer discrepancies in thyroid tumor diagnosis, resulting in difficulty in cytologic-histologic correlation studies and comparisons of data in the literature, will be highlighted. These reasons underlying such observer variations may also be applied to the diagnostic criteria of thyroid FNA cytology. Because the majority of thyroid malignancies in the current diagnostic schema do not recur or metastasize (20, 21), and a significant proportion of PTCs is proposed to be renamed NIFTP (precursor benign tumor) (10), the author of this chapter recommends applying stricter diagnostic criteria and retaining a more conservative attitude in the diagnosis of thyroid carcinomas. This is because there are several thyroid tumors currently classified as carcinomas, including papillary microcarcinoma, intrathyroidal PTC, encapsulated follicular variant PTC, and minimally invasive FTC, whose recurrence rates are less than 5% after initial surgery and cancer specific death rates are at negligible levels (1, 22, 23).

4. Diagnostic Algorithm for Thyroid FNA Cytology (Figure 2)

Assessment of cellularity and specimen adequacy is the first step in evaluation of FNA cytology specimens. Only adequate specimens must be processed for further cytological evaluation; however, special care must be paid to rare atypical cells in compromised specimens (sparse cellularity, air-drying artifact, bloody sample, poor fixation, or crush artifact) (please refer to Chapter 5). Thus, in such cases, assessment of the presence of atypical cells should be indicated as inadequate, followed by a statement pointing out the presence of atypical cells, clarifying that PTC cannot be ruled out, and that the specimen may be categorized into the low-risk indeterminate category (Figure 2), such as indeterminate B: others in the Japanese system or AUS (PTC type atypia in suboptimal specimen) in the American system (please refer to Chapters 2 and 5). If rare, but conclusive, malignant cells are found in a poor(low quality) specimen, the specimen maybe classified in the suspicious for malignancy, but not malignancy, category (Figure 2). In adequate smear samples, the following features are searched for: nuclear atypia (24, 25) (presence or absence of papillary carcinoma type nuclear atypia, neuroendocrine carcinoma type nuclear features, high-grade nuclear features, and atypical lymphocytes) (Figures 3-4), and architectural abnormalities, such as nuclear crowding and overlapping in follicular or trabecular clusters due to loss of cellular polarity, and dispersed cells or microfollicles due to loss of cellular cohesiveness (Figures 5-7). The microfollicle is emphasized in the Bethesda text book and the microfollicle consists of groups of 6-12 follicular cells in a small circle; sometimes with a small amount of thick luminal colloid (Figures 6 and 7) (24). These features are further graded depending on morphological features (mild, moderate, and marked) into benign, low-risk indeterminate, suspicious for malignancy, and malignancy categories for the PTC lineage (Figures 3 and 4), and benign, low-risk

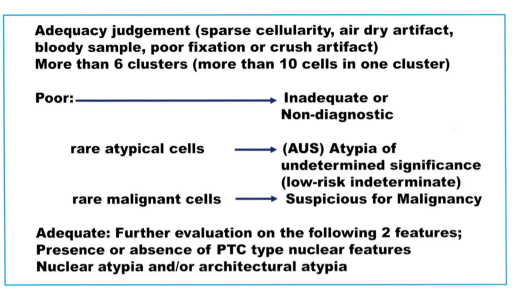

Figure 2. An adequate sample must contain at least 6 clusters composed of more than 10 cells. Special care must be paid to the possible presence of rare atypical cells in compromised specimens. In such cases, the assessment for the presence of atypical cells should be pointed out as being inadequate, followed by a statement indicating the presence of atypical cells or in the low-risk indeterminate category, such as indeterminate B: others in the Japanese system or AUS (PTC type atypia in suboptimal specimen) in the American system. If rare, but conclusive, malignant cells are found in a poor specimen, then the specimen should be classified into the suspicious for malignancy category.

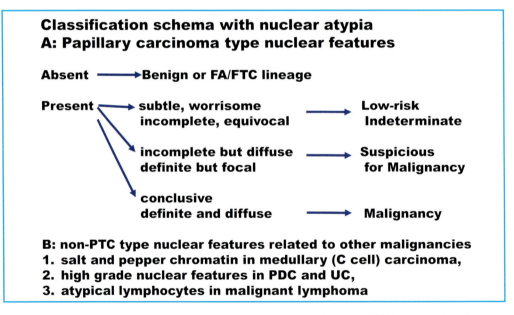

Figure 3. The next step is an assessment of the presence or absence of PTC type nuclear features. These are graded into four classes (negative, worrisome, definite but focal, and definite). Other types of nuclear features related to thyroid malignancy may also be evaluated here. They are 1) salt and pepper chromatin in medullary (C cell) carcinoma (please refer to Chapters 15 and 16), 2) high grade nuclear features in PDC and UC (Please refer to Chapter 21), and 3) atypical lymphocytes in malignant lymphoma (please refer to Chapter 14).

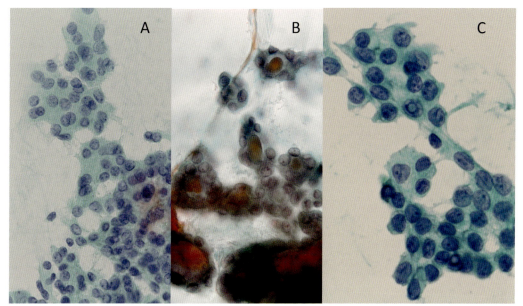

Figure 4. Papillary thyroid carcinoma type nuclear features. A: Subtle PTC type nuclear features, including nuclear enlargement and nuclear irregularity with questionable grooves. B: Incomplete PTC type nuclear features, such as pale (ground glass) nuclear chromatin with distinct small nucleoli in addition to nuclear enlargement. C: Fully developed PTC type nuclear features are seen, such as nuclear grooves and intranuclear cytoplasmic pseudo inclusions. (Conventional smear, Papanicolaou stain, A and B: x200, C: x400)

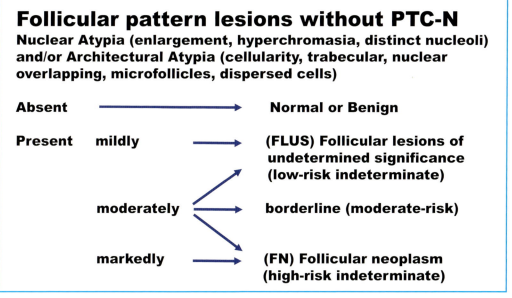

Figure 5. Follicular pattern lesions without PTC type nuclear features are graded into three classes, benign, low-risk indeterminate (FLUS in the American or indeterminate A1, favorable benign in the Japanese system), and high-risk indeterminate category (indeterminate A3, favorable malignant in the Japanese system or FN in the American, Thy 3f in the British or TIR3B in the Italian systems).

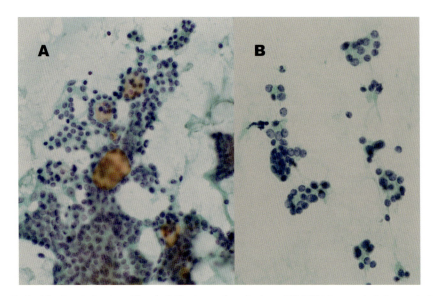

Figure 6. Architectural abnormalities in follicular pattern lesions (FA/FTC lineage). A: Large trabecular clusters show nuclear crowding and overlapping with small round nuclei. Cellular cohesion is fairly preserved and isolated cells are minimally found. Few macro-follicles containing colloid (orange red) are also seen. B: There are small clusters forming microfollicles with distorted cellular polarity. Note papillary thyroid carcinoma type nuclear features are not seen. (Conventional smear, Papanicolaou stain, A: x200, B: x400).

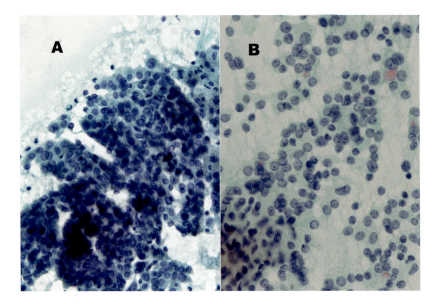

Figure 7. Architectural abnormalities in follicular pattern lesions (FA/FTC lineage). A: Nuclear crowding and overlapping are markedly seen in 3-dimensional, thick trabecular clusters. B: Predominantly dispersed cells are shown as a loss of cellular cohesiveness. Few micro-follicles containing colloid (orange red) are also seen. (Conventional smear, Papanicolaou stain, A: x200, B: x400).

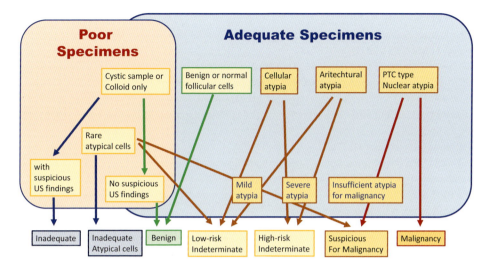

Figure 8. Algorithms for thyroid FNA cytology assessment, composed of three steps: 1) adequate judgement, 2) nuclear atypia, and 3) architectural abnormality.

indeterminate, and high-risk indeterminate categories in the FA/FTC lineage (Figures 6-7) (please refer to the scoring system by Kameyama in Chapter 20) (8, 25). These algorithms, shown in Figures 2, 3 and 5, are summarized in Figure 8.

Sample preparation, fixation, and/or staining methods may require some modifications for evaluation of these morphological features, an example of which is specimen adequacy for more than 180-320 follicular cells in LBC samples in comparison to more than 6 cell clustes in conventional smear (24, 26); please refer to Chapter 27 for liquid based cytology and Chapter 31 for different staining methods.

References

1. Haugen BR, Alexander EK, Bible KC, et al. American Thyroid Association management guidelines for adult patients with thyroid nodules and differentiated thyroid cancer. Thyroid 2015; 26:1-134.
2. Park JH, Yoon SO, Son EJ, et al. Incidence and malignancy rates of diagnoses in the Bethesda system for reporting thyroid aspiration cytology: an institutional experience. Korean J Pathol 2014; 48:133-9.
3. Hyeon J, Ahn S, Shin JH, et al. The prediction of malignant risk in the category 'atypia of undetermined significance/follicular lesion of undetermined significance' of the Bethesda System for Reporting Thyroid Cytopathology using subcategorization and BRAF mutation results. Cancer Cytopathol 2014; 122:368-76.
4. Zhu Y, Dai J, Lin X, et al. Fine needle aspiration of thyroid nodules: Experience in a Chinese population. J Basic Clin Med 2015; 4:65-9.
5. Takezawa N, Sakamoto A, Komatsu K, et al. Cytological evaluation of the "indeterminate" category by the Bethesda System for Reporting Thyroid Cytopathol. J Jpn Soc Clin Cytol 2014; 53:251-6 (in Japanese with English abstract).
6. Maekawa M, Hirokawa M, Yanase Y, et al. Cytology of follicular thyroid tumors, quality assurance, and differential diagnosis. J Jpn Soc Clin Cytol 2010; 48-54 (in Japanese with English abstract).
7. Yamao N, Hirokawa M, Suzuki A, et al. Analysis of atypia of undetermined significance (AUS)/follicular lesion of undetermined significance (FLUS) in the Bethesda system for reporting thyroid cytopathology. J Jpn Soc Clin Cytol 2014; 53:342-8 (in Japanese with English abstract).
8. Kameyama K, Sasaki E, Sugino K, et al. The Japanese Thyroid Association reporting system of thyroid aspiration cytology and experience from a high-volume center, especially in indeterminate category. J Basic

Clin Med 2015; 4:70-4.
9. Sugino K, Kameyama K, Ito K. Characteristics and outcome of thyroid cancer patients with indeterminate cytology. J Basic Clin Med 2015; 42:92-8.
10. Nikiforov YE, Seethala RR, Tallini G, et al. Nomenclature revision for encapsulated follicular variant of papillary thyroid carcinoma: A paradigm shift to reduce overtreatment of indolent tumors. JAMA Oncol, 2016 Apr 14. doi: 10.1001/jamaoncol.2016.0386 [Epub ahead of print]
11. Williams ED. Guest Editorial: Two proposals regarding the terminology of thyroid tumors. Int J Surg Pathol 2000; 8:181-3.
12. Liu Z, Zhou G, Nakamura M, et al. Encapsulated follicular thyroid tumor with equivocal nuclear changes, so-called well-differentiated tumor of uncertain malignant potential: a morphological, immunohistochemical, and molecular appraisal. Cancer Sci 2011; 102:288-94.
13. Lloyd RV, Erickson LA, Casey MB, et al. Observer variation in the diagnosis of follicular variant of papillary thyroid carcinoma. Am J Surg Pathol 2004; 28:1336-40.
14. Kakudo K, Katoh R, Sakamoto A, et al. Thyroid gland: international case conference. Endocrine Pathol 2002; 13:131-4.
15. Hirokawa M, Carney JA, Goellner JR, et al. Observer variation of encapsulated follicular lesions of the thyroid gland. Am J Surg Pathol 2002; 26:1508-14.
16. Strickland KC, Howitt BE, Marquesee E, et al. The impact of non-invasive follicular variant of papillary thyroid carcinoma on rates of malignancy for fine-needle aspiration diagnostic categories. Thyroid 2015; 25:987-92.
17. Faquin WC, Wong LQ, Afrogheh AH, et al. Impact of reclassifying noninvasive follicular variant of papillary thyroid carcinoma on the risk of malignancy in the Bethesda system for reporting thyroid cytopathology. Cancer Cytopathol 2015 Oct 12. doi: 10.1002/cncy.21631. [Epub ahead of print]
18. Maletta F, Massa F, Torregrossa L et al. Cytological features of "noninvasive follicular thyroid neoplasm with papillary-like nuclear features" and their correlation with tumor histology. Hum Pathol 2016, doi: 10.1016/j.humpath.2016.03.014. [Epub ahead of print]
19. Cipriani NA, Nagar S, Kaplan SP, et al. Follicular thyroid carcinoma: How have histologic diagnosis changed in the last half-century and what are the prognostic implications? Thyroid 2015; 25:1209-16.
20. Geffredo P, Cheung K, Roman SA, et al. Can minimally invasive follicular thyroid cancer be approached as a benign lesion? Ann Surg Oncol 2013; 20:767-72.
21. Piana S, Frasoldati A, Di Felice E, et al. Encapsulated well-differentiated follicular-patterned thyroid carcinomas do not play a significant role in the fatality rates from thyroid carcinoma. Am J Surg Pathol 2010; 34:868-72.
22. Kakudo K, Bai Y, Liu Z, et al. Classification of thyroid follicular cell tumors: with special reference to borderline lesions. Endocr J 2012; 59:1-12.
23. Kakudo K, Bai Y, Liu Z, et al. Encapsulated papillary thyroid carcinoma, follicular variant: A misnormer. Pathol Int 2012; 62:155-60.
24. Ali SZ, Cibas ES (ed). The Bethesda system for reporting thyroid cytopathology. Definitions, criteria and explanatory notes. Springer, New York, USA, 2010, pp1-166.
25. Kakudo K, Kameyama K, Miyauchi A, et al. Introducing the reporting system for thyroid fine-needle aspiration cytology according to the new guidelines of the Japan Thyroid Association. Endocr J 2014; 61: 539-52.
26. Michael CM, Pang Y, Pu RT et al: Cellular adequacy for thyroid aspirates prepared by ThinPrep: how many cells are needed? Diagn Cytopathol 2007; 35:792-97.

Chapter 2

Comparison of Diagnostic Systems: The American, British, Italian, and Japanese Reporting Systems of Thyroid FNA Cytology

Kennichi Kakudo, Zhiyan Liu and Kaori Kameyama

1. **History of Diagnostic Systems in Different Countries**

In the 2000s, the most popular reporting system of thyroid fine needle aspiration (FNA) cytology was the one recommended by the Papanicolaou society published in 1996 (1). It had a single indeterminate category (Follicular Neoplasm: FN), with many cytopathologists modifying it to their own institutional systems, which may have led to significant problems for clinical doctors on how to decide the clinical management of their patients. In 2008, the National Cancer Institute of the United States proposed a new reporting system for thyroid FNA cytology, the American (so-called Bethesda) system, in which standardization of terminologies, clinical managements and risks of malignancy were established (2). This diagnostic system sub-classified the indeterminate category into low-risk (AUS/FLUS) and high-risk (FN) categories (2, 3). Following this recommendation, the United Kingdom Royal College of Pathologists (the British system) (4) and Italian Societies of Endocrinology and the Italian Society for Anatomic Pathology and Cytology joint with the Italian Division of the International Academy of Pathology (the Italian system) (5) updated their diagnostic schema to be comparable with the American system. These were again updated in 2014 (6, 7). The Japan Thyroid Association (JTA) published its clinical guidelines for thyroid nodules in 2013 (8), which included a reporting system for thyroid cytology (the Japanese system), based on diagnostic systems used in high volume thyroid centers in Japan (9, 10). This system is characterized by more self-explanatory terminologies, and its principle of sub-classification (follicular pattern and papillary carcinoma lineages) of the indeterminate category, differing from other systems.

2. **Differences among the Four National Systems (Table 1)**

All four national reporting systems are comparable with one another, as shown in Table 1 (11, 12). However, there are slight, but significant, differences among them. First, cystic samples with fewer than 6 follicular cell clusters are classified into the non-diagnostic (Inadequate) category in the American system (2, 3). It is because the 2015 ATA guideline does not recommend FNA cytology to purely cystic nodule therefore cystic cytology samples in the American system usually have solid part suspicious for PTC. On the contrary, these samples are classified into benign category in the Japanese system (9), because majority of them are from pure cystic nodules. Repeat examination of all cystic samples with fewer than 6 follicular cell clusters is not justified in the TIR 1C category in the Italian system (6, 11) and the Thy 1C category in the British systems (7) due to its extremely low-risk nature (equal to or less than benign category). (Please refer to Supplemental Chapter 3) It is also stated in the 2015 ATA guideline, although an FNA specimen found to have abundant colloid and few epithelial cells may be considered nondiagnostic, this is also likely a benign biopsy. Second, the American system recommends limiting the percentage of cases diagnosed as AUS/FLUS (low-risk indeterminate category) to less than 7%, stating that overuse of this low-risk category as a wastebasket should be avoided (2). These strict target numbers for the low-risk and high-risk categories were not emphasized in the other reporting systems, although a proportion of less than 20% of indeterminate diagnoses was recommended by the Papanicolaou society in 1996, which has been maintained as a common standard in all systems (1). The third characteristic is the different diagnostic criteria of the high-risk indeterminate (TIR 3B) category in the Italian system compared with the American and British systems. A significant degree of nuclear atypia serves as an inclusion criterion of the high-risk category (TIR 3B), and the risk of malignancy of the low-risk category (TIR 3A) in the Italian system was reported to be slightly lower (5-10%) than those (5-15%) of the American and British systems (6, 11) (please refer to Supplemental Chapter 1). The fourth is the manner in dividing the indeterminate category. In the Japanese system, the indeterminate category is divided into the follicular adenoma (FA)/follicular carcinoma (FTC) lineage and the PTC lineage, differing in principle from the other three diagnostic systems, where the indeterminate category is divided into low-risk (TIR 3A in the Italian, Thy3a in the British, and AUS/FLUS in the American systems) and high-risk (TIR 3B in the Italian, Thy 3b in the British, and FN in the American systems) categories, regardless of presence or absence of PTC type nuclear features (PTC-N). This difference was further demonstrated when a significant number of PTC type malignancies were found in both the low-risk and high-risk categories in the Italian, British, and American systems (2-7), whereas the majority of PTC cases were found in the indeterminate B: others (PTC-lineage) category in the Japanese system (9, 13-15). Sugino *et al.* reported that the risk of malignancy in the indeterminate A category was 283/779 (36.3%), and only 61/235 cases (26.0%) of PTC were classified as indeterminate A. On the other hand, they reported that while the risk of malignancy in the indeterminate B (Others) category was 202/270 (74.8%), and the majority of PTC cases (174/235, 64.4%) were classified into the indeterminate B (15) category. In the Japanese system, the distinction between PTC type and FTC type malignancies can be more accurately achieved in cytology due to application of stricter criteria for PTC-N in both the histological and cytological diagnoses by Asian pathologists (16-22).

Encapsulated non-invasive follicular pattern lesions with subtle (incomplete and questionable) nuclear changes of PTC are traditionally classified into the benign category in Asia, either as hyperplastic nodules or follicular adenomas (17-22). This diagnostic attitude by Asian pathologists has helped accommodate a recent reclassification and renaming of the non-invasive encapsulated follicular variant of PTC into the benign precursor tumor category NIFTP (non-invasive follicular thyroid neoplasm with papillary-like nuclear features) by Nikiforov *et al.* (23), as is the case with previously proposed borderline tumor terminologies, such as well-differentiated tumor of uncertain malignant potential (WDT-UMP) by Williams (24) and well-differentiated tumor with uncertain behavior (WDT-UB) by Liu *et al.* (20, 25) (please refer to Chapters 1 and 6).

3. **How to Subclassify Indeterminate Thyroid Nodules, and the Principle of the Japanese System (Figure 1)**

The American, Italian, and British systems subclassify the indeterminate category into low-risk and high-risk categories (Table 1). Their morphological criteria were established regardless of presence or absence of PTC type nuclear features. As a result, a significant proportion of the malignancies in both the low-risk and high-risk categories are PTCs (2-7). There are a number of explanations as to why PTCs are found in the follicular pattern lesions of the indeterminate category (FN in the American system, Thy 3f in the British system, and TIR 3B in the Italian system). The most accepted explanation is that this is due to the lax criteria for PTC-N in the histological diagnosis of encapsulated non-invasive follicular variant PTC; the presence of subtle PTC-N in this variant is not uncommon, and may lead to diagnosis of FN rather than PTC by cytology (2-4). The authors of this chapter believe it is important to separate the two different lineages (FA/FTC and PTC) using stricter criteria for PTC type

Table 1. Comparison of the Italian, British, American (Bethesda), and Japanese reporting systems of thyroid cytopathology

Diagnostic Category/ National Systems/ Risk of Malignancy	Itary	Risk of Malignancy by Fadda et al reference No. 9	British	American (Bethesda)	Risk of Malignancy by Ali et al reference No. 2	Japanese (Japan Thyroid Association)	Risk of Malignancy after triage by Kakudo et al reference No.7
Non Diagnostic	TIR 1	Not Defined	Thy 1	I. Non Diagnostic	Not Defined	Inadequate (Non-Diagnostic)	<10%
Non-Diagnostic-Cystic	TIR 1C	Low	Thy 1c:	I. Non Diagnostic	Not Defined		
Non-Neoplastic/Benign	TIR 2	<3%	Thy 2/Thy 2c	II. Benign	0-3%	Normal or Benign	<1%
Low-Risk Indeterminate Lesion	TIR 3A	<10%	Thy 3a: Neoplasm Possible-Atypia/Non-Diagnostic	III. (AUS/FLUS) Atypia of Undetermined Significance /Follicular Lesion of Undetermined	5-15%	Indeterminate A: Follicular Neoplasms (Follicular Pattern Lesions) A1: Favor Benign, A2: Borderline, A3: Favor Malignant B: Others (Non-Follicular Pattern Lesions and PTC	A1: 5-15%, A2: 15-30%, A3: 40-60%, B: 40-60%
High-Risk Indeterminate Lesion	TIR 3B	15-30%	Thy 3f: Neoplasm Possible-Suggesting Follicular Neoplasm	IV. (FN/SFN) Follicular Neoplasm /Suspicious for Follicular Neoplasm	15-30%		
Suspicious of Malignancy	TIR 4	60-80%	Thy 4: Suspicious of Malignancy	V. Suspicious of Malignancy	60-75%	Malignancy Suspected (Not Conclusive for Malignancy)	>80%
Malignant	TIR 5	>95%	Thy 5: Diagnostic of Malignancy	VI. Malignant	97-99%	Malignancy	>99%

nuclear features, because the two types of well-differentiated follicular cell carcinomas have different molecular alterations in their carcinogenesis, which should be useful for molecular diagnosis. In addition, encapsulated follicular variant PTCs that have subtle PTC-N belong to the FA/FTC lineage, and do not harbor BRAF mutation or RET/PTC rearrangements (20, 26, 27) (please refer to Chapters 6 and 29). This distinction should also be useful for deciding clinical management, because their treatment strategies are different (28).

In the Japanese system, follicular pattern lesions without PTC type nuclear features (Indeterminate A: Follicular Neoplasm) are further sub-classified into A1: favor benign, A2: borderline, and A3: favor malignant (Figure 1), with a scoring system developed by Kameyama *et al*. (14) using three parameters (cellularity, nuclear overlapping, and nuclear atypia). Several studies from Japan have reported successful stratification of resection rates and risks of malignancy using this system (13-15, 29). Cases with PTC type nuclear features are also risk-stratified into three categories (Figure 1), Indeterminate B (40-60% risk), Malignancy suspected (more than 80% risk), and Malignancy (more than 99% risk), using strict criteria of PTC type nuclear features. With use of these criteria, Kameyama *et al*. were successful in differentiating PTC and FTC in their indeterminate categories (14).

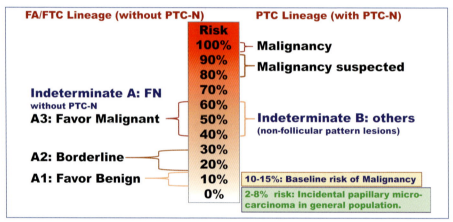

Figure 1. Risks of malignancy in Indeterminate A (Follicular Neoplasm: FA/FTC Lineage) and B (Others: PTC Lineage). On the left side, follicular pattern lesions without PTC type nuclear features (Indeterminate A: Follicular Neoplasm) are sub-classified into A1: favor benign, A2: borderline, and A3: favor malignant. Their risks of malignancy were reported to be 5-15%, 15-30%, and 40-60% using three parameters (cellularity, nuclear overlapping, and nuclear atypia). On the right side, cases with PTC type nuclear features are also risk-stratified into three categories, Indeterminate B (40-60% risk), Malignancy suspected (more than 80% risk), and Malignancy (more than 99% risk). These numbers are higher than those of the other three reporting systems, because strict criteria of PTC type nuclear features were applied for the cytological diagnosis, not just the histological diagnosis.

4. **Clinical Management of Patients with Indeterminate Nodules**

The American and Italian systems recommend a diagnostic lobectomy for all patients with high-risk (FN in the American system and TIR 3B in the Italian system) indeterminate nodules (1-4, 6, 30). In this regard, FNA may be thought of as a screening test selecting patients for surgery with higher probability of malignancy, although this clinical management has been reported to result in overtreatment for the majority (more than 75%) of patients, because they had benign nodules. Advising diagnostic surgery for all patients with high-risk indeterminate nodules may result in a high proportion (60-80%) of surgery and a 15-30% risk of malignancy in surgically-treated patients with high-risk indeterminate nodules (31-

33). It should be noted that all cases with indeterminate thyroid nodules (Thy 3a, Thy 3f, and Thy 4) in the British system are referred to so-called multidisciplinary team discussions to determine more appropriate clinical management (5, 7). In the JTA clinical guidelines, patients with indeterminate thyroid nodules are also recommended to undergo further triage with other clinical tests to minimize unnecessary diagnostic surgeries for those who actually have benign nodules (8, 9). This is a completely different approach from the clinical management of the American and Italian systems. If all patients with indeterminate cytology are advised to undergo diagnostic surgery immediately and unselectively, then the efforts of sub-classification of indeterminate A (FN), as in the Japanese system, or the use of multidisciplinary meetings, as in the British system, should not be necessary. Alternatively, emphasis should be placed on stricter diagnostic criteria of the high-risk (FN) category to reduce the proportion of this category and to avoid diagnostic surgery in patients with benign follicular pattern lesions (34, 35). Abele and Levine suggested that compared with their experience of 5%, the 15% national rate of the high-risk indeterminate category (FN) was in large part due to overdiagnosis (34), and a stricter approach is essential if patients with high-risk indeterminate nodules are sent to the operation room immediately and unselectively. The Japanese and British systems have set up a different strategy to reduce the overtreatments of patients, demonstrating that integrated clinical examination and watchful follow-up of thyroid nodules can spare many patients with benign nodules from diagnostic surgery. The authors of this chapter believe that this process may also assuage cytopathologists' anxiety over how to reduce the rate of missing FTC type malignancies in the benign category (9). This is because FTC cases with mild cellular abnormality and the absence of an altered architectural pattern, cell crowding, and/or a microfollicle formation may be placed in the indeterminate A1 (FN: favor benign), and these patients can be followed up without surgical intervention and be advised to undergo diagnostic surgery only when other clinical tests reveal malignant characteristics. This ultimately helps reduce missed diagnoses of FTC cases with mild cellular abnormality (please refer to Chapters 19 and 20).

5. **Which Reporting System Has Better Performance?**

The performance of these reporting systems likely depends on the manner of triaging patients with thyroid nodules as well as the decision making process of clinical management of patients with indeterminate nodules. Reports from Asian countries have demonstrated that the application of strict triage criteria preoperatively using integrated clinical tests for patients with indeterminate cytology may result in a low resection rate and a high proportion of malignancies in patients with indeterminate cytology (13-15, 22, 29). In clinical practice, if avoidance of missing a malignancy is the highest priority, as opposed to minimization of patient overtreatment, diagnostic surgery should be advised for patients with indeterminate nodules, because histological examination is ultimately necessary to determine whether the nodule is benign or malignant. Under such circumstances, higher resection rates and lower malignant risks have been reported in those with indeterminate nodules (31, 34, 35). Whatever reporting system is chosen to be used, the clinical management of patients with thyroid nodules is ultimately decided between the clinical doctors (endocrinologists and endocrine surgeons) and the patient, which significantly impacts the resection rates of thyroid nodules and their risks of malignancy. Although these numbers are measures of performance, they are dependent on the clinical guidelines applied to the patients. Thus, the thyroid FNA cytology reporting system remains only one of the decisive factors for obtaining a good performance in clinical practice of thyroid tumors. The increased role of conservative management using molecular testing and clinical/radiologic risk stratification is emphasized in the most recent edition of 2015 American Thyroid Association clinical guidelines, and all international diagnostic systems for reporting thyroid cytology come close more and more, and, I believe, they will have only negligible differences soon (28).

Conclusion

An alternative approach for establishing good performance in thyroid cytology is a second opinion consultation with experts to establish more definitive diagnoses. This textbook, Thyroid FNA Cytology, Differential Diagnoses and Pitfalls, is designed to provide helpful consultation and guarantees better performance in the differential diagnoses of difficult cases. It also presents high quality evidence and helpful instructions on how to avoid the pitfalls of cytology practice, regardless of the reporting system used.

References

1. The Papanicolaou Society of Cytopathology Task Force on Standards of Practice. Guidelines of the Papanicolaou Society of Cytopathology for the examination of fine-needle aspiration specimens from thyroid nodules. Diagn Cytopathol 1996; 15:84-9. (also simultaneously published in Mod Pathol 1996; 9:710-5)
2. Baloch ZW, LiVolsi VA, Asa SL, et al. Diagnostic terminology and morphologic criteria for cytologic diagnosis of thyroid lesions: a synopsis of the National Cancer Institute Thyroid Fine-Needle Aspiration State of the Science Conference. Diagn Cytopathol 2008; 36:425-37.
3. Ali SZ and Cibas ES (ed). The Bethesda system for reporting thyroid cytopathology. Definitions, criteria and explanatory notes. Springer, New York, USA, 2010, 1-166.
4. Fadda G, Basolo F, Bondi A, et al. Cytological classification of thyroid nodules. Proposal of the SIAPEC-IAP Italian consensus working group. Pathologica 2010; 102:405-6.
5. Lobo C, McQueen A, Beale T, et al. The UK royal college of pathologists' thyroid fine-needle aspiration diagnostic classification: is a robust tool for the clinical management of abnormal thyroid nodules. Acta Cytol 2011; 55:499-506.
6. Nardi F, Basolo F, Crescenzi A, et al. Italian consensus for the classification and reporting of thyroid cytology. J Endocrinol Invest 2014; 37:593-9.
7. Perros P, Colley S, Boelaert K, et al. Guidelines for the management of thyroid cancer Third edition British Thyroid Association Chapt 5.1 pages 19-24; Clin Endocrinol 2014; 81, Suppl S1.
8. Japanese Thyroid Association Guidelines for Clinical Practice for the Management of Thyroid Nodules in Japan 2013; pp1-277, Nankodo Publishing Co. Tokyo, Japan (in Japanese).
9. Kakudo K, Kameyama K, Miyauchi A, et al. Introducing the reporting system for thyroid fine-needle aspiration cytology according to the new guidelines of the Japan Thyroid Association. Endocr J 2014; 61:539-52.
10. Kakudo K, Kameyama K, Miyauchi A. History of thyroid cytology in Japan and reporting system recommended by the Japan Thyroid Association. J Basic Clin Med 2013; 2:10-5.
11. Fadda G, Rossi ED. The 2014 Italian reporting system for thyroid cytology: Comparison with the national reporting systems and future directions. J Basic Clin Med 2015; 4:46-51.
12. Bongiovanni M, Kakudo K, Nobile A. Performance comparison in the "follicular neoplasm" category between the American, British, Italian, and Japanese system for reporting thyroid cytology. J Basic Clin Med 2015; 4:42-5.
13. Fujisawa T, Morimitsu E, Hirai T, et al. Fine needle aspiration cytology of follicular tumor, proposal for our subclassification. J Jpn Soc Clin Cytol 2010; 49:42-7 (in Japanese with English abstract).
14. Kameyama K, Sasaki E, Sugino K, et al. The Japanese Thyroid Association reporting system of thyroid aspiration cytology and experience from a high-volume center, especially in indeterminate category. J Basic Clin Med 2015; 4:70-4.
15. Sugino K, Kameyama K, Ito K. Characteristics and outcome of thyroid cancer patients with indeterminate cytology. J Basic Clin Med 2015; 4:92-8.
16. Lloyd RV, Erickson LA, Casey MB, et al. Observer variation in the diagnosis of follicular variant of papillary thyroid carcinoma. Am J Surg Pathol 2004; 28:1336-40.

17. Kakudo K, Katoh R, Sakamoto A, et al. Thyroid gland: international case conference. Endocrine Pathol 2002; 13:131-4.
18. Hirokawa M, Carney JA, Goellner JR, et al. Observer variation of encapsulated follicular lesions of the thyroid gland. Am J Surg Pathol 2002; 26:1508-14.
19. Liu J, Singh B, Tallini G, et al. Follicular variant of papillary carcinoma. A clinicopathologic study of a problematic entity. Cancer 2006; 107:1255-64.
20. Liu Z, Zhou G, Nakamura M, et al. Encapsulated follicular thyroid tumor with equivocal nuclear changes, so-called well-differentiated tumor of uncertain malignant potential: a morphological, immunohistochemical, and molecular appraisal. Cancer Sci 2011; 102:288-94.
21. Chan JK. Strict criteria should be applied in the diagnosis of encapsulated follicular variant of papillary thyroid carcinoma. Am J Clin Pathol 2002; 117:16-8.
22. Y Zhu, Dai J, Lin X, et al. Fine needle aspiration of thyroid nodules: experience in a Chinese population. J Basic Clin Med 2015; 4:65-9.
23. Nikiforov Y, Seethala RR, Tallini G, et al. Nomenclature revision for encapsulated follicular variant of papillary thyroid carcinoma: A paradigm shift to reduce overtreatment of indolent tumors. JAMA Oncol, 2016, doi: 10.1001/jamaoncol.2016.0386 [Epub ahead of print].
24. Williams ED. Guest editorial: Two proposals regarding the terminology of thyroid tumors. Int I Surg Pathol 2000; 8:181-3.
25. Kakudo K, Bai Y, Liu Z, et al. Encapsulated papillary thyroid carcinoma, follicular variant: A misnomer. Pathol Int 2012; 62:155-60.
26. Rivera M, Ricarte-Hilho J, Knauf J, et al. Molecular genotyping of papillary thyroid carcinoma follicular variant according to its histological subtypes (encapsulated vs infiltrative) reveals distinct BRAF and RAS mutation patterns. Mod Pathol 2010; 23:1191-200.
27. Howitt BE, Paulson VA, Barletta JA. Absence of BRAF V600E in non-infiltrative, non-invasive follicular variant of papillary thyroid carcinoma. Histopathol 2015; 67:579-82.
28. Haugen BR, Alexander EK, Bible KC, et al. American Thyroid Association management guidelines for adult patients with thyroid nodules and differentiated thyroid cancer. Thyroid 2015; 26:1-134.
29. Maekawa M, Hirokawa M, Yanase Y, et al. Cytology of follicular thyroid tumors, quality assurance, and differential diagnosis. J Jpn Soc Clin Cytol 2010; 49:48-54 (in Japanese with English abstract).
30. Takami H, Ito Y, Okamoto T, et al. Revisiting the guidelines by the Japanese Society of Thyroid Surgeons and Japan Association of Endocrine Surgeons: a gradual move towards consensus between Japanese and Western practice in the management of thyroid carcinoma. World J Surg 2014; 38:2002-10.
31. Theoharis CG, Schofield KM, Hammers L, et al. The Bethesda thyroid fine-needle aspiration classification system: year 1 at an academic institution. Thyroid 2009; 19:1215-23.
32. Ohori NP, Schoedel KE. Variability in the atypia of undetermined significance/follicular lesion of undetermined significance diagnosis in the Bethesda system for reporting thyroid cytopathology: sources and recommendation. Acta Cytol 2011; 55:492-8.
33. Bongiovanni M, Crippa S, Baloch Z, et al. Comparison of 5-tired and 6-tired diagnostic systems for the reporting of thyroid cytopathology: a multi-institutional study. Cancer Cytopathol 2012; 120:117-25.
34. Strickland KC, Howitt BE, Marqusee E, et al. The impact of noninvasive follicular variant of papillary thyroid carcinoma on rates of malignancy for fine-needle aspiration diagnostic categories. Thyroid 2015; 25:987-92.
35. Abele JS, Levine RA. Diagnostic criteria and risk-adapted approach to indeterminate thyroid cytodiagnosis. Cancer Cytopathol 2010; 118:415-22.
36. Renshaw AA, Gould EW. Reducing indeterminate thyroid FNAs. Cancer Cytopathol 2015; 123:237-43.

Chapter 3

Pitfalls in the Diagnosis of Papillary Thyroid Carcinoma

Xin Jing and Claire W. Michael

Clinical History

A 10 year-old male presented with a two-year history of an enlarged neck, which was concerning for thyroid mass. He denied weight change, chills, excessively warm, diarrhea, constipation, sweatiness, anxiety, and palpitations. His mother stated that he had difficulty keeping up with his siblings and tired a little more easily.

Clinical Tests

TSH measured 1.6 (reference range: 0.30-5.50 mU/L), thyroid peroxidase antibody measured 35 (reference range: 0-30 IU/mL), and free T4 measured 1.39 (0.76-1.70 ng/dL).

Ultrasound Findings

The right thyroid contained a complex cyst measuring 2.1 cm (transverse) x 3.2 cm (superior-inferior) x 1.3 cm (anterior-posterior). Color Doppler demonstrated vascularity in the periphery. Central vascularity was not evident. Multiple non-shadowing punctate echoes were present throughout the complex cyst (Figure 1).

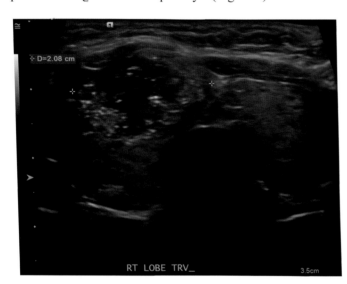

Figure 1. Ultrasound examination of the neck reveals a right thyroid nodule.

Cytological Findings

An ultrasound-guided fine needle aspiration (FNA) of the right thyroid nodule was performed with preparations of Diff-Quik- and Papanicolaou-stained conventional smears. Review of the Diff-Quik-stained conventional smears showed a cellular aspirate consisting of lymphocytes and follicular cells, which were arranged as single cells and/or irregular fragments/sheets (Figure 2). Some of the latter had a syncytial configuration with unevenly distributed nuclei (Figure 3). Various shaped nuclei (round, oval, or elongated) and nuclear enlargement were evident. Some cells contained abundant cytoplasm, mimicking Hurthle cells (Figure 4). Detailed nuclear features were better appreciated upon examining the Papanicolaou-stained conventional smears, including an irregular nuclear membrane, pale chromatin, and distinct nucleoli (Figures 5 and 6). In addition, intranuclear grooves were occasionally seen (Figure 7). However, no intranuclear pseudoinclusions (NCI) were identified.

Differential Diagnoses
1. Benign hyperplastic nodule
2. Lymphocytic (Hashimoto's) thyroiditis
3. Follicular neoplasm/Hurthle cell neoplasm
4. Suspicious for papillary thyroid carcinoma (PTC)
5. PTC, including its variants

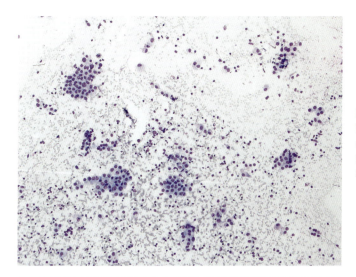

Figure 2. The aspirate is cellular with background lymphocytes, and single and irregular sheets of follicular cells. (Conventional smear, Diff-Quik stain, x100)

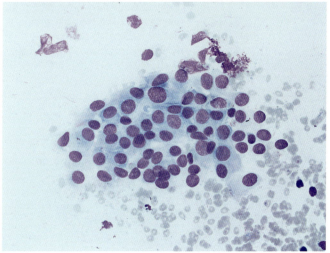

Figure 3. Syncytial sheets with unevenly distributed nuclei. (Conventional smear, Diff-Quik stain, x400)

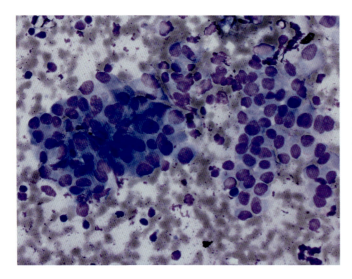

Figure 4. Various shaped nuclei (round, oval, or elongated) and nuclear enlargement are evident. Some cells contain abundant cytoplasm, mimicking Hurthle cells. (Conventional smear, Diff-Quik stain, x400)

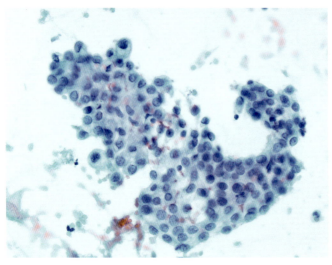

Figures 5 and 6. Irregular nuclear membrane, pale chromatin and distinct nucleoli are appreciated. (Conventional smear, Papanicolaou stain, x400)

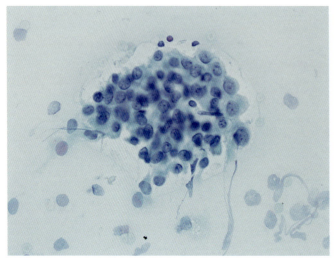

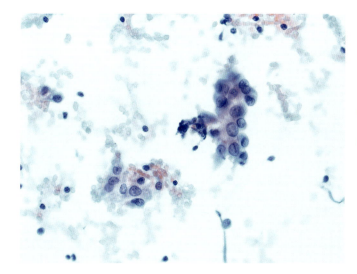

Figure 7. Intranuclear grooves are noted. (Conventional smear, Papanicolaou stain, x400)

Discussions

It has been widely accepted that FNA is a useful triage method in distinguishing neoplastic/malignant nodules from non-neoplastic/benign nodules of thyroid. Greater than 90% of diagnostic accuracy has been reported while utilizing FNA to detect PTC (1). Cytomorphological features associated with PTC have been well defined and The Bethesda System for Reporting Thyroid Cytopathology (TBSRTC) provides diagnostic criteria of PTC along with imaging illustrations and explanations. Briefly, the cytomorphological features of PTC include hypercellularity, papillae and/or syncytial tissue fragments, nuclear enlargement, oval or irregular shaped nuclei with crowding/overlapping/molding, intranuclear longitudinal grooves and NCIs, powdery chromatin, marginally located micronucleoli, psammoma bodies, and multinucleated giant cells (please refer to Chapters 4 and 5) (Tables 1 and 2) (2). It is noteworthy to mention that none of these features itself is specific for PTC. We have encountered benign hyperplastic nodule with monolayer sheets and/or papillary fragments of follicular cells, intranuclear grooves, and/or rarely NCIs; Hurthle cell-containing nodules (i.e. Hashimoto's thyroiditis and Hurthle cell neoplasm) with NCIs; and benign hyperplastic nodule with suboptimal preparation of smears showing foci of pale nuclei that mimic pale nuclei with powdery chromatin. Similarly, Kini reported three aspirates obtained from Hashimoto's thyroiditis that contained NCIs (3) (please refer to Chapter 13). Faquin *et al.* identified nuclear enlargement, nuclear grooves, fine chromatin, and distinct nucleoli, as well as rare nuclear crowding and NCI in cyst-lining cells (4) (please refer to Chapters 5 and 7). Other investigators also suggested that the presence of occasional intranuclear grooves should be interpreted as a non-specific finding (5-7). Overall, extreme cautions should be excised in the assessment of specimens with single or a few of the PTC-related features in order to avoid misinterpretation of these specimens as PTC. In addition, it is not uncommon that NCIs may be easily appreciated in other malignant neoplasms involving the thyroid, i.e., medullary thyroid carcinoma and metastatic melanoma to the thyroid. (please refer to Chapters 15 and 16)

There are limited literatures focusing on diagnostic pitfalls associated with FNA cytology of PTC. Generally, the presence of overlapping cytological features between PTC and non-PTC, as well as the over-interpretation of certain PTC-associated features are contributing factors to misdiagnosis of PTC. We previously performed a retrospective review of 22 thyroid aspirates with a histology-proven false diagnosis of PTC and identified several pitfalls attributed to the misdiagnosis. The pitfalls included misinterpretation of papillary-like tissue fragments and/or monolayer sheets with honeycomb arrangement as syncytial fragments/sheets (please refer to Figure 6 in the Chapter 4), over-interpretation of suboptimal intranuclear grooves or rare NCIs, while other PTC-associated features were minimal or absent, and misinterpretation of the elongated or spindle cells that actually represented atypical cyst lining cells (8) (please refer to Chapter 7). Others have reported cases of histology-proven Hashimoto thyroiditis being over-interpreted as PTC (please refer to Chapter 13). The authors of these studies demonstrated the pitfalls leading to over-diagnosis of PTC, including powdery chromatin, occasional nuclear grooves or pseudoinclusions, and a paucity of background lymphocytes. Furthermore, it was indicated that appreciation of lymphocytes infiltrating follicular groups is a helpful approach to avoid over-diagnosis of Hashimoto thyroiditis as PTC (9, 10). In addition, one study retrospectively reviewed three cases in which cytologic evaluation raised suspicion PTC and the subsequent thyroidectomy revealed solitary papillary hyperplastic nodule. The retrospective review of the FNA specimens showed worrisome cytologic findings including broad flat sheets, 3-dimensional clusters, nonbranching papillae with transgressing vessels, as well as mild to moderate nuclear pleomorphism and occasional intranuclear grooves. The authors pointed out that the presence of short nonbranching papillae, watery and inspissated colloid plus lack of NCIs may be useful features of distinguishing solitary papillary hyperplastic nodule from PTC (11). Last but not the least, Pusztaszeri *et al*. reported a case of histology-proven primary Langerhans cell histiocytosis of the thyroid in which FNA specimen was interpreted as suspicious for PTC due to the finding of cells with nuclear enlargement, pale chromatin, and prominent nuclear grooves (12).

Besides aforementioned over-interpretation phenomenon, under-interpretation of variants of PTC poses a challenge to practicing cytopathologist as the classic features associated with PTC may appear subtle in some of these variants (please refer to Chapters 6, 9 and 10). Among all variants of PTC, the follicular variant is the most common one, in which FNA smear may display predominantly architectural atypia manifested by a microfollicular pattern, while PTC-associated nuclear features are inconspicuous. It is not uncommon that such variant is interpreted as follicular neoplasm rather than PTC (please refer to Chapters 4 and 6). Nonetheless, there has been an on-going discussion of reclassifying non-invasive follicular variant of PTC, which however, is beyond the scope of current discussion (please refer to Chapters 4-6).

Histological Diagnosis

A total thyroidectomy was subsequently performed. Gross examination of the right thyroid lobe revealed a 2.6 cm nodule, which abutted the anterior and isthmus margins (Figure 8). Microscopic examination demonstrated morphological features consistent with PTC, mixed follicular and Hurthle cell variant (Figure 9).

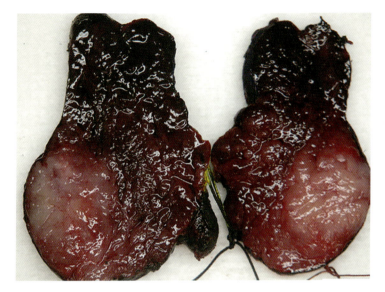

Figure 8. Gross examination of the right thyroid lobe revealed a 2.6 cm nodule.

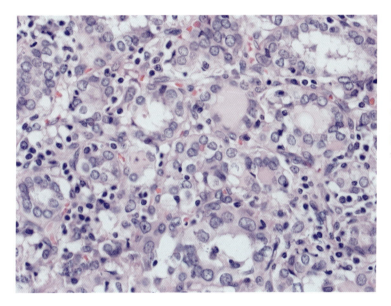

Figure 9. Microscopic examination identified morphological features of PTC, follicular and Hurthle cell variants. (H&E stain, x400)

Table 1. Differentiating features between PTC and benign non-neoplastic thyroid nodules

Features	PTC	BFH	LT/HT
Papillary-like fragments	syncytial arrangement with nuclear crowding/overlapping/molding	honeycomb arrangement with evenly spaced nuclei	honeycomb arrangement with evenly spaced nuclei
Syncytial-type sheets	moderate to abundant, diffuse	rare, focal	rare, focal
Microfollicles	prominent in FV variant	minor portion	minor portion
Hurthle cells	may be present	may be present	may be present
Lymphocytes	may be present	may be present	prominent, polymorphous population
Colloid	various amounts, may show a bubble-gum appearance	various amounts, homogenous, hard or watery	various amounts, homogenous, hard or watery
Psammomata bodies	may be present	rare	may be present
Multinucleated giant cells	may be present, numerous nucleoli	rare	may be present, few nucleoli
Nuclei	oval, elongate or irregular shaped, variation in size, markedly enlarged, Irregular contour, pale chromatin	uniformed round or oval-shaped, slightly enlarged, smooth contour, fine chromatin	uniformed round or oval-shaped, slightly enlarged, smooth contour, fine chromatin
Intranuclear grooves	thick/longitudinal, accompanied by other architectural/nuclear atypia	isolated, thin and/or incomplete	isolated, thin and/or incomplete
Intranuclear pseudoinclusion	Present along with other architectural/nuclear atypia	rare and an isolated finding	rare and an isolated finding

PTC: papillary thyroid carcinoma; BFH: benign follicular nodule; LT/HT: Lymphocytic/Hashimoto's thyroiditis; FV: follicular variant

Table 2. Differentiating features between PTC and other neoplastic/malignant thyroid nodules

Features	PTC	FN/HN	MTC
Architecture	papillae and/or syncytial sheets, single cell	microfollicles, trabeculae, single cells	various, commonly dispersed single cell
Cells	enlarged cells with various amount of cytoplasm may have histocytoid or squamoid appearance	microfollicles seen in FV Hurthle cell type may show transgressing vessels uniformed, normal to slightly enlarged Hurthle cells may show marked pleomorphism	plasmacytoid, spindled, small blue cell, etc.,
Nuclei	oval, elongate or irregular shaped, variation in size, markedly enlarged, irregular contour, pale chromatin	uniformed round or oval-shaped, slightly enlarged, smooth contour, fine chromatin. Hurthle cells may show size variation and prominent nucleoli	round, oval or spindled, salt and pepper chromatin, inconspicuous nucleoli
Intranuclear grooves	thick/longitudinal, accompanied by other architectural/nuclear atypia	isolated, thin and/or incompleteay	none
Intranuclear pseudoinclusion	present along with other architectural/nuclear atypia	rare and an isolated finding	common
Background materials	bubble-gum colloid may present	scant amount or no colloid	amyloid may present
Positive immunostaining	TTF1 and thyroglobulin	TTF1 and thyroglobulin	calretinin, synaptophysin, chromogranin, CD56, CEA

PTC: papillary thyroid carcinoma; FN/HN: follicular/Hurthle cell neoplam; MTC: medullary thyroid carcinoma; FV: follicular variant

References

1. Renshaw AA. Accuracy of thyroid fine-needle aspiration using receiver operator characteristic curves. Am J Clin Pathol 2001; 116(4):477-82.
2. Auger M SE, Yang GCH, Sanchez MA, et al. Papillary thyroid carcinoma and variants. In: The Bethesda system for reporting thyroid cytopathology: definitions, criteria and explanatory notes [Internet]. New York: Springer; 2010. p91-115.
3. Kini SR. Thyroid cytopathology: an atlas and text. 1st ed. Philadelphia: Lippincott Williams & Wilkins; 2008. p196-210.
4. Faquin WC, Cibas ES, Renshaw AA. "Atypical" cells in fine-needle aspiration biopsy specimens of benign thyroid cysts. Cancer 2005; 105(2):71-9.
5. Gould E, Watzak L, Chamizo W, Albores-Saavedra J. Nuclear grooves in cytologic preparations. A study of the utility of this feature in the diagnosis of papillary carcinoma. Acta Cytol 1989; 33(1):16-20.
6. Rupp M, Ehya H. Nuclear grooves in the aspiration cytology of papillary carcinoma of the thyroid. Acta Cytol 1989; 33(1):21-6.
7. Francis IM, Das DK, Sheikh ZA, et al. Role of nuclear grooves in the diagnosis of papillary thyroid carcinoma. A quantitative assessment on fine needle aspiration smears. Acta Cytol 1995; 39(3):409-15.
8. Jing X, Michael CW. Potential pitfalls for false suspicion of papillary thyroid carcinoma: a cytohistologic review of 22 cases. Diagn Cytopathol 2012; 40(Suppl 1):E74-9.
9. Haberal AN, Toru S, Ozen O, et al. Diagnostic pitfalls in the evaluation of fine needle aspiration cytology of the thyroid: correlation with histopathology in 260 cases. Cytopathol 2009; 20(2):103-8.
10. Harvey AM, Truong LD, Mody DR. Diagnostic pitfalls of Hashimoto's/lymphocytic thyroiditis on fine-needle aspirations and strategies to avoid overdiagnosis. Acta cytologica 2012; 56(4):352-60.
11. Khurana KK, Baloch ZW, LiVolsi VA. Aspiration cytology of pediatric solitary papillary hyperplastic thyroid nodule. Arch Pathol Lab Med 2001; 125(12):1575-8.
12. Pusztaszeri MP, Sauder KJ, Cibas ES, et al. Fine-needle aspiration of primary Langerhans cell histiocytosis of the thyroid gland, a potential mimic of papillary thyroid carcinoma. Acta Cytologica 2013; 57(4):406-12.

Chapter 4

Risk Stratification of Cases with Papillary Thyroid Carcinoma Type Nuclear Features into Low-risk, High-risk, and Malignancy Categories

Zhiyan Liu and Kennichi Kakudo

Brief Clinical Summary

The patient was a 23-year-old female with a one-month history of a thyroid nodule in her left lobe. She was referred to our hospital for further check-up.

Ultrasound

A thyroid nodule with rich vascularity in the left lobe was detected on ultrasound (Figure 1). The nodule was 1.1 cm in diameter. Irregular margin and calcification were observed, suggesting tumor invasion into the thyroid parenchyma.

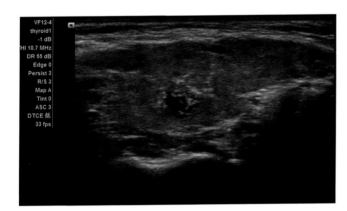

Figure 1. Ultrasound image, showing a solid tumor with an irregular margin and calcification.

Cytological Findings

At low magnification, a moderate number of follicular cell clusters were seen in the conventional smear HE-stained samples (Figures 2-5). It consisted of tightly cohesive three-dimensional and monolayer clusters. Papillary fragments with or without vascular cores were present (Figure 2). At high magnification (Figure 3), the tumor cells were medium-sized and had large nuclei with fine powdery chromatin. There were nuclear grooves in a moderate number and also several definite nuclear cytoplasmic inclusions (NCI) (red arrows in Figure 3). Cellular syncytial sheets, cellular swirls sheet (Figure 4), nuclear crowding, overlapping, molding and loosely cohesive isolated dispersed cells could be seen as shown in the Figure 5. Multinucleated giant cells were present in the Figures 2 and 5. Neither colloid, cystic change, psammoma bodies nor necrosis was identified in the smear background.

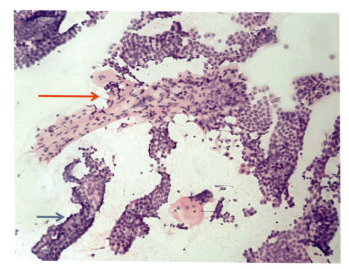

Figure 2. Showing true papillae with fibrovascular cores (red arrow), which is rare and not a major diagnostic criterion for PTC. Macrofollicles or sheets and microfollicles could also be found in PTC. Identification of architecture is the first step at low magnification and evaluation of PTC-N is critical for the ultimate diagnosis of PTC at high magnification.

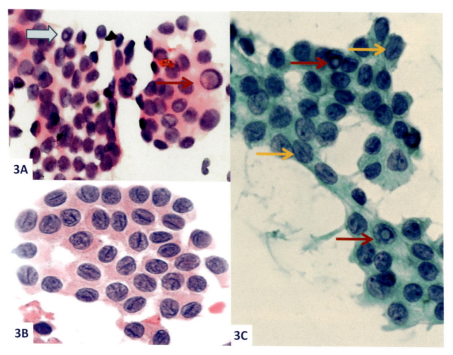

Figure 3. Identification of the architecture is the first step and evaluation of PTC-N is critical for the ultimate diagnosis of PTC. Overlapping and optically clear crowded nuclei are shown in this cluster. Nuclear cytoplasmic inclusions are indicated by red arrows (A and C). The one that could not be regarded as a diagnostic inclusion is marked with a thick arrow (A). Marked nuclear grooves are seen in B and C (yellow arrow).

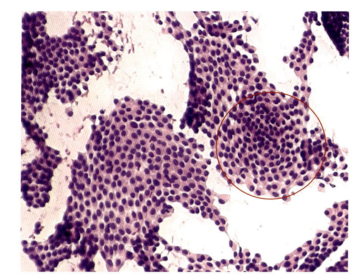

Figure 4. Macrofollicles, syncytial sheets or monolayers are found. A red circle indicates a cellular swirls pattern sheet.

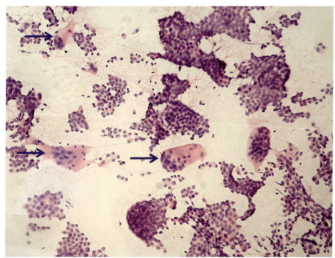

Figure 5. A minor diagnostic criterion of PTC: Blue arrows indicate multinucleated giant cells with multiple nuclei.

List of Differential Diagnoses
1. Benign, atypical follicular adenoma
2. Benign, atypical follicular cells in Hashimoto thyroiditis
3. Benign, suspicious for hyalinizing trabecular adenoma
4. Indeterminate B, others, PTC cannot be ruled out (AUS by the Bethesda system)
5. Suspicious for non-invasive follicular thyroid neoplasm with papillary-like nuclear features
6. Suspicious for conventional PTC
7. Malignant, conventional PTC

Differential Diagnosis

Thyroid FNA samples that contain numerous epithelial cells relative to the trace amount of colloid raise the possibility of a neoplasm (Figures 2, 4, and 5). Such samples should be carefully screened for the papillae, syncytial sheets, nuclear features of PTC (fine chromatin, nuclear grooves, and NCIs), and psammoma bodies (1). The diagnostic features observed frequently in the cytological smear of conventional PTC are listed in Table 1 (please refer to Supplemental Chapter 5). If these are absent, then the differential diagnoses for these lesions include follicular neoplasm, cellular adenomatous nodule, and other non-follicular cell neoplasms (2). Atypical follicular adenoma can be ruled out by the papillary growth pattern (Figure 2), syncytial sheets (Figure 4), and fully developed papillary thyroid carcinoma type nuclear changes (PTC-N) (Figure 3) of tumor cells. Hashimoto thyroiditis can be ruled out by absence of lymphocytes in the smear background and characteristic oxyphilic change of degenerated follicular cells, although occasional nuclear grooves and fake pseudoinclusions can be found in Hashimoto thyroiditis (please refer to Chapters 3 and 13). Pseudo-papillary growth in hyperplastic adenomatous nodule (Figures 6A and 6B) should not be miss-interpreted as true papillary clusters, the nuclei of which are round and regular, although nuclear grooves could be found occasionally (Figure 6C). For differential diagnosis of hyalinizing trabecular adenoma, please refer to Chapter 12.

Explanatory Notes

The diagnosis of PTC relies heavily on PTC-N, however, the interpretation of what constitutes PTC-N varies among pathologists (2-7). It is noteworthy to mention that none of these features itself is specific for PTC, and strict criteria should be applied when evaluating the PTC-N. It is because the evaluation of PTC-N is undoubtedly subjective. Nishigami *et al*. reported that the nuclei of PTC are usually larger and more irregular than those of normal follicular cell, and those of borderline tumor (such as non-invasive encapsulated follicular variant of PTC, NIFTP, or well differentiated tumor of uncertain malignant potential: WDT-UMP) are between them (8). On the other hand, there are PTCs with mild nuclear changes, and Renshaw pointed out that the cases of PTC that lack marked nuclear enlargement, pale chromatin, and NCIs are significantly more difficult to be recognized than those that have these features (9). These two facts are the main reasons why we need indeterminate categories and a suspicious for malignancy category in addition to the malignancy category in reporting system of thyroid cytology. As the low-risk indeterminate category, Atypia of Undetermined Significance (AUS) in the Bethesda system, has a 5-15% risk of PTC type malignancy and the high-risk PTC type indeterminate category (Suspicious for Malignancy) has a 60-75% risk of PTC type malignancy (10, 11), the authors of this chapter recommend that risk stratification into the low-risk, high-risk, and malignancy categories should be performed more objectively. Only cellar clusters of nuclear enlargement and crowding, which have prominent nuclear grooves and easily detectable NCIs, should be classified to PTC type malignancy. Without any one of these features, it should be classed into either low-risk or high-risk category depending on the degree of these features. (please refer to Figure 4 of Chapter 1)

Table 1. Diagnostic features of papillary thyroid carcinoma

Architecture of the tissue fragments	Papillary pattern, with or without complex branching, containing central fibrovascular cores (Figure 2)
	Papillary-like pattern, without visible central cores but appearing as finger-like progresses (Figure 3)
	Monolayered with or without branching
	Syncytial without architecture patterns or appear as three-dimensional balls, onionskin pattern or cellular swirls pattern (Figure 4, Red circle)
Cellularity	Variable; overwhelmingly cellular to scant in tumors with desmoplasia, or with cystic change
Cells	Wide range of sizes and shapes
	Small, medium-sized to very large
	Round, cuboidal, short columnar, enlongated; polygonal, spindle shaped
	Cell borders well-to-poorly defined
	N/C ratios variable
Cytoplasm	Variable; pale
Nuclei	Variably crowded or overlapped
Nucleus	Pleomorphic in size and shape, round, oval, oblong
	With smooth or irregular nuclear membranes
	Pale and dusty chromatin with powdery to finely granular
	Longitudinal nuclear grooves
	Nuclear pseudoinclusions, larger than one third of nuclear diameter with distinctive sharp contour by a rim of condensed chromatin
Psammoma body	Often presented
	Naked or incorporated in syncytial tissue fragments of neoplastic cells displaying PTC-N
	Single or multiple within any given tissue fragments
	Naked psammoma bodies not of diagnostic importance
Calcification	Often presented and not specific
Osseous metaplasia	Often presented and not specific
Squamous metaplasia	Often presented and not specific
Multinucleated giant cells	Nearly always present; varies in numbers and size (Figure 5)
Background	Usually clean without necrosis
	Histiocytes indicating cystic changes
	Lymphocytic infiltration ±
	Variable colloid, pale to dense, often stringy
Immunoprofile	Reactive with Thyroglobulin, TTF-1, cytokeratin 19, HBME-1 and Galectin 3

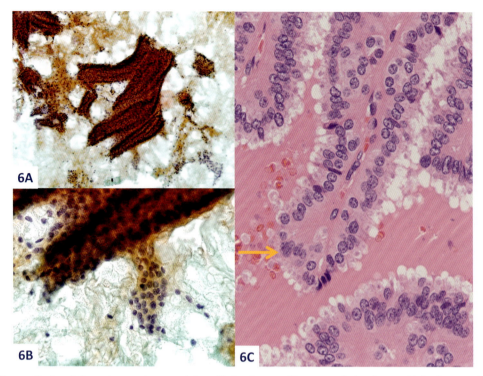

Figure 6. A cellular adenomatous nodule with benign papillary growth is shown. Note the regular round nuclei without PTC-N. A few grooves are present (yellow arrow). (6A and 6B: Papanicolaou stain and 6C: HE stain; 6A, x40; 6B, x200; and 6C, x400)

Histological Diagnosis: PTC, Classic Type, pT1b, ex0, pN0 (0/5)

A 1.2 cm nodule with an irregular margin was found in the left lobe of the thyroid gland on cut section. It was a non-encapsulated nodule with an irregular margin and invasive growth into thyroid parenchyma was found. Histologically, it was a papillary growth patterned tumor, and numerous papillae composed of tumor cells with PTC-N were observed (Figures 7, 8). These tumor cells had oval nuclei with nuclear grooves and NCIs, which was corresponding to the cytological observation, as shown in Figure 3. Crowded and overlapped nuclei with powdery (ground glass) appearance were also observed (Figures 7, 8). Multinucleated giant cells were present (Figure 8), which was corresponding to the giant cells shown in Figure 5. Central neck lymph node dissection was carried out and no metastatic carcinoma was identified in the five dissected lymph nodes histologically.

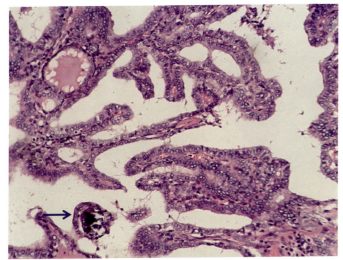

Figure 7. Papillary architecture with central fibrovascular cores supports an atypical epithelial proliferation in this low magnification. A psammoma body indicated by the blue arrow presents within a papillary cluster. (HE stain, x100)

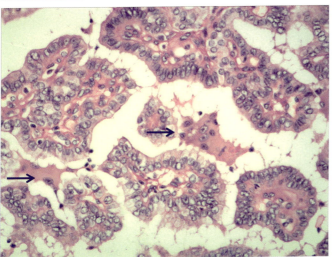

Figure 8. Giant cells with multiple nuclei are observed between papillary clusters (blue arrows). These papillary clusters are covered with malignant follicular cells with powdery chromatin. (HE stain, x200)

Take Home Message

Nuclear grooves are present in nearly all cases of PTC, but they may be sparse in up to 25% of cases (10-12). They are often run parallel to the long axis of the oval nuclei, giving a "coffee bean" appearance (Figure 3B). The chromatin pattern of PTC is unique among thyroid lesions, and represents an important diagnostic feature (11, 12). The pale chromatin of PTC is distinctly different from that of normal follicular cell nuclei, and has been interpreted as a "ground glass" or "powdery chromatin" feature. These chromatin differences are much more easily appreciated using ethanol-fixed Papanicolaou-stained preparations than air-dried Diff-Quik preparations and HE staining (Figure 3) (please refer to Chapter 31). The presence of NCIs is highly suggestive of PTC, particularly when in combination with other characteristic nuclear features (Figures 3A and 3C). NCIs are found in more than 90% of PTC aspirates, although they may be present in a small number of cells. Strict criteria should be used to identify a NCI, because both air-dried and ethanol-fixed preparations can result in artifacts and nonspecific structures that mimic the nuclear inclusion. The NCIs of PTC are large, often occupying one third or more of the nuclear area, more optically clear than the surrounding chromatin, and share the tinctorial properties of the cytoplasm bounded by a distinct membrane and surrounded by a thin condensed rim of basophilic chromatinic material (Figure 3A). The structure indicated by the thick arrow in Figure 3 should not be regarded as a diagnostic NCI. A schematic illustration of PTC-N is shown on the cover page.

References:

1. Kaushal S, Iyer VK, Mathur SR, et al. Fine needle aspiration cytology of medullary carcinoma of the thyroid with a focus on rare variants: a review of 78 cases. Cytopathology 2011; 22:95-105.
2. Liu Z, Zhou G, Nakamura M, et al. Encapsulated follicular thyroid tumor with equivocal nuclear changes, so-called well-differentiated tumor of uncertain malignant potential: a morphological, immunohistochemical, and molecular appraisal. Cancer Sci 2011; 102:288-94.
3. Rosai J, DeLellis RA, Carcangiu ML, eds. Tumors of the thyroid and parathyroid glands. Maryland: ARP PRESS; 2014.
4. Chan JK. Strict criteria should be applied in the diagnosis of encapsulated follicular variant of papillary thyroid carcinoma. Am J Clin Pathol 2002; 117:16-8.
5. Rivera M, Tuttle RM, Patel S, et al. Encapsulated papillary thyroid carcinoma: a clinico-pathologic study of 106 cases with emphasis on its morphologic subtypes (histologic growth pattern). Thyroid 2009; 19:119-27.
6. Rivera M, Ricarte-Filho J, Patel S, et al. Encapsulated thyroid tumors of follicular cell origin with high grade features (high mitotic rate/tumor necrosis): a clinicopathologic and molecular study. Hum Pathol 2010; 41:172-80.
7. Piana S, Frasoldati A, Di Felice E. Encapsulated well-differentiated follicular-patterned thyroid carcinomas do not play a significant role in the fatality rates from thyroid carcinoma. Am J Surg Pathol 2010; 34:868-72.
8. Nishigami K, Liu Z, Taniguchi E, et al. Cytological features of well-differentiated tumors of uncertain malignant potential: Indeterminate cytology and WDT-UMP. Endocr J 2012; 59:483-7.
9. Renshaw AA, Wang E, Haja J, et al: Fine needle aspiration of papillary thyroid carcinoma: distinguishing between cases that performed well and those performed poorly in the College of American Pathologists Nongynecologic cytology program. Arch Pathol Lab Med 2006; 130:452-5.
10. Cibas ES, Ali SZ. The Bethesda System for Reporting Thyroid Cytopathology. Am J Clin Pathol 2009; 132:658-65.
11. Ali S, Cibas E. The bethesda system for reporting thyroid cytopathology. New York, NY: Springer; 2009.
12. Kini SR. Thyroid Cytopathology. Wolters Kluwer; 2015.

Chapter 5

Diagnostic Criteria of AUS/FLUS in the Bethesda Reporting System and the Low-risk Indeterminate Category

Yubo Ren, Zhiyan Liu and Kennichi Kakudo

Brief Clinical Summary

The patient was a 49-year-old female who had a one-year history of multiple thyroid nodules in the bilateral thyroid lobes. She was referred to Liaocheng People's Hospital for further examination. Her TSH level was 37 IU/L (reference range: 0.270-4.200 IU/L), anti-TG antibody was 234 IU/L (reference range: <4.11 IU/L) and anti-peroxidase antibody was 598 Ku/L (reference range: 0-34.0 Ku/L) by serological tests. The FT3 and FT4 levels were 5.4 pmol/L (reference range: 3.67-10.43 pmol/L) and 6.2 pmol/ L (reference range: 12-22 pmol/ L), respectively.

Ultrasound

A solid hypoechoic nodule with an irregular margin and measuring 0.3 cm in diameter was identified in the right lobe (Figure 1). No calcification was observed in the nodule.

Cytological Findings:

A small number of follicular cell clusters were observed in bloody Papanicolaou-stained conventional smears (Figures 2-4). The follicular cells were arranged in syncytial clusters or microfollicles in the background of lymphocyte-rich smears (Figures 2 and 3). Condensed colloid and multinucleated giant cells are shown in Figure 3. These follicular cells had large nuclei with small conspicuous nucleoli (yellow arrow in Figure 3). Squamous metaplastic features of the follicular cells were observed, such as polygonal cells with abundant dense cytoplasm (Figure 4). Occasional nuclear grooves and small distinct nucleoli (yellow arrow in Figure 4) could be observed, but no definite nuclear cytoplasmic inclusions were identified. Crush (mechanical) artifacts and fibrin clot artifacts in the smear resulted in pseudocomplexity and made detailed cytomorphological evaluation difficult (1-4). No cystic change, psammoma bodies, or necrosis was identified (Figures 2-4).

List of Differential Diagnoses
1) Inadequate
2) Benign, Hashimoto thyroiditis
3) AUS/FLUS (atypia of undetermined significance/follicular lesion of undetermined significance, low-risk indeterminate category)
4) Follicular neoplasm (high-risk indeterminate category)
5) Suspicious for malignancy, papillary thyroid carcinoma (PTC), follicular variant
6) Malignancy, PTC, conventional type

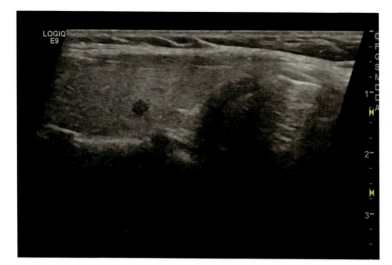

Figure 1. A hypoechoic small mass with an irregular margin (Ultrasound).

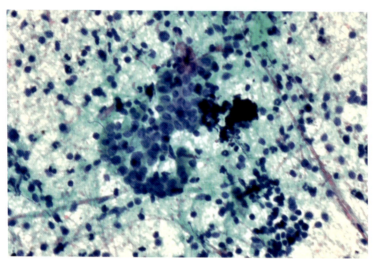

Figure 2. Nuclear crowding in a follicular cell cluster arranged in syncytial sheets. The inflammatory background shows numerous lymphocytes and granulocytes. (Conventional smear, Papanicolaou stain, x200)

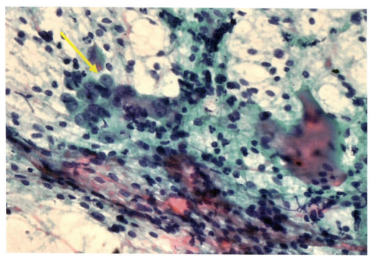

Figure 3. Follicular cells entrapped in fibrin clots demonstrate pseudocomplexity and nuclear crowding in the 3-dimensional microfollicular architecture. Oval nuclei have vesicular chromatin and distinct nucleoli (yellow arrow). Condense colloid (right), irregularly shaped lymphocytes, and fibrin streaking of a poor quality smear sample are observed in the background. (Conventional smear, Papanicolaou stain, x200)

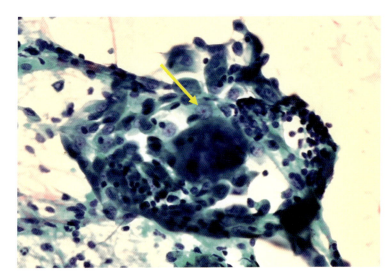

Figure 4. Abundant dense cytoplasm of the follicular cells suggesting oxyphilic change or squamous metaplasia. These polygonal-shaped cells with cyanophilic cytoplasm have large vesicular nuclei and distinct nucleoli (yellow arrow). Note small lymphocytes are present within the epithelial clusters. (Conventional smear, Papanicolaou stain, x400)

Differential Diagnosis

Differential diagnoses include atypical follicular cells in Hashimoto thyroiditis, follicular adenoma, follicular variant PTC (well-differentiated tumor with uncertain malignant potential or non-invasive encapsulated follicular thyroid neoplasm with papillary-like nuclear features), and conventional PTC.

Hashimoto thyroiditis may be considered due to the lymphocyte infiltration observed in the smear background as well as the cytoplasmic density of the follicular cells, although the characteristic oxyphilic change of degenerated follicular cells was not obvious (2-4). Mild nuclear enlargement, irregularity of nuclear shape with small conspicuous nucleoli (Figures 3 and 4), and nuclear crowding (Figure 2) in follicular pattern lesions are worrisome nuclear features of follicular neoplasm (high-risk indeterminate category) and/or PTC type malignancy. However, these nuclear changes, as shown in Figures 2 to 4, were subtle and not diagnostic nuclear features for PTC type malignancy (please refer to Chapters 3 and 4). The cellularity of this sample was not sufficient for diagnosis of the follicular neoplasm category (3, 4). Although nuclear grooves were occasionally observed, intranuclear cytoplasmic inclusions were completely lacking. Therefore, AUS (incomplete nuclear features suggestive of PTC) may be the most suitable category, and repeat FNA cytology may be warranted for clinical management. It is also acceptable to classify this sample into the indeterminate B, others category in the Japanese system, or the low-risk indeterminate category (TIR3A in the Italian system or Thy 3a in the British system) (please refer to Chapter 2). The sample was sparsely cellular with a lymphocyte-rich background. Nuclear enlargement, crowding, grooves, irregularity, and molding were minimal. It is also acceptable to classify this case as pattern B (incomplete nuclear changes) of suspicious for malignancy in the Bethesda system (3, 4). However, a conclusive diagnosis of malignancy, such as conventional PTC, should not be made because of the compromised specimen, sparse cellularity, and subtle cytological features, although histology at resection later confirmed PTC.

Histological Diagnosis: Papillary microcarcinoma and Hashimoto thyroiditis

A 0.3-cm sclerotic lesion with an irregular infiltrative margin was identified in the background of Hashimoto thyroiditis (Figure 5). The lesion was a follicular pattern tumor, with no papillary growth observed (Figures 5 and 6). Mildly increased nuclear size and an irregular nuclear contour, similar to the cytological findings, were observed (Figure 6). The nuclei were hyperchromatic, and ground-glass nuclei (pale chromatin) and overlapping were not obvious. Although no nuclear cytoplasmic inclusions or typical nuclear grooves were observed, the invasive growth pattern in the sclerotic background suggested a diagnosis of infiltrative type follicular variant PTC. No enlarged lymph nodes suggestive of metastasis were found during surgery, and prophylactic lymph node dissection was not performed.

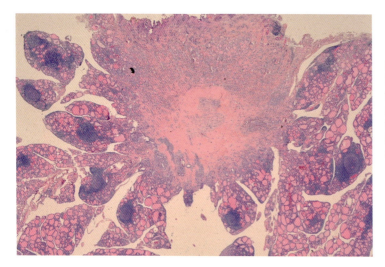

Figure 5. A 0.3-cm sclerotic lesion with an irregular margin was identified in the thyroid parenchyma of Hashimoto thyroiditis, showing invasion into the thyroid capsule and cut margin. (HE stain, x40)

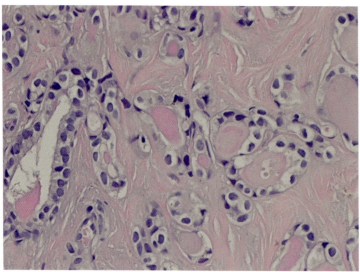

Figure 6. A follicular pattern tumor with sclerotic stroma and no papillary growth. Mildly increased nuclear size and irregular nuclear contour similar to the cytological findings are observed. (HE stain, x200)

Exploratory Note

Approximately 20% to 30% of thyroid FNA cytology assessments lead to clinically inconclusive diagnoses (inadequate, indeterminate, or suspicious for malignancy), resulting in a diagnostic dilemma for clinicians (1-8). The National Cancer Institute (NCI) hosted the NCI Thyroid FNA State of the Science Conference in 2007 and published a textbook on the Bethesda System for Reporting Thyroid Cytopathology (TBSRTC) in 2010 (3). This system proposed to dividing the indeterminate category into two sub-categories: low-risk indeterminate (AUS/FLUS) and high-risk indeterminate (Follicular Neoplasm). The AUS/

FLUS category is a low-risk category that exhibits borderline atypia of uncertain significance (3-7) (please refer to Chapter 2). It is reserved for aspirates that contain follicular cells, C cells, or lymphocytes with architectural and/or nuclear atypia that is more pronounced than that observed in normal/benign lesions, yet is not sufficient to be classified into the follicular neoplasm (high-risk indeterminate category), suspicious for malignancy, or malignant category (3-7).

Definition of AUS/FLUS and the Bethesda Scenarios

This category is for cases that do not fulfill the criteria for either the benign or high-risk indeterminate category (please refer to Chapters 3, 4, 6, 19, and 20). The AUS/FLUS category is the low-risk indeterminate category of the American (Bethesda) system (please refer to Chapter 2), and it is composed of heterogeneous diseases. The textbook by Ali and Cibas has outlined nine scenarios for which the diagnosis of AUS/FLUS category is appropriate, as summarized in Table 1 (3-7). The diagnosis of AUS/FLUS is established by the presence of either architectural atypia (loss of cellular polarity and loss of cellular cohesiveness) or nuclear atypia (insufficient nuclear atypia for the suspicious for malignancy category). Nuclear crowding and overlapping in 3-dimensional follicular cell clusters, known as architectural atypia, are often observed in follicular adenoma, follicular carcinoma, and poorly differentiated carcinoma (please refer to Chapters 19, 20, and 21). In addition to cases in the high risk indeterminate category, architectural atypia or pseudocomplexity may be found in poorly prepared specimens due to air-drying, mechanical (crush) artifacts (Figures 2-4), poor fixation, or excess blood in the specimen (Figure 7). Mild nuclear atypia, such as nuclear enlargement (Figure 4), nuclear crowding (Figure 2), pale chromatin (ground-glass nuclei) (Figure 4), and nuclear grooves may be found in patients with Hashimoto thyroiditis (please refer to Chapter 13), subacute thyroiditis (please refer to Chapter 11), regenerating follicular cells, and cyst-lining cells (Figure 8) (please refer to Figure 11 of Chapter 7) (9). PTC type nuclear features may be seen in only a small proportion of cells, with a predominance of benign-appearing follicular cells (Figure 9) (please refer to Chapter 6). Nuclear atypia may be seen in patients treated with external radiation, radioactive iodine, or thyroid suppressive agents (Table 1) (1-5). Air-drying artifacts often create serious problems in alcohol-fixed Papanicolaou stain samples, leading to suboptimal nuclear detail (nuclear enlargement, irregularity, and hyperchromasia) (Figure 10A). The authors of this chapter emphasize that repeat FNA examination is the best approach for obtaining a more definite diagnosis (Figure 10B) in such AUS/FLUS cases; VanderLaan has also suggested this approach (11). As the case shown in Figure 10, repeat FNA cytology often resolves the indeterminate AUS/FLUS diagnosis into a more definitive category, either benign or malignant, in the majority of cases (7-15).

Table 1. Most common scenarios for which AUS/FLUS interpretation is appropriate (modified from the Bethesda system for reporting thyroid cytopathology) (3, 4)

A) Architectural atypia
  a) Follicular cells of uncertain significance
    1) Predominance of microfollicles, trabeculae or crowded groups of follicular cell clusters in sparsely cellular aspirate with scant colloid.
    2) Predominance of microfollicles in a single slide with benign macrofollicles and flat sheets in other slides.
  b) Oncocytic (Hurthle) follicular cells of uncertain significance
    1) In a paucicellular smear, predominance of Hurthle cell clusters in a background lacking lymphocytes and normal follicular cells.
    2) Cellular aspirate comprised exclusively of Hurthle cells in patients with Hashimoto thyroiditis or multinodular adenomatous goiter.
  c) Atypia secondary to preparation artifact
    1) Nuclear and cytoplasmic enlargement in air-dried samples.
    2) Falsely crowded or observation of microfollicles in excess bloody or microclotting samples.
B) Nuclear atypia
  a) Worrisome nuclear features of PTC in predominantly benign-appearing samples
    1) Only few follicular cells with nuclear atypia suggestive of PTC in a hypocellular smear.
    2) Only few follicular cells with nuclear atypia suggestive of PTC in a cellular background that has an otherwise benign appearance (please refer to Chapters 4 and 6).
    3) Mild nuclear atypia, such as nuclear enlargement, nuclear crowding, and powdery chromatin (ground glass nuclei), but without conclusive nuclear features for PTC, such as frequent nuclear grooves, irregularity, and inclusions (please refer to Chapters 4 and 6).
    4) Atypia in Hashimoto chronic thyroiditis (please refer to Chapter 13).
  b) Atypia in cyst-lining cells
    1) Nuclear grooves, prominent nucleoli, elongated nuclei and cytoplasm, and/or intranuclear cytoplasmic inclusions may be observed in flat sheets in an otherwise predominantly benign-appearing sample.
  c) Secondary atypia of follicular cells
    1) Nuclear atypia may be observed in patients treated with external radiation, radioactive iodine, or thyroid suppressive agents.
  d) Atypical lymphocytes insufficient for diagnosis of malignant lymphoma
    1) Immature atypical lymphocytes in Hashimoto thyroiditis.
  e) Atypia secondary to preparation artifact
    1) Nuclear enlargement, irregularity and hyperchromasia in air-dried samples.
  f) Not otherwise specified

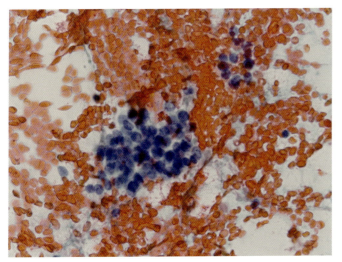

Figure 7. Follicular lesion of undetermined significance. Nuclear crowding and overlapping of small hyperchromatic nuclei are observed in this 3-dimensional follicular cell cluster, which is matted in blood. Extensive blood and a thick smear resulted in poor fixation and shrinkage of the follicular cells, leading to suboptimal nuclear detail. Note the microfollicular cluster in the upper right. Subsequent surgery revealed an adenomatous hyperplastic nodule. (Papanicolaou, x400)

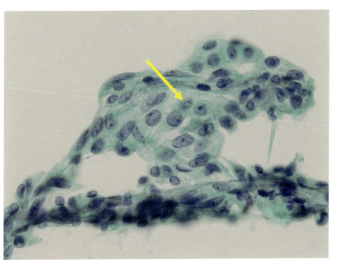

Figure 8. Atypia of undetermined significance. Cyst-lining cells in a flat sheet have wide cytoplasm and elongated irregular nuclei with distinct nucleoli. Note the possible intranuclear cytoplasmic inclusion (yellow arrow). A tight cohesive flat sheet and absence of nuclear crowding/overlapping permits the maintenance of a conservative diagnosis of AUS/FLUS (low-risk indeterminate), rather than suspicious for malignancy or malignancy. Subsequent surgery revealed cystic degeneration in the adenomatous nodule. (Papanicolaou stain, x400)

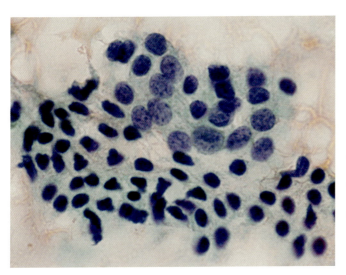

Figure 9. Atypia of undetermined significance. Benign appearing macrofollicular sheet of follicular cells with small condensed nuclei (lower half) and a small group of cells in the upper field displays some nuclear features suggestive of papillary carcinoma including nuclear enlargement and paler chromatin. (Conventional smear, Papanicolaou stain, x1000)

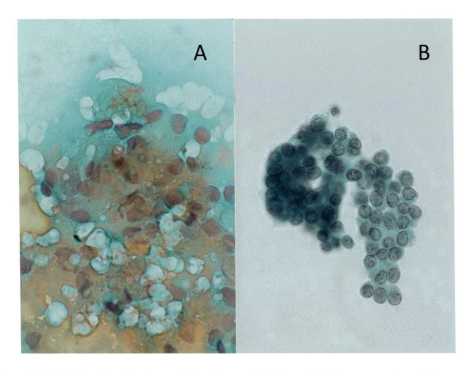

Figure 10. (A) Suboptimal nuclear detail with an air-drying artifact in a sparsely cellular smear. Nuclear irregularity is a worrisome nuclear feature of papillary carcinoma. Repeat FNA cytology was requested under a diagnosis of atypia (air dry artifact). A repeat FNA examination demonstrated nuclear crowding and overlapping in 3-dimensional cellular clusters, pale chromatin suggesting diagnosis of papillary carcinoma (B). Subsequent surgery demonstrated a conventional type papillary thyroid carcinoma. (Conventional smear, Papanicolaou stain, x400)

Controversies in AUS/FLUS

AUS/FLUS is the most controversial category in TBSRTC, with a reported rate ranging 0.7-18% and the risk of malignancy in surgically treated patients ranging widely, from 6% to 48% (5, 11, 16-21). This is likely due to the differing application of diagnostic criteria among cytopathologists, and significant observer disagreements have been reported for this category (16-22). The most common malignancy diagnosed at surgery in patients with AUS/FLUS nodules is follicular variant PTC (9, 10, 16, 18, 21-28). The subtle nuclear features of NIFTP (encapsulated follicular variant PTC was renamed to non-invasive follicular thyroid neoplasm with papillary-like nuclear features) contribute to the poor reproducibility and observer variability in malignancy rate (please refer to Chapter 6) (26-30). It is also worth noting that a compromised specimen, such as those including sparse cellularity, air-drying artifacts, bloody samples, poor fixation, or crush artifacts, is an additional and important predisposing condition for the AUS/FLUS category (3-7). Therefore, significant overlap of cytological features and observer disagreement may occur between the AUS/FLUS and inadequate categories. The distinction between an "Inadequate" and "AUS/FLUS" specimen rests on the subjective judgment of the cytopathologist, based on the assessment of the entire sample and the extent of artifact presence (4). It has also been pointed out that the AUS/FLUS category overlaps significantly with the suspicious for malignancy and other categories (19). As a result, observer disagreement has been very high in the AUS/FLUS category in many reports (16-22, 24, 31). It is important for cytopathologists to refine the cytological criteria of AUS/FLUS, and to minimize the use of this controversial category (10, 32). To promote standardization of the diagnostic criteria of AUS/FLUS interpretation, Bongiovanni has introduced reference images available on the home page of the Papanicolaou Society of Cytopathology (www.papsociety.org), as well as other useful educational materials in his review (5). The authors of this chapter believe that routine cytologic-histologic correlation studies and measurement of their quality in surgically-treated patients are the most useful data for cytopathologists to refine the diagnostic criteria and to place cases in more definitive categories (19, 21. 23, 33). This feedback of malignancy probability is also important for clinical doctors, aiding clinical management decisions for patients with thyroid nodules.

Sub-categories in AUS/FLUS

The risk of malignancy in patients with AUS/FLUS nodules has not been well established, and a wide range (6-48%) has been reported from Western countries. This is because only a subset (30.3-52.5%) of patients undergoes diagnostic surgery, and the outcome of most patients remains unknown (3, 4, 18, 19). In those patients in whom high-risk features are identified by other clinical tests, a higher risk of malignancy (69%) at resection was reported in a study from Korea (33), and an extremely high risk of malignancy (88.6%) was reported in a study from Japan after triage of patients with other clinical tests (34). Thus, the reported risk of malignancy in the literature for AUS/FLUS diagnosis determined by cytologic-histologic correlation is most likely an overestimation (19). Renshaw reported several cellular patterns in the AUS/FLUS category and concluded that different cell patterns carry different risks of malignancy (Table 2) (35, 36). The presence of nuclear features of PTC in the indeterminate category has been reported to be true PTC at histology and carries a higher risk of malignancy (21, 22, 26, 29, 33, 35-44). This is why the Japanese system classifies this indeterminate category separately (Indeterminate B) from follicular pattern lesions without PTC type nuclear features (Indeterminate A) (please refer to Chapter 2). Furthermore, cases of PTC lineage are separately handled from the FA/FTC lineage in the Japanese system because PTC accounts for the vast majority (more than 90%) of thyroid malignancies in the Japanese population, and confirmation or denial of PTC type malignancy is achieved more efficiently by molecular techniques using FNA samples (38, 45, 46). Further qualification of the AUS/FLUS category with different cellular patterns would be beneficial for further refining this heterogeneous category (5, 32, 36, 38, 42, 44, 46).

Rates of AUS/FLUS and Risk of Malignancy

As with the diagnostic categories of undetermined significance in other organs, the authors of the TBSRTC were concerned that AUS/FLUS may be potentially overused, and they recommended that the diagnoses of AUS/FLUS should be in the range of approximately 7% of all thyroid FNA diagnoses (3). The authors have further stated that AUS/FLUS is a category of last resort, and should not be used indiscriminately (4). It is important for cytopathologists to reduce the rates of indeterminate (inadequate, low-risk indeterminate, high-risk indeterminate and suspicious for malignancy) categories to minimize diagnostic surgery for patients with indeterminate nodules. Address of possible technical issues is warranted in institutions with high rates of indeterminate diagnoses. If corrected, the incidence of indeterminate diagnoses, including AUS/FLUS, should decrease (19). Abele and Levine discussed the diagnostic criteria of the indeterminate category and suggested that the national rate of 15% results in large part from overdiagnosis, and proposed in detail how to reduce the rates of indeterminate categories (1). Concerning the diagnostic criteria of AUS/FLUS, VanderLaan *et al*. analyzed more than 5000 thyroid FNAs that had been handled by seven cytopathologists and found that the higher the cytopathologist's AUS/FLUS rate, the lower the rate of malignancy in that AUS/FLUS cohort (21). Singh *et al.* and Renshaw and Gould analyzed the cellular patterns of the AUS/FLUS category and demonstrated the inclusion of heterogeneous diseases carrying different risks of malignancy (Table 2) (17, 36). From these observations, Renshaw proposed in detail how to reduce the rates of the indeterminate categories (36), and Singh *et al.* proposed their diagnostic schema and concluded that the AUS/FLUS category can be eliminated by providing appropriate management (32).

Table 2. Cellular patterns in the indeterminate categories and proposed reported systems by Renshaw, Singh and Wang, and diagnostic categories in the American, Italian, British and Japanese systems

Cell patterns by Renshaw/ reporting systems (36)	Modified Bethesda by Renshaw (7,8)	Proposed system by Singh and Wang (32)	American/ Italian/British systems	Category in Japanese system
<100 Follicular cells, all in a few tight microfollicles, not trapped in blood	AUS	Microfollicular lesion	FLUS/TIR3A/ Thy 3a	Indeterminate, A1: favor benign
Discrete area of 5 to 6 clustered microfollicles, background benign	AUS	Microfollicular lesion	FLUS/TIR3A/ Thy 3a	Indeterminate, A1: favor benign
Follicular cells, trapped in blood, variable architecture	Favor benign	Suboptimal specimen due to excess blood but suggestive of microfollicular lesion	FLUS/TIR3A/ Thy 3a	Inadequate, Benign or A1: favor benign (depend on quality of sample)
<100 Cells, all Hurthle cells	AUS	Hurthle cell nodule	FLUS/TIR3A/ Thy 3a	Indeterminate, A1: favor benign
Numerous Hurthle cells with dysplasia	AUS	Hurthle cell neoplasm	FN (Hurthle cell type)/ TIR3B/ Thy 3b	Indeterminate, A1-3 (depend on cellular and structural atypia)
Numerous Hurthle cells, no dysplasia, usually in flat sheets	Favor benign	Hurthle cell lesion	FLUS/TIR3A/ Thy 3a	Indeterminate, A1-3 (depend on cellular and structural atypia)
Numerous Hurthle cells in 1 slide in a background of Hashimoto thyroiditis	Favor Benign	Hurthle cell lesion	AUS/TIR3A/ Thy 3a	Benign
Focal features of papillary carcinoma, usually <100 cells	AUS	Follicular lesion with focal features suggestive of but not diagnostic for PTC	AUS/TIR3A/ Thy 3a	Indeterminate, B

Table 2 (*Continued*). Cellular patterns in the indeterminate categories and proposed reported systems by Renshaw, Singh and Wang, and diagnostic categories in the American, Italian, British and Japanese systems

Cytologic atypia other than features of papillary carcinoma and not in microfollicles	AUS	Not defined	AUS/TIR3A/Thy 3a	Indeterminate, A1-3 (depend on cellular and structural atypia)
Air-dry artifact	Favor benign	Suboptimal specimen due to air dry	AUS/TIR3A/Thy 3a	Inadequate, Benign or Indeterminate, B (depend on quality of sample)
Hashimoto thyroiditis atypia (elongated dark and smudgy nuclei, no papillary features)	Favor benign	Benign follicular lesion	AUS/TIR3A/Thy 3a	Benign or Indeterminate, B (depend on cellular atypia)
Atypical cyst lining cells	Favor benign	Follicular lesion with focal features suggestive of, but not diagnostic for PTC	AUS/TIR3A/Thy 3a	Benign or Indeterminate, B (depend on cellular atypia)
Radiation atypia (isolated, elongated dark nuclei often with nucleoli)	Favor benign	Follicular lesion with focal features suggestive of, but not diagnostic for PTC	AUS/TIR3A/Thy 3a	Indeterminate, B
Numerous microfollicles with or without cytological atypia but no features of papillary carcinoma	FN/SFN	Microfollicular follicular neoplasm	FN/TIR3B/Thy 3b	Indeterminate, A1-3 (depend on cellular and structural atypia)
Numerous dysplastic Hurthle cells	Suspicious for Hurthle cell neoplasia	Hurthle cell neoplasm	FN (Hurthle cell type)/TIR3B/Thy 3b	Indeterminate, A1-3 (depend on cellular and structural atypia)
Numerous microfollicles with nuclear features of papillary carcinoma	Suspicious papillary carcinoma, rule out FN	Suspicious for PTC	Suspicious for Malignancy	Malignancy
Numerous dysplastic Hurthle cells with nuclear features of papillary carcinoma	Suspicious papillary carcinoma, rule out Hurthle cell neoplasia	Suspicious for PTC	Suspicious for Malignancy	Malignancy

Take Home Message

The 2015 American Thyroid Association clinical guidelines recommend a repeat FNA cytology, ultrasound, or molecular tests for further risk assessment instead of a diagnostic surgery for patients with an AUS/FLUS nodule. Repeat FNA cytology often resolves poor sample quality and allows a more definite diagnosis in the majority of cases. Although the terms of AUS and FLUS are synonymous in the TBSRTC, the authors of this chapter believe that the AUS and FLUS subcategories should be separately reported and not combined into one category, because their clinical managements and risks of malignancy are different. In cases with worrisome PTC type nuclear features, a higher risk of malignancy (>40%) has been reported in surgically treated patients.

References

1. Abele JS, Levine RA. Diagnostic criteria and risk-adapted approach to indeterminate thyroid cytodiagnosis. Cancer Cytopathol 2010; 118:415-22.
2. Kini SR. Thyroid Cytopathology: An Atlas and Text. 2nd ed. Philadelphia:Wolters Kluwer Health; 2015.
3. Cibas ES, Ali SZ. The Bethesda System for Reporting Thyroid Cytopathology. Am J Clin Pathol 2009; 132:658-65.
4. Ali SZ and Cibas ES (ed). The Bethesda system for reporting thyroid cytopathology. Definitions, criteria and explanatory notes. Springer, New York, USA, 2010, p1-166.
5. Bongiovanni M, Krane JF, Cibas ES, et al. The atypical thyroid fine-needle aspiration: past, present, and future. Cancer Cytopathol 2012; 120:73-86.
6. Nayar R, Ivanovic M. The indeterminate thyroid fine-needle aspiration: experience from an academic center using terminology similar to that proposed in the 2007 National Cancer Institute Thyroid Fine Needle Aspiration State of the Science Conference. Cancer 2009; 117:195-202.
7. Faquin WC, Baloch ZW. Fine-needle aspiration of follicular patterned lesions of the thyroid: Diagnosis, management, and follow-up according to National Cancer Institute (NCI) recommendation. Diagn Cytopathol 2010; 38:731-9.
8. Haugen BR, Alexander EK, Bible KC, et al. American Thyroid Association management guidelines for adult patients with thyroid nodules and differentiated thyroid cancer. Thyroid 2015; 26:1-134.
9. Faquin WC, Cibas ES, Renshaw AA. "Atypical" cells in fine-needle aspiration biopsy specimens of benign thyroid cysts. Cancer Cytopathol 2005; 105:71-9.
10. Utsun H, Astarci HM, Altunkaya C, et al. Fine-needle aspiration of follicular patterned lesions of the thyroid: diagnosis, management, and follow-up according to thyroid Bethesda system. Acta Cytol 2012; 56:361-9.
11. VanderLaan PA, Marqusee E, Krane JF. Clinical outcome for atypia of undetermined significance in thyroid fine-needle aspirations. Should repeated FNA be the preferred initial approach? Am J Clin Pathol 2011; 135:770-5.
12. Yassa L, Cibas ES, Benson CB, et al. Long-term assessment of a multidisciplinary approach to thyroid nodule diagnostic evaluation. Cancer Cytopathol 2007; 111:508-16.
13. Sullivan PS, Hirschowitz SL, Fung PC, et al. The impact of Atypia/Follicular Lesion of Undetermined Significance and repeat fine-needle aspiration: 5 years before and after implementation of the Bethesda system. Cancer Cytopathol 2014; 122:866-72.
14. Yoo MR, Gweon HM, Park AY, et al. Repeat diagnosis of Bethesda category III Thyroid nodules: What to do next? PLoS One 2015; 10(6):e0130138.
15. Brandler TC, Aziz MS, Coutsouvelis C, et al. Young investigator challenge: Atypia of undetermined significance in thyroid FNA: Standardized terminology without standardized management-Acloser look at repeat FNA and quality measures. Cancer Cytopathol 2016; 124:37-43.
16. Layfield LJ, Cibas ES, Gharib H, et al. Thyroid Aspiration Cytology: Current Status. CA Cancer J Clinicians 2009; 59:99-110.
17. Shi Y, Ding X, Klein M, et al. Thyroid Fine-needle aspiration with atypia of undetermined significance. A necessary or optional category? Cancer Cytopathol 2009; 117:298-304.
18. Marchevsky AM, Walts AE, Bose S, et al. Evidence-based evaluation of the risks of malignancy predicted by thyroid fine-needle aspiration biopsies. Diagn Cytopathol 2010; 38:252-9.
19. Ohori NP, Schoedel KE. Variability in the atypia of undetermined significance/follicular lesion of

undetermined significance diagnosis in the Bethesda system for reporting thyroid cytopathology: Sources and recommendations. Acta Cytol 2011; 55:492-8.
20. Cochand-Priollet B, Schmitt FC, Totsch M, et al. The Bethesda terminology for reporting thyroid cytopathology: from theory to practice in Europe. Acta Cytol 2011; 55:507-11.
21. VanderLaan PA, Krane JF, Cibas ES. The frequency of 'atypia of undetermined significance' interpretation is negatively correlated with histologically proven malignant outcomes. Acta Cytol 2011; 55:512-7.
22. Mathur A, Najafian A, Schneider EB, et al. Malignancy risk and reproducibility associated with atypia of undetermined significance on thyroid cytology. Surgery 2014; 156:1471-6.
23. Kierman CM, Broome JT, Solorzano CC. The Bethesda system for reporting thyroid cytopathology: A single-center experience over 5 years. Ann Surg Oncol 2014; 21:3522-7.
24. Muddegowda PH, Srinivasan S, Lingegowda JB, et al. Spectrum of cytology of neck lesions: comparative study from two centers. J Clin Diagn Res 2014; 8:44-5.
25. Park VY, Kim EK, Kwak JY, et al. Malignancy risk and characteristics of thyroid nodules with two consecutive results of atypia of undetermined significance or follicular lesion of undetermined significance on cytology. Eur Radiol 2015; 25:2601-7.
26. Jung YY, Jung S, Kee HW, et al. Significance of subcategory atypia of undetermined significance/follicular lesion of undetermined significance showing both cytological and architectural atypia in thyroid aspiration cytology. Acta Cytol 2015; 59:370376.
27. Strickland KC, Howitt BE, Marquesee E, et al. The impact of non-invasive follicular variant of papillary thyroid carcinoma on rates of malignancy for fine-needle aspiration diagnostic categories. Thyroid 2015; 25:987-92.
28. Faquin WC, Wong LQ, Afrogheh AH, et al. Impact of reclassifying noninvasive follicular variant of papillary thyroid carcinoma on the risk of malignancy in the Bethesda system for reporting thyroid cytopathology. Cancer Cytopathol 2015 Oct 12. doi: 10.1002/cncy.21631. [Epub ahead of print]
29. Wu HH, Jones JN, Grzybicki DM, et al. Sensitive cytologic criteria for the identification of follicular variant of papillary thyroid carcinoma in fine-needle aspiration biopsy. Diagn Cytopathol 2003; 29:262-6.
30. Nishigami K, Liu Z, Taniguchi E, et al. Cytological features of well-differentiated tumors of uncertain malignant potential: indeterminate cytology and WDT-UMP. Eendocr J 2012; 59:483-7.
31. Cibas ES, Baloch ZW, Fellegra G, et al. A prospective assessment defining limitations of thyroid nodule pathologic evaluation. Ann Int Med 2013; 159:325-32.
32. Singh RS, Wang HH. Eliminating the "atypia of undetermined significance/follicular lesion of undetermined significance" category from the Bethesda System for Reporting Thyroid Cytopathology. Am J Clin Pathol 2011; 136:896-902.
33. Park JH, Yoon SO, Son EJ, et al. Incidence and malignancy rates of diagnoses in the Bethesda system for reporting thyroid aspiration cytology: an institutional experience. Korean J Pathol 2014; 48:133-9.
34. Takezawa N, Sakamoto A, Komatsu K, et al. Cytological evaluation of the "indeterminate" category by the Bethesda System for Reporting Thyroid Cytopathol. J Jpn Soc Clin Cytol 2014; 53:251-6. (in Japanese with English abstract)
35. Renshaw AA. Focal features of papillary carcinoma of the thyroid in fine needle aspiration material are strongly associated with papillary carcinoma at resection. Am J Clin Pathol 2002; 118:208-10.
36. Renshaw AA, Gould EW. Reducing indeterminate thyroid FNAs. Cancer Cytopathol 2015; 123:237-43.
37. Weber D, Brainard J, Chen L. Atypical epithelial cells, cannot exclude papillary carcinoma, in fine needle aspiration of the thyroid. Acta Cytol 2008; 52:320-4.
38. Hyeon J, Ahn S, Shin JH, et al. The prediction of malignant risk in the category 'atypia of undetermined significance/follicular lesion of undetermined significance' of the Bethesda System for Reporting Thyroid Cytopathology using subcategorization and BRAF mutation results. Cancer Cytopathol 2014; 122:368-76.
39. Olson MT, Clark DP, Erozan YS, et al. Spectrum of risk of malignancy in subcategories of 'atypia of undetermined significance'. Acta Cytol 2011; 55:518-25.
40. Krane JF, VanderLaan PA, Faquin WC, et al. The atypia of undetermined significance/follicular lesion of

undetermined significance: malignant ratio: a proposed performance measure for reporting in the Bethesda System for thyroid cytopathology. Cancer Cytopathol 2012; 120:111-6.
41. Wu HH, Inman A, Cramer HM. Subclassification of 'atypia of undetermined significance' in thyroid fine-needle aspirates. Diagn Cytopathol 2014; 42:23-9.
42. Park HJ, Moon JH, Yom CK, et al. Thyroid 'atypia of undetermined significance' with nuclear atypia has high rates of malignancy and BRAF mutation. Cancer Cytopathol 2014; 122:512-20.
43. Zhu Y, Dai J, Lin X, et al. Fine needle aspiration of thyroid nodules: experience in a Chinese population. J Basic Clin Med 2015; 4:65-9.
44. Yoon JH, Kwon HJ, Kim EK, et al. Subcategorization of atypia of undetermined significance/follicular lesion of undetermined significance (AUS/FLUS): a study applying thyroid imaging reporting and data system (TIRADS). Clin Endoclinol (Oxf) 2015 Dec 7. doi: 10.1111/cen.12987. [Epub ahead of print]
45. Kakudo K, Kameyama K, Miyauchi A, et al. Introducing the reporting system for thyroid fine-needle aspiration cytology according to the new guidelines of the Japan Thyroid Association. Endocr J 2014; 61:539-52.
46. Kakudo K, Kameyama K, Takano T. Thyroid fine needle aspiration cytology: current and future. Proposal of a new diagnostic system for reporting thyroid cytology. J Basic Clin Med 2915; 4:110-4.

Chapter 6

The New Tumor Entity "NIFTP (Non-invasive Follicular Thyroid Neoplasm with Papillary-like Nuclear Features)" and Conventional Papillary Carcinoma

Zhiyan Liu, Shinya Satoh and Kennichi Kakudo

Brief Clinical Summary

The patient was a 72-year-old female who has a history of stroke. During follow up, she was found to have a nodule in the right lobe of the thyroid. She was referred to our hospital for a further check-up, and under ultrasound guidance, a fine needle aspiration (FNA) was performed for the 18 mm thyroid nodule (Figure 1).

Ultrasound Findings

Ultrasound detected a well-circumscribed nodule in the right lobe of the thyroid (Figure 1). The nodule was solid with minor cystic change. Neither irregular margin suggestive of invasion into thyroid parenchyma nor invasion to thyroid capsule was found. No calcification was identified in the nodule. A clinical diagnosis of a benign adenomatous nodule was made based on the ultrasound images.

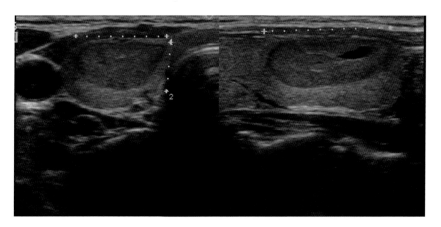

Figure 1. Ultrasound images show a well-demarcated thyroid nodule.

Cytological Findings:

A moderate number of follicular cells in follicular pattern clusters were seen in the Papanicolaou-stained conventional smear (Figures 2-6). No macrophages suggesting cystic change were noted in the smear background. These follicular cell clusters appeared in loosely cohesive with moderate nuclear overlapping (Figures 2-4) or in large trabecular clusters (Figure 5). Many isolated cells with ill-defined pale cytoplasm were also noted (Figure 4). The tumor cell nuclei were irregular in shape (Figures 3 and 5), and moderately enlarged, and they had a few grooves with fine powdery chromatin (Figures 2-6). Nuclear crowding, overlapping, and molding were conspicuous as shown in the Figure 5. A definite nuclear cytoplasmic inclusion (NCI) body was found in only one sample (Figure 6), but small questionable nuclear inclusions or vacuoles (red arrows in Figures 3 and 4) and a few of nuclear grooves (yellow arrows in Figures 3 and 4) were worrisome nuclear features, suggesting papillary thyroid carcinoma (PTC) type malignancy. Nucleoli were small and inconspicuous. Neither psammoma bodies nor necrosis was identified in the smear background.

List of Differential Diagnoses
1. Benign, follicular adenoma
2. Benign, atypical follicular adenoma (FA)
3. Benign, Hashimoto thyroiditis
4. Indeterminate A, follicular neoplasm (FN by the Bethesda system, TIR 3B by Italian system or Thy 3f by British system)
5. Indeterminate B, others, PTC cannot rule out (AUS by the Bethesda system, TIR 3A by the Italian system or Thy 3a by the British system)
6. Suspicious for PTC, follicular variant
7. Malignant, PTC, follicular variant
8. Malignant, PTC, conventional

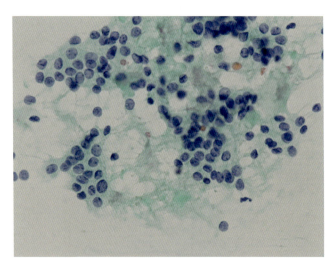

Figure 2. Moderate nuclear enlargement is seen in microfollicular or loosely arranged clusters. (Conventional smear, Papanicolaou stain, x400)

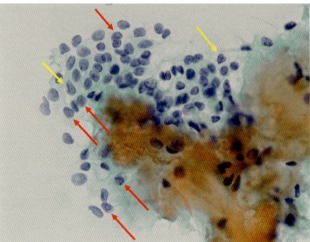

Figure 3. Small nuclear vacuoles (red arrows) and grooves (yellow arrows) are shown in loosely cohesive follicular cells. (Conventional smear, Papanicolaou stain, x400)

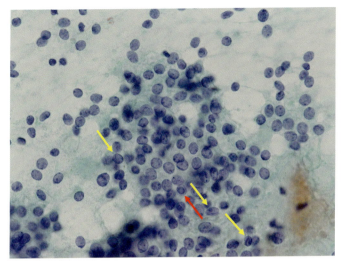

Figure 4. Note a small nuclear vacuole or inclusion (red arrow) and grooves (yellow arrows) in a loosely cohesive large cluster of follicular cells. Numerous isolated cells are also seen in the smear background. (Conventional smear, Papanicolaou stain, x400)

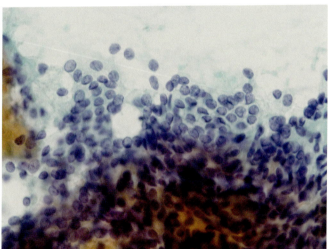

Figure 5. A large follicular cell cluster forms trabecular arrangement. Nuclear crowding, molding and irregularity are shown. (Conventional smear, Papanicolaou stain, x400)

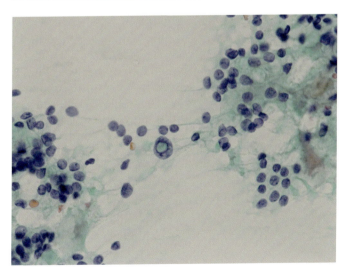

Figure 6. A large nucleus with a cytoplasmic inclusion is shown in the center. This is the only nuclear inclusion identified in the samples. (Conventional smear, Papanicolaou stain, x400)

Differential Diagnosis:
Differential diagnoses include atypical FA, atypical follicular cells in Hashimoto thyroiditis, conventional PTC, follicular variant PTC, well differentiated tumor of uncertain malignant potential (WDT-UMP), NIFTP, and follicular thyroid carcinoma (FTC).

Hashimoto thyroiditis can be ruled out by the absence of lymphocytes in the smear background. Characteristic oxyphilic change (Hurthle) of follicular cells in Hashimoto thyroiditis is absent (please refer to Chapter 13).

Moderate nuclear enlargement, nuclear shape irregularity, and small nuclear vacuoles in this case were worrisome nuclear features of PTC type malignancy. NCIs are seen in more than 80% of conventional PTC (please refer to Chapters 3 and 4), however, they are not specific for PTC type malignancy because they are also seen in C cell (medullary) carcinomas (please refer to Chapters 15 and 16), benign hyalinizing trabecular adenomas (please refer to Chapter 12), and in some cases of adenomatous nodules and FA (please refer to Chapters 3 and 4). The NCI of PTC are larger than one third of the nuclear diameter and have distinctive sharp contour by a rim of condensed chromatin (please refer to Chapters 3 and 4), which was rarely found in this case. The minimum number of NCIs necessary for a PTC diagnosis is uncertain because the threshold varies among observers and a significant observer variation exists. For PTC, NCIs should be observed in many tumor cells and is found easily when examining. However those nuclear changes as shown in the Figures 3 and 4 are incomplete nuclear features for PTC type malignancy. Therefore it may be appropriate to classify this case in either indeterminate B, others, PTC cannot be ruled out (AUS by the Bethesda system, TIR 3A by the Italian system or Thy 3a by the British system) or indeterminate A, follicular neoplasm (FN by the Bethesda system, TIR 3B by the Italian system or Thy 3f by the British system). It is also acceptable but not advisable to classify it in suspicious for PTC (TIR 4 or Thy 4), follicular variant, or pattern B of suspicious for malignancy by the Bethesda system, because it's clinical management is usually different from that of indeterminate categories. A conservative approach of classifying cases with mild PTC-N, which are intermediate between the indeterminate category and suspicious categories, into indeterminate category is recommended. Classification of NIFTP or WDT-UMP in suspicious for malignancy category has been reported in a high proportion from several academic centers (1-4), and it should be minimized because of benign nature of this lesion. One typical NCI (Figure 6) is not sufficient for a diagnosis of malignant. A diagnosis of malignancy, such as conventional PTC, should not be applied to this case.

Histological Diagnosis: NIFTP (non-invasive follicular thyroid neoplasm with papillary-like nuclear features), WDT-UMP (well differentiated tumor of uncertain malignant potential), or non-invasive encapsulated follicular variant papillary carcinoma of the thyroid

An 18 mm well-circumscribed nodule was found in the right lobe of the thyroid gland (Figure 7). Small areas of hemorrhage and cystic change were noted on the cut surface (Figure 7). It was a capsulated, follicular patterned lesion with thin a fibrous capsule (Figures 8A and 8B). Neither invasive growth beyond the tumor capsule (Figure 8) nor papillary growth was identified (Figures 8-10). Moderately increased nuclear size and an irregular nuclear contour similar to the cytological features were well demonstrated in the histological samples (Figures 8-10). An irregular nuclear contour and ground glass (powdery chromatin) nuclei were more clearly shown in the Figures 9 and 10. Incomplete NCIs or degenerative vacuoles were seen as indicated with blue arrows in the Figures 9 and 10. No enlarged lymph nodes suggesting metastasis were found during surgery, and prophylactic lymph node dissection was not carried out.

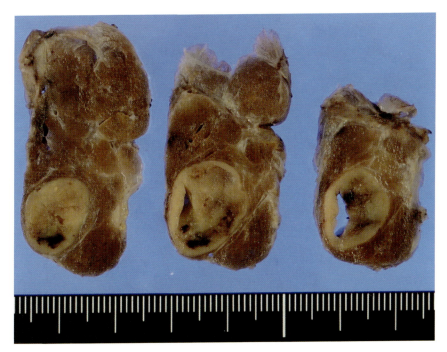

Figure 7. Gross appearance of the thyroid tumor (cut surface after formalin fixation), showing an encapsulated nodule, 18 mm in diameter, ivory-white in color, and solid with hemorrhage and cystic change.

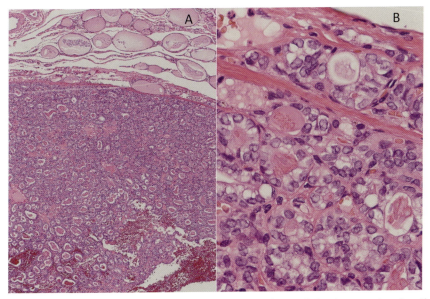

Figure 8. Low (A, x100) and high (B, x400) magnifications of the tumor, showing the well encapsulation by a thin fibrous capsule. Note follicular but not papillary growth pattern. These follicles are composed of atypical follicular cells with large irregular nuclei.

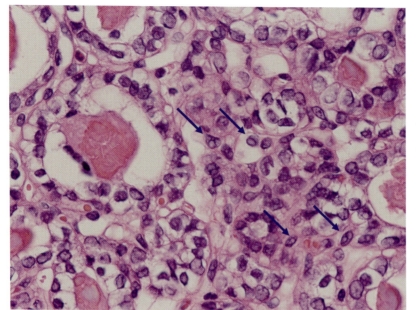

Figure 9. Incomplete nuclear inclusions or vacuoles are indicated by blue arrows. Note the irregular nuclear contour and hyperchromatic nuclear chromatin (x400).

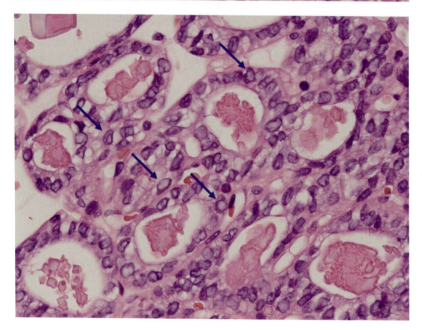

Figure 10. Blue arrows indicate nuclear vacuoles in irregular nuclei. Note the pure follicular growth pattern (x400).

Explanatory Notes:

PTC is a malignant follicular cell tumor characterized by distinctive nuclear features. Follicular variant PTC (FVPTC) is the most common sub-type of PTC, which is characterized by PTC type nuclear features (PTC-N) and a follicular (non-papillary) growth pattern. There are debates on diagnostic criteria of this variant and observer variation between benign FA and malignant FVPTC has been reported to be significant (5-7). The Memorial Sloan-Kettering Cancer Center group has clarified that there are three sub-types of FVPTC that have different genetic profiles and different biological behaviors (8-10). None of the 57 cases of non-invasive encapsulated sub-type of FVPTC developed recurrence or metastasis after surgery with an average follow up time of 9.5 years (10). The encapsulated group of FVPTC did not contain BRAF mutations and 36% of them had RAS mutations similarly as FA or FTC (9). The benign biological nature of the non-invasive encapsulated FVPTC after lobectomy without radioactive iodine treatment has been confirmed by several other groups (11-13) and NIFTP has been proposed to replace cancer terminology to avoid overtreatment to this possible precursor lesion of malignant invasive encapsulated FVPTC (12). This case probably belonged to this spectrum of thyroid tumor with benign behavior. Synonyms include encapsulated FVPTC, atypical adenoma, WDT-UMP (15), and well differentiated tumor with uncertain behavior (11, 16). This group of thyroid tumors typically shows cells with nuclear enlargement and chromatin clearing, but nuclear grooves and NCIs are less common than observed in conventional PTC. Nishigami *et al.* analyzed cytological features of WDT-UMP and have concluded that WDT-UMP belongs to intermediate category between PTC and FA morphologically, and this is one of the reasons why some NIFTP or WDT-UMP cases are found more in the indeterminate category (17). It has been confirmed by other studies that a large number of PTCs in the indeterminate categories are low grade PTC or benign non-invasive encapsulated FVPTC (1-4, 18). Therefore, it is important for cytopathologists and cytotechnologists to understand that the worrisome nuclear features of PTC should be classified into either low-risk or high-risk indeterminate categories and only those of definite PTC-N should be classified into the malignant category to reduce false positive diagnoses and unnecessary surgical treatments to this biologically benign tumor with incomplete PTC-N (please refer to Chapters 1, 4, and 6).

Take Home Message:
A conservative approach to evaluate PTC-N is recommended for the cases with focal or limited nuclear changes. Incomplete or worrisome nuclear features of PTC do not represent a diagnostic feature of high-risk thyroid carcinoma or advanced stage PTC, but in most cases, they represent an indicator of early stage neoplastic lesions, such as benign FA, precursor tumors (NIFTP) of low malignant potential or early stage (T1 or T2) thyroid carcinomas, which can be followed clinically without immediate surgical treatments when no other clinical tests indicate high-risk malignant features.

References

1. Strickland KC, Howitt BE, Marquesee E, et al. The impact of non-invasive follicular variant of papillary thyroid carcinoma on rates of malignancy for fine-needle aspiration diagnostic categories. Thyroid 2015; 25:987-92.
2. Liu X, Medici M, Kwong N, et al. Bethesda categorization of thyroid nodule cytology and prediction of thyroid cancer type and prognosis. Thyroid 2015; [Epub ahead of print]
3. Faquin WC, Wong LQ, Afrogheh AH, et al. Impact of reclassifying noninvasive follicular variant of papillary thyroid carcinoma on the risk of malignancy in the Bethesda system for reporting thyroid cytopathology. Cancer Cytopathol 2015 Oct 12. doi: 10.1002/cncy.21631. [Epub ahead of print]
4. Maletta F, Massa F, Torregrossa L et al. Cytological features of "noninvasive follicular thyroid neoplasm with papillary-like nuclear features" and their correlation with tumor histology. Hum Pathol 2016, doi: 10.1016/j.humpath.2016.03.014. [Epub ahead of print]
5. Kakudo K, Katoh R, Sakamoto A, et al. Thyroid gland: international case conference. Endocrine Pathol 2002; 13:131-4.
6. Hirokawa M, Carney JA, Goellner JR, et al. Observer variation of encapsulated follicular lesions of the thyroid gland. Am J Surg Pathol 2002; 26:1508-14.
7. Lloyd RV, Erickson LA, Casey MB, et al. Observer variation in the diagnosis of follicular variant of papillary thyroid carcinoma. Am J Surg Pathol 2004; 28:1336-40.
8. Liu J, Singh B, Tallini G, et al. Follicular variant of papillary carcinoma. A clinicopathologic study of a

problematic entity. Cancer 2006; 107:1255-64.
9. Rivera M, Ricarte-Filho J, Knauf J, et al. Encapsulated papillary thyroid carcinoma: A clinic-pathologic study of 106 cases with emphasis on its morphologic subtypes (histologic growth pattern). Mod Pathol 2010; 23:1191-200.
10. Ganly I, Wang L, Tuttle RM, et al. Invasion rather than nuclear features correlates with outcome in encapsulated follicular tumors: further evidence for the reclassification of the encapsulated papillary thyroid carcinoma follicular variant. Hum Pathol 2015; 46:657-64.
11. Liu Z, Zhou G, Nakamura M, et al. Encapsulated follicular thyroid tumor with equivocal nuclear changes, so-called well-differentiated tumor of uncertain malignant potential: a morphological, immunohistochemical, and molecular appraisal. Cancer Sci 2011; 102:288-94.
12. Vivero M, Kraft S, Barletta JA. Risk stratification of follicular variant of papillary thyroid carcinoma. Thyroid 2013; 23(3):273-9.
13. Rosario PW, Penna GC, Calsolari MR. Noninvasive encapsulated follicular variant of papillary thyroid carcinoma: is lobectomy sufficient for tumours >/=1 cm? Clin Endocrinol (Oxf) 2014; 81(4):630-2.
14. Nikiforov YE, Seethala RR, Tallini Gi, et al. Nomenclature revision for encapsulated follicular variant of papillary thyroid carcinoma: A paradigm shift to reduce overtreatment of indolent tumors. JAMA Oncol 2016; 2:1023-9.
15. Williams ED. Guest editorial: Two proposals regarding the terminology of thyroid tumors. Int I Surg Pathol 2000; 8:181-3.
16. Kakudo K, Bai Y, Liu Z, et al. Encapsulated papillary thyroid carcinoma, follicular variant: A misnomer. Pathol Int 2012; 62:155-60.
17. Nishigami K, Liu Z, Taniguchi E, et al. Cytological features of well-differentiated tumors of uncertain malignant potential: Indeterminate cytology and WDT-UMP. Endocrine J 2012; 59:483-7.
18. Rago T, Scutari M, Latrofa F, et al. The large majority of 1520 patients with indeterminate thyroid nodule at cytology have a favorable outcome, and a clinical risk score has a high negative predictive value for a more cumbersome cancer disease. J Clin Endocrinol Metab 2014: 99:3700-7.

Chapter 7

Cyst or Cystic Papillary Carcinoma

Kayoko Higuchi

Clinical Summary

A 66-year-old female presented with hoarseness and an anterior neck mass measuring 10 cm in diameter. She noticed the mass 9 months ago, and the mass had been increasing in size. Palpation demonstrated that it was smooth, lobulated, and elastic-hard. Cystic papillary carcinoma was suspected based on the lesion's ultrasound (US), computed tomography (CT), and fine-needle aspiration biopsy (FNA) findings. Total thyroidectomy and lymph node dissection were performed.

Clinical Tests

Blood tests revealed that the patient's levels of free triiodothyronine (T3) and thyroxine (T4) were normal, but her thyroglobulin level was devated to 125 (normal level: ~33.7) ng/ml.

Ultrasound and CT Findings

With neck US, a multilocular cyst measuring 10 cm in diameter was found in the right thyroid. In addition, an irregularly shaped solid nodule of 2.4 cm in size was observed on the cyst wall. The nodule exhibited heterogeneous contents and many dot-like echogenic foci, which were suggestive of microcalcification (Figure 1A). Color Doppler demonstrated vascular structures within the nodule (Figure 1B).

A contrast-enhanced CT scan revealed a multilocular cystic mass with an enhanced irregularly shaped mural nodule in the right lobe of the thyroid (Figure 2). The mural nodule contained fine calcifications and was consistent with papillary carcinoma.

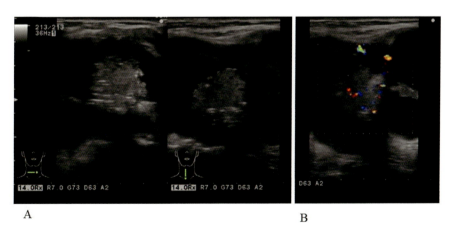

Figure 1. Ultrasound images of the right neck. A: A multilocular cyst measuring 10 cm in diameter is shown in the right thyroid. An irregularly shaped solid nodule of 2.4 cm in size is demonstrated in the cyst, which contains heterogeneous contents and many dot-like echogenic foci, suggestive of microcalcifications. B: Color Doppler demonstrates vascular structures within the nodule.

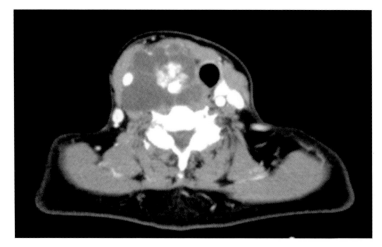

Figure 2. CT image of the neck. Contrast-enhanced CT shows a multilocular cystic mass with an enhanced irregularly shaped mural nodule in the right lobe of the thyroid. The mural nodule contains fine calcifications, consistent with papillary carcinoma.

Cytological Findings

The aspirates of the cyst were bloody, and contained a few of tumor cell clusters and numerous macrophages with or without hemosiderin, which obscured the malignant cells (Figure 3). No colloid material was observed in the smear background. The tumor cells were isolated cells with thickened cytoplasm and sharp cytoplasmic borders, and formed small papillary clusters and scalloped ball-like clusters (Figures 4, 5, and 6). The cytoplasm of many tumor cells was vacuolated. The degree of vacuolation varied from cell to cell (Figure 7). The aspiration specimens from the mural nodule were cellular and contained syncytial epithelial sheets and papillary clusters of typical papillary carcinoma cells with powdery chromatin (Figure 8). Figures 9A-9D of the tumor cells detected in a liquid-based cytology (LBC) specimen show: a syncytial epithelial sheet (Figure 9A); a monolayered tumor cell cluster in which the cells exhibited thickened dome-shaped cytoplasm (suggestive of squamous metaplasia) (Figure 9B); a small papillary cluster of vacuolated tumor cells (Figure 9C); and a tumor cell cluster containing a psammoma body (Figure 9D). Figure 10 shows a cancer cell cluster that displays squamous and regenerative changes.

List of Differential Diagnoses
1. Cystic papillary carcinoma
2. Cystic nodular goiter
3. Cystic anaplastic carcinoma
4. Branchial cleft cyst of the neck
5. Other benign cysts

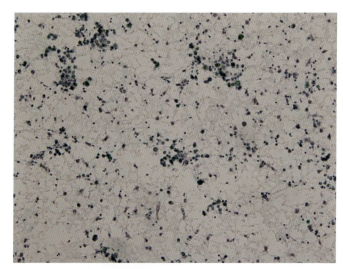

Figure 3. FNA smear of the cystic fluid. The aspirates of the cyst are bloody and contain many macrophages. Malignant cells are not distinct and colloid material is absent. (Papanicolaou stain, x200)

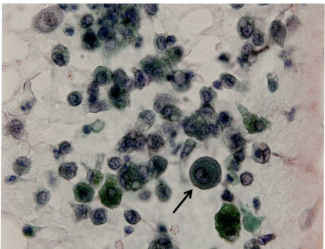

Figure 4. FNA smear of the cystic fluid with only a few tumor cells. The tumor cells are isolated with thickened cytoplasm and sharp cytoplasmic borders. Many histiocytes with or without hemosiderin are also observed. (Papanicolaou stain, x1000)

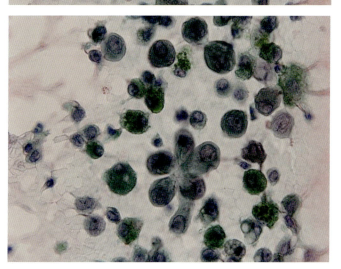

Figue 5. FNA smear of the cystic fluid showing small papillary clusters of the hobnail-shaped tumor cells. (Papanicolaou stain, x1000)

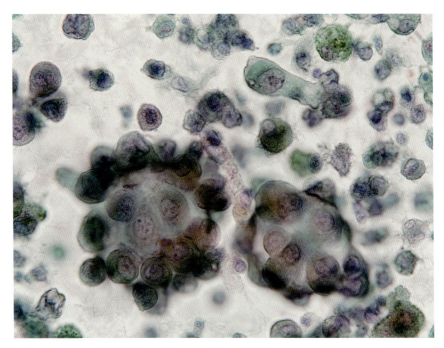

Figure 6. FNA smear of the cystic fluid showing the tumor cells arranged in scalloped ball-like clusters. (Papanicolaou stain, x1000)

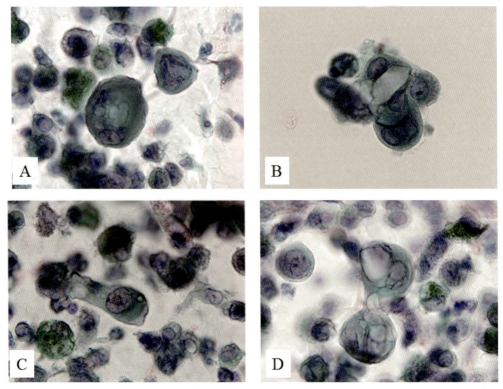

Figure 7. FNA smear of the cystic fluid. The cytoplasm of many tumor cells is vacuolated. The number of vacuoles varies among the cells. (Papanicolaou stain, x1000)

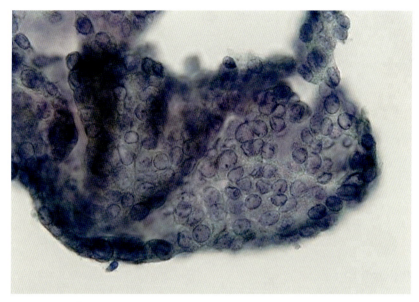

Figure 8. FNA smear of aspirates from the mural nodule showing syncytial papillary clusters of typical papillary carcinoma cells with powdery chromatin. (Papanicolaou stain, x1000)

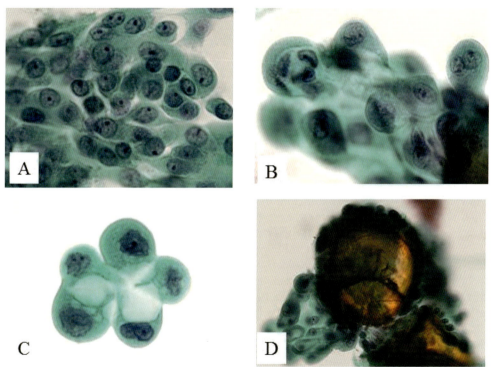

Figure 9. Liquid-based smear of aspirates from the mural nodule. A: A syncytial epithelial sheet of papillary carcinoma cells; B: A monolayered tumor cell cluster in which the cells exhibit thickened dome-shaped cytoplasm (suggestive of squamous metaplasia); C: A small papillary cluster of vacuolated tumor cells; D: Tumor cell cluster containing psammoma bodies. (Papanicolaou stain, x1000)

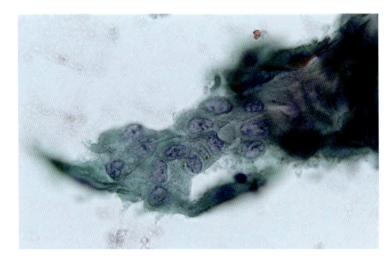

Figure 10. FNA smear of aspirates from the mural nodule. A cancer cluster exhibits squamous and regenerative changes. (Papanicolaou stain, x1000)

Differential Diagnosis

The most common cystic lesion of the thyroid is cystic nodular goiter, and thus, the incidence of carcinoma in thyroid cysts is generally low (1). On the contrary, the most common malignant neoplasm of the thyroid that exhibits cystic changes is papillary carcinoma, and its incidence is reported to be as high as 16.6%. The aspirates from the cystic portion of the cystic papillary carcinoma often contain few neoplastic cells. In such cases, it is extremely difficult to differentiate cystic papillary carcinoma from cystic nodular goiter (2, 3). In addition, the specimens can be poorly cellular or cellular, but contain many histiocytes. When mural nodules are found in cystic lesions, both the lesion and cystic fluid should be subjected to aspiration biopsy examinations. The tumor cells of cystic papillary carcinoma exhibit some characteristic features in addition to the findings shared by all forms of papillary carcinoma (4, 5) (please refer to Chapters 3 and 4). For example, isolated tumor cells often have a thickened cytoplasm with clear borders. The nuclei of these cells are larger and have a higher nuclear-cytoplasmic ratio than histiocytes. Scallop-shaped ball-like clusters and small papillary clusters consisting of hobnail-shaped thick tumor cells are also features of cystic papillary carcinoma. Furthermore, the tumor cells frequently have a vacuolar cytoplasm, and hence resemble vacuolated histiocytes, therefore, they should not be mistaken for histiocytes (5). In cystic nodular goiter, the follicular epithelium of the cyst wall can exhibit regenerative changes and be composed of monolayered sheets consisting of large atypical cells with dense cytoplasm and large irregular nuclei with enlarged nucleoli. Such cases should not be mistaken for papillary carcinoma (Figure 11) (Please refer to Figure 8 of Chapter 5) (6). In cystic degeneration of anaplastic carcinoma, necrotic debris and highly atypical large neoplastic cells are found (please refer to Chapter 32, mini-test case 2). Branchial cleft cysts can also develop within the thyroid. In such cases, the aspirates may contain squamous cells with or without keratinization, but these cells are mature and have typical morphological features (please refer to Chapter 32, mini-test case 8) (7).

Gross and Histological Diagnosis:

Macroscopically, a cystic mass measuring up to 10 cm in diameter with an irregularly shaped mural nodule was found in the right lobe of the thyroid. A loupe image illustrated that the cyst wall was fibrous and thick (Figure 12). High power images demonstrated that the mural nodule contained both papillary and follicular structures (Figure 13). Some tumor cells displayed hobnail-shaped eosinophilic cytoplasm, which protruded into the cystic lumen

(Figure 14). The tumor cells also lined the cyst wall and occasionally displayed squamous metaplasia (Figure 15).

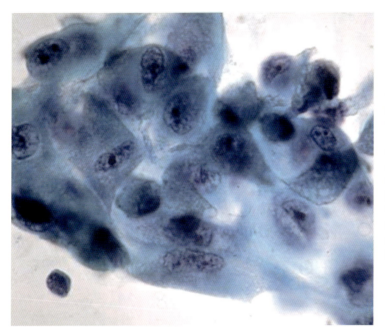

Figure 11. FNA smear of aspirates from cystic nodular goiter. Follicular cyst wall epithelial cells exhibiting regenerative changes are shown. They are large atypical cells with dense cytoplasm. In addition, they have large irregular nuclei with enlarged nucleoli and are arranged in monolayered sheets. (Papanicolaou stain, x1000)

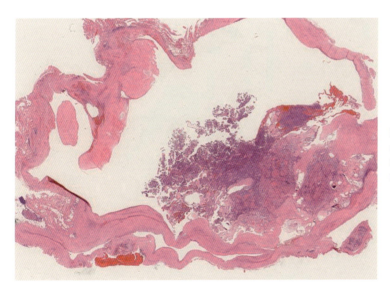

Figure 12. Histological section showing the fibrous and thick wall of the cyst. (H&E stain, x3.5).

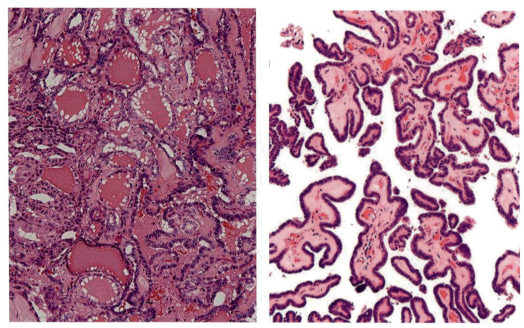

Figure 13. Histological sections. The mural nodule consists of both follicular and papillary proliferations of tumor cells. (H&E stain, x200)

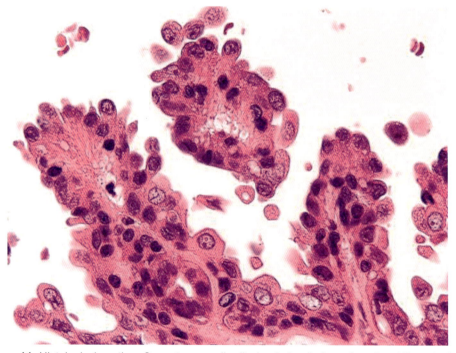

Figure 14. Histological section. Some tumor cells display hobnail-shaped eosinophilic cytoplasm, protruding into the cystic lumen. (H&E stain, x1000)

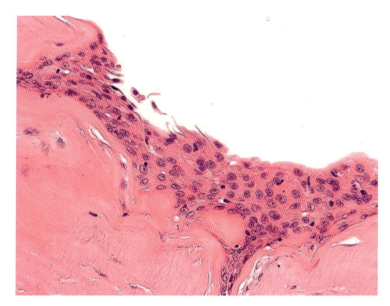

Figure 15. Histological section. Tumor cells line the cyst wall and occasionally display squamous metaplasia. (H&E stain, x400)

References

1. Miller JM, Zafar S, Karo JJ. The cystic thyroid nodule. Diagn Radiol 1974; 110:257-62.
2. Goellner JR, Johnson DA. Cytology of cystic papillary carcinoma of the thyroid. Acta Cytol 1982; 26:797-808.
3. Ali SZ, Cibas ES. The Bethesda System for Reporting Thyroid Cytopathology: Definitions, Criteria, and Explanatory Notes. New York, NY, Springer, 2009.
4. Kini SR. Chapter 17. Cysts and cystic lesions of the thyroid. In Thyroid cytopathology: an atlas and text. 2nd ed. Philadelphia, Lippincott Williams & Wilkins. 2015, 10630-11098/15102 (e-book version).
5. Renshaw AA. "Histiocytoid" cells in fine-needle aspirations of papillary carcinoma of the thyroid. Frequency and significance of an under-recognized cytologic pattern. Cancer Cytopathol 2002; 96:240-3.
6. Faquin WC, Cibas ES, Renshaw AA. Atypical cells in fine-needle aspiration biopsy specimens of benign thyroid cysts. Cancer 2005; 105:71-9.
7. Lim-Tio SW, Judson R, Busmanis I, et al. An intra-thyroidal branchial cyst: a case report. Aust N Z J Surg 1992; 62:826-8.

Chapter 8

Tall Cell Variant of Papillary Thyroid Carcinoma vs. Conventional Papillary Thyroid Carcinoma

Miyoko Higuchi

Case Report
   A 62-year-old female with a neck mass visited our hospital. She had a history of total thyroidectomy with left cervical lymph node dissection because of papillary thyroid carcinoma (PTC) six years ago. Ultrasonographically, the mass was located in the subcutaneous tissue, measuring 8.2 mm x 7.8 mm x 5.1mm (Figure 1). It was hypoechoic and slightly lobulated. The margin was ill-defined and irregular, indicating infiltrative growth. Aspiration cytology of the mass revealed PTC. Thyroglobulin in the needle wash-out fluid rinsed with 0.5 mL of saline solution after smearing was 1335.0 ng/mL (please refer to Chapter 23). Needle tract implantation was suggested, and the mass was resected (please refer to Chapter 26).

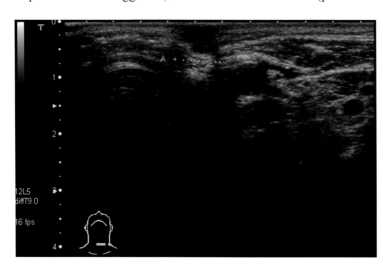

Figure 1. A hypoechoic mass with ill-defined margin is located in the subcutaneous tissue. (Ultrasound B-mode)

Cytologic Findings
   The aspirated material was highly cellular. There were no inflammatory cells, psammoma bodies, or colloid materials in the background. The atypical cells presented solid, trabecular, papillary, and monolayered patterns (Figure 2). The nuclei were arranged in a line at the periphery of the papillary clusters (Figure 3). Follicular pattern was not observed. The atypical cells were round, tall columnar, or spindle in shape, and the N/C ratio was not high. The cytoplasm was abundant, and deeply stained in lightgreen. Cytoplasmic elongation toward an outside of the cell clusters was observed (Figure 4). Nuclear (intranuclear) cytoplasmic inclusions (NCI) and nuclear grooves were present, but powdery chromatin was not apparent.

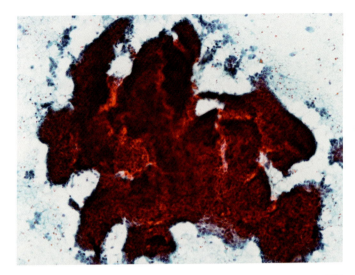

Figure 2. The atypical cells exhibit a papillary pattern. (Papanicolaou stain, x40)

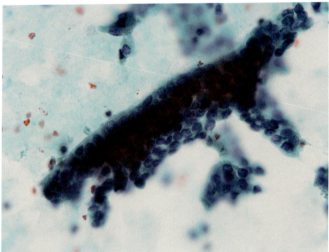

Figure 3. The nuclei are arranged in a line at the periphery of the trabecular clusters (Papanicolaou stain, ×400)

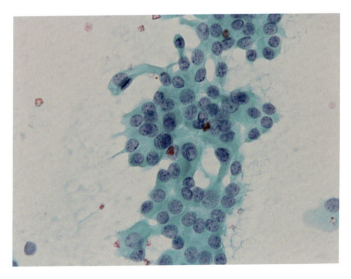

Figure 4. Cytoplasmic elongation toward the outside of the cell clusters. (Papanicolaou, x400)

Histologic Findings

The PTC was located in the dermis and subcutaneous adipose tissue (Figure 5). The carcinoma cells showed trabecular or papillary growth. Most of the carcinoma cells were tall columnar cells that were more than three times as tall as their width (Figure 6). The cytoplasm was abundant and moderately eosinophilic. The nuclei were slightly elongated, and showed the features consistent with papillary carcinoma except for ground glass appearance. Ki-67 (please refer to Chapter 28) labeling index was 10% in the hot-spot areas observed under ×400 magnification.

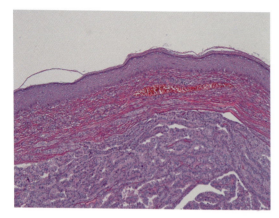

Figure 5. Papillary carcinoma is located in the dermis, and shows papillary or trabecular growth. (H&E stain, x40)

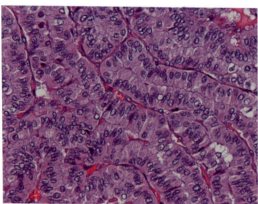

Figure 6. Papillary carcinoma cells are tall, and the cytoplasm is eosinophilic. (H&E stain, x400)

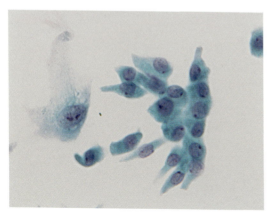

Figure 7. The atypical cells are columnar in shape. Some of them are spindle-like. (LBC, SurePath, Papanicolaou stain, x400)

Differential Diagnosis

The tall cell variant (TCV) is an aggressive form of PTC that comprises 10% of all PTCs (1). This variant usually extends extrathyroidal tissue, and tends to occur in elderly patients (2). The tall cells are more than three times as tall as their width, and should occupy 50% or more of papillary carcinoma cells to make the diagnosis of tall cell variant (3). They often show eosinophilic cytoplasm and a papillary growth pattern. The nuclei are elongated, and have features characteristic of conventional PTC, such as NCIs, nuclear grooves, and a ground glass appearance.

Because of its association with aggressive clinical features, preoperative cytological diagnosis of TCV is clinically important. But, it is not easy to identify TCV via fine needle aspiration cytology, because there is an overlap between TCV and conventional PTC, and the carcinoma cells with features of conventional PTC can be seen in TCV cases.

The smears of TCV are usually cellular, and the colloid, and inflammatory cells including lymphocytes, and foamy cells are infrequently observed (1). Psammoma bodies are extremely rare. The carcinoma cells predominantly show papillary and trabecular pattern, but branching papillary and monolayered sheet pattern that are seen in conventional PTC are infrequent. Follicular arrangement is not usually observed.

The most important finding indicating TCV is the morphology to be related to tall columnar cells. The carcinoma cells are elongated to columnar in shape, and they occasionally look like spindle cells. They are more often polygonal (4). The cytoplasm is deeply stained in lightgreen, and the cell border is distinct (1). The carcinoma cells with the cytoplasmic elongation toward an outside of the cell clusters are called tail-like cells or tadpole cells (5). The N/C ratio of the carcinoma cells in TCV is lower than that in conventional PTC because of abundant cytoplasm (Table 1). Lee *et al.* and Suzuki *et al.* described that the tall cell configurations were more easily recognized in liquid-based-cytology smears than conventional smears (Figure 7) (please refer to Chapter 27) (6, 7).

The TCV of PTC represents the nuclear features of conventional PTC, but the nuclei have less powdery chromatin and more granular chromatin (4). Multiple NCIs within the same nucleus called "soap bubble appearance" are frequently observed in TCV of PTC, but rarely in conventional PTC (8).

Differential diagnoses of the carcinoma composed of tall cells in thyroid FNA include Warthin tumor-like PTC, cribriform variant of PTC (please refer to Chapter 9), columnar cell variant of PTC (please refer to Chapter 10), and metastatic colonic adenocarcinoma. In Warthin tumor-like PTC, the cytoplasm is more abundant and oxyphilic, and numerous lymphocytes are present in the background. Cribriform variant of PTC occurs in younger patients and the tumors are ultrasonographically well-demarcated (9). Cytologically, the chromatin is granular and foamy cells are seen in the background. The presences of peculiar nuclear clearing, morules, and hyaline materials indicate the cribriform variant of PTC (10). Columnar cell variant of PTC is more aggressive and the cytological findings are similar to those of metastatic colonic adenocarcinoma (please refer to Chapter 10). Both of the carcinomas reveal spindle-shaped nuclei and a granular chromatin pattern (11).

Table 1. Cytological features of the tall cell variant of papillary carcinoma

Cellularity
    Usually very cellular
Background
    Infrequent colloid, infrequent inflammatory cells (lymphocytes, foam cells),
    Very rare psammoma bodies
Arrangement
    Predominantly papillary pattern and trabecular pattern,
    Infrequent branching papillary pattern and monolayered sheet pattern, infrequent follicular pattern
Cells
    Lower N/C ratio, elongated to columnar in shape (tail-like cells or tadpole cells), spindle-like, polygonal
Cytoplasm
    Abundant, dense staining, well-defined cell border
Nucleus
    Eccentric, round to oval in shape
    Multiple intranuclear cytoplasmic inclusions within the same nucleus (soap bubble appearance)
    Nuclear grooves, irregular nuclear membrane, more granular chromatin (infrequent powdery chromatin)
    Mitotic figures

References

1. Guan H, Vandenbussche CJ, Erozan YS, et al. Can the tall cell variant of papillary thyroid carcinoma be distinguished from the conventional type in fine needle aspirates? A cytomorphologic study with assessment of diagnostic accuracy. Acta Cytol 2013; 57:534-42.
2. Cameselle-Teijeiro J, Febles-Pérez C, Cameselle-Teijeiro JF, et al. Cytologic clues for distinguishing the tall cell variant of thyroid papillary carcinoma. A case report. Acta Cytol 1997; 41(4 Suppl):1310-6.
3. DeLellis RA, Lloid RV, Heitz PU, et al. WHO classification of tumours, Pathology & Genetics, Tumours of Endocrine Organs. IARC Press, Lyon, 2004.
4. Bocklage T, DiTomasso JP, Ramzy I, et al. Tall cell variant of papillary thyroid carcinoma: cytologic features and differential diagnostic considerations. Diagn Cytopathol 1997; 17:25-9.
5. Gamboa-Domínguez A1, Candanedo-González F, Uribe-Uribe NO, et al. Tall cell variant of papillary thyroid carcinoma. A cytohistologic correlation. Acta Cytol 1997; 41:672-6.
6. Lee SH, Jung CK, Bae JS, et al. Liquid-based cytology improves preoperative diagnostic accuracy of the tall cell variant of papillary thyroid carcinoma. Diagn Cytopathol 2014; 42:11-7.
7. Suzuki A, Hirokawa M, Higuchi M, et al. Cytological characteristics of papillary thyroid carcinoma on LBC specimens, compared with conventional specimens. Diagn Cytopathol 2015; 43:108-13.
8. Solomon A, Gupta PK, LiVolsi VA, et al. Distinguishing tall cell variant of papillary thyroid carcinoma from usual variant of papillary thyroid carcinoma in cytologic specimens. Diagn Cytopathol 2002; 27:143-8.
9. Fujimoto T, Hirokawa M, Ota H, et al. Characteristic sonographic features of cribriform papillary thyroid carcinoma for differentiation from other thyroid nodules. J Med Ultrason (2001) 2015; 42:83-7.
10. Hirokawa M, Maekawa M, Kuma S, et al. Cribriform-morular variant of papillary thyroid carcinoma--cytological and immunocytochemical findings of 18 cases. Diagn Cytopathol 2010; 38:890-6.
11. Ylagan LR, Dehner LP, Huettner PC, et al. Columnar cell variant of papillary thyroid carcinoma. Report of a case with cytologic findings. Acta Cytol 2004; 48:73-7.

Chapter 9

Cribriform Variant of Papillary Thyroid Carcinoma

Ayana Suzuki

Case Report

The case was a 21-year-old female. She was found to have nodules in her anterior neck by a medical checkup. As aspiration cytology was suspicious for malignancy, she was referred to our hospital for surgical therapy. Ultrasonographic examination revealed two nodules in the thyroid. The nodule located in the left lobe measured 8 mm x 5 mm x 7 mm. It was slightly hypoechoic, homogeneous, irregular-shaped, and not associated with fine strong echoes. The border of the mass was well-defined (Figure 1). Color Doppler ultrasound showed that it was hypovascular. The ultrasound interpretation was a malignancy, and the cribriform variant of papillary thyroid carcinoma (CV-PTC) was suspected by aspiration cytology. Another nodule located in the right lobe, measuring 11 mm x 3 mm x 6 mm, was interpreted as a benign nodule by ultrasonographic and cytological examinations. She underwent a left thyroid lobectomy including isthmus with central neck dissection. Colonic examination performed after the microscopic diagnosis of CV-PTC did not detect any abnormalities. A test for *APC* gene mutation was not permitted. Her parents had no history of polyposis coli and thyroid tumors.

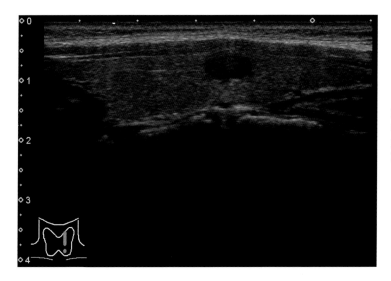

Figure 1. A hypoechoic mass with well-defined border is present. (Ultrasound B-mode image)

Cytological Findings

Aspirated material was cellular. There were a small number of foamy histiocytes in the background. Colloid materials were not observed. Carcinoma cells appeared as papillary or cribriform clusters. The cribriform clusters exhibited slit-like empty spaces and anastomosing bars (Figure 2). Papillary clusters partially showed nuclear palisading. Some clusters contained small hyaline materials. Carcinoma cell nests with eddy formation were scattered (Figure 3). Most of the carcinoma cells were tall columnar and their N/C ratios were low. Isolated carcinoma cells were spindle or elongated in shape. The cytoplasm was weakly stained with lightgreen, even in the carcinoma cells forming morules. Metaplastic cytoplasm showing dense cytoplasm was not observed. Tail-like cytoplasmic elongation was observed at the periphery of the cell clusters (Figure 4). The nuclei were round, oval or short spindle, and exhibited nuclear grooves and nuclear cytoplasmic inclusions (NCIs). The nuclear chromatin was not ground glass-like, but granular (Figure 5). Some morular cells showed peculiar nuclear clearing that occupied most of the nuclei and directly surrounded by a nucleoplasm (Figure 6).

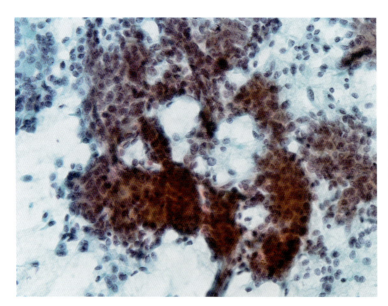

Figure 2. The cribriform clusters showing slit-like empty spaces and anastomosing bars are seen. There are no colloid materials in the lumen and background. (Papanicolaou, x100)

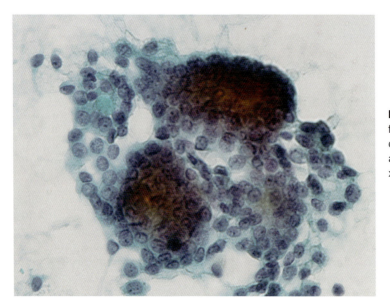

Figure 3. Two eddy formations, called "morule", composed of carcinoma cells are seen. (Papanicolaou, x400)

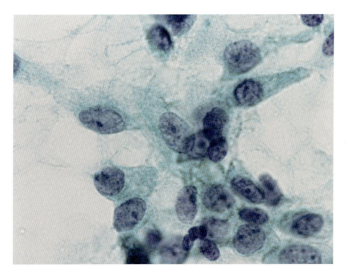

Figure 4. The carcinoma cells exhibit tail-like cytoplasmic elongation. (Papanicolaou, x1000)

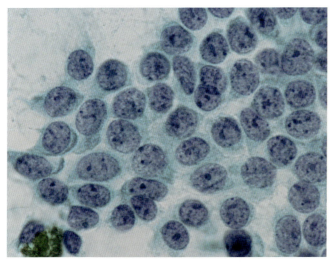

Figure 5. The nuclear chromatin is not ground glass, but granular. (Papanicolaou, x1000)

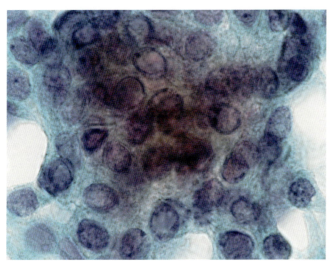

Figure 6. Some nuclei show peculiar nuclear clearing that occupies most of the nuclei and is directly surrounded by a nucleoplasm. (Papanicolaou, x1000)

Pathological Findings

The tumor was located in the left lobe, and it measured 7 mm x 5 mm. On cut surface, it was solid and lobulated (Figure 7). It was well-encapsulated and did not invade the surrounding thyroid tissue. Microscopically, the carcinoma cells showed cribriform (Figure 8), papillary, solid and follicular pattern. The cribriform pattern was formed by anastomosing bars and arches of carcinoma cells without intervening stroma. There was no colloid in the lumen. The morules were scattered in the solid area. Papillary area was composed of tall columnar carcinoma cells. The cytoplasm was slightly eosinophilic. The nuclei were round to spindle, and represented cytoplasmic inclusions (Figure 9). Peculiar nuclear clearing was observed in some of the morular cells (Figure 10). The chromatin pattern was granular. A ground glass pattern consistent with classic papillary carcinoma was not observed. There were no psammoma bodies. No lymphnode metastasis was found. Immunohistochemically, the carcinoma cells showed nuclear and cytoplasmic positivity for beta-catenin (Figure 11). Thyroglobulin was almost negative (Figure 12). Estrogen receptor (ER) was positive except for morular cells (Figure 13).

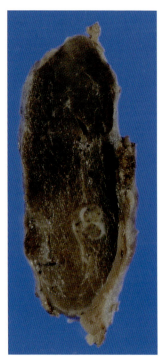

Figure 7. An encapsulated and lobulated tumor is present in the thyroid.

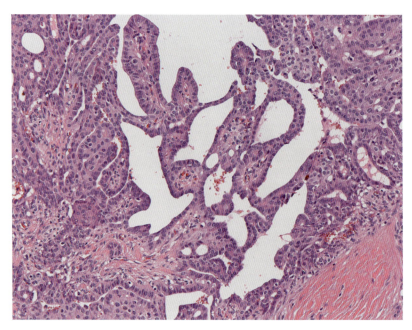

Figure 8. Cribriform structure composed of anastomosing bars and arches of carcinoma cells are seen. There are no colloid materials in the lumen. (HE, x100)

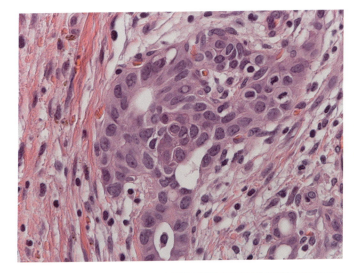

Figure 9. The nuclei are dark, and an intranuclear cytoplasmic inclusion is noticed. (HE, x400)

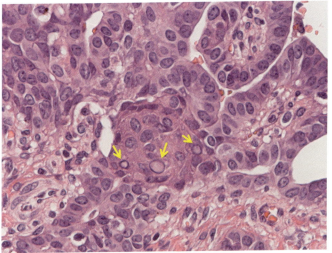

Figure 10. Peculiar nuclear clearings (arrows) are seen. (HE, x400)

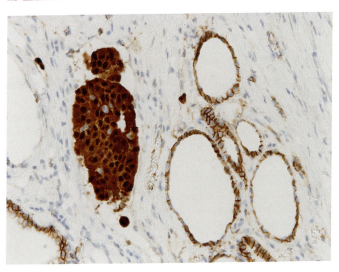

Figure 11. Beta-catenin displays membranous positivity in normal follicular cells (right). By contrast, the carcinoma cells (left) show nuclear and cytoplasmic positivity for beta-catenin. (Beta-catenin immunostaining, x200)

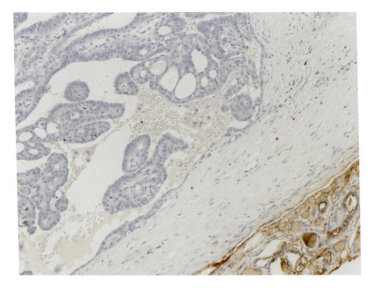

Figure 12. The carcinoma cells do not express thyroglobulin, but normal follicular cells are positive (right lower). (Thyroglobulin immunostaining, x100)

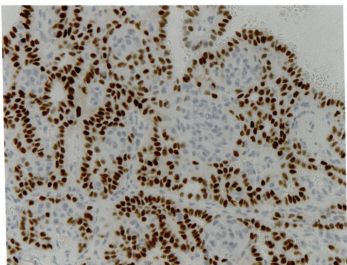

Figure 13. The carcinoma cells are positive for the estrogen receptor, except for morular cells. (Estrogen receptor immunostaining, x200)

Differential Diagnoses

CV-PTC is rare and constitutes less than 0.5% of all PTCs. CV-PTC typically affects young adults with a female predominance, showing a female-to-male ratio of 17:1 (Table 1) (1). It is commonly associated with familial adenomatous polyposis (FAP) and has a germline mutation in the adenomatous polyposis coli (*APC*) gene (2-3). However, sporadic form without FAP has been reported.

The preoperative diagnosis of CV-PTC is important. As CV-PTC with FAP usually displays multifocal nodules, total thyroidectomy is required. On the contrary, lobectomy is sufficient for sporadic cases because of solitary nodule and excellent prognosis. In addition, the fact that colonic polyposis may be detected after the diagnosis of CV-PTC indicates the necessity of preoperative colonoscopy and/or *APC* gene analysis (1). Therefore, aspiration cytology bears an important responsibility in the management of this variant.

Table 1. Clinical features of CV-PTC

Age	Young adults
Gender	Female predominance (F/M ratio, 17:1)
Genetic background	*APC* gene abnormality (not all)
Focus	Multifocal in FAP-associated cases
	Solitary in non-FAP-associated cases
Prognosis	Excellent
Nodal metastasis	10-20%

This variant is histologically characterized by an intricate blending of cribriform, follicular, papillary, trabecular, and solid patterns with the morules (Table 2). The cribriform pattern is formed by anastomosing bars and arches of carcinoma cells without intervening stroma and resembles ductal carcinoma of the breast. The lumen of the cribriform pattern is usually devoid of colloid. The carcinoma cells showing papillary growth are tall columnar cells, and the nuclei frequently display pseudostratification. Trabecular arrangement may be reminiscent of hyalinizing trabecular tumor. Amongst thyroid carcinomas, the morules appear limited to this variant. The nuclear chromatin is fine granular and ground glass appearance is obscure. Peculiar nuclear clearing characteristic of this variant tends to be observed in the morules (4). According to the report by Hirokawa et al., the cytology of CV-PTC is characterized by 1) hypercellularity, 2) papillary arrangement composed of tall columnar cells, 3) cribriform pattern, 4) morules, 5) spindle cells, 6) obscure ground-glass nuclei, 7) peculiar nuclear clearing, 8) foamy or hemosiderin-laden histiocytes, 9) hyaline materials, and 10) no colloid in the background (5).

A papillary arrangement is frequently seen in CV-PTC. However, the finding is not important for the diagnosis of CV-PTC, because it is common in conventional PTC. Cribriform structure is characterized by slit-like empty spaces and anastomosing bars within cell clusters (6). Insular carcinoma and follicular neoplasm may also present cribriform pattern. In such tumors, the spaces are small in size, round, and contain colloid (please refer to Figure 11 of Chapter 20). In contrast, the spaces seen in CV-PTC are larger in size, not round, and do not contain any colloid. Tall columnar cells are easily identified in CV-PTC as carcinoma cells showing nuclear palisading and low N/C ratio. Tail-like cytoplasmic elongation is also consistent with tall columnar cells (6). Tall columnar cells are also seen in the tall cell variant and columnar cell variants of PTC (please refer to Chapters 3, 8 and 10). Pseudostratified nuclei, hyperchromasia, and nuclear atypia are helpful in distinguishing columnar cell variant from CV-PTC. The distinction of columnar cells between CV-PTC and the tall cell variant is difficult (please refer to Table 1 of Chapter 10). The age of the patient may be useful. The latter occurs in elder persons. Morules are cell clusters with eddy formations (6-7). They may mimic squamous metaplasia. Compared with squamous metaplasia, the cytoplasm of carcinoma cells forming the morules is not densely stained. The spindle cells singly appear in the background (8).

Similar to conventional PTC, CV-PTC presents NCIs and nuclear grooves. However, a ground glass appearance is rare. The chromatin seen in CV-PTC is granular, and it mimics that of follicular neoplasm or medullary carcinoma. The presence of peculiar nuclear clearing is very useful for the diagnosis of CV-PTC (7). It is identified as pale-staining area is occupying most of the nuclei, and usually accompanied by condensed chromatin at the periphery of the nuclei. It is distinguished from NCIs by cytoplasmic staining and sharp circumscription with the nuclear membrane.

Immunocytochemical staining is very useful in diagnosing CV-PTC (please refer to Chapter 28). When this variant is suspected, we routinely stain for beta-catenin (Figure 14), ER (Figure 15), and progesterone receptor (PgR). Beta-catenin reveals nuclear and cytoplasmic immunoreactivity (9-10). In contrast, conventional PTC reacts with the cell membrane against the antibody. CV-PTC shows strong nuclear positivity for ER and PgR, except for morular cells (11). Conventional PTC is almost negative for these receptors.

Table 2. Pathological features of CV-PTC

Gross	Well-demarcated or encapsulated
	Solid, infrequently and focally cystic
Microscopy	
Growth pattern	Cribriform, trabecular, solid, papillary, follicular
	Morules (characteristic)
Cell shape	Tall columnar, cuboidal, round, spindle
Cytoplasm	Moderately abundant, eosinophilic
Nuclei	Peculiar nuclear clearing (characteristic)
	Fine granular chromatin
	Obscure ground glass appearance
Colloid	Absent
Psammoma bodies	Very rare
Immunohistochemistry	
Thyroglobulin	Almost negative
Beta-catenin	Nuclear and cytoplasmic positivity
ER, PgR	Positive except for morules

Table 3. Cytological differential diagnoses of the cribriform variant and conventional papillary thyroid carcinoma

	Cribriform Variant	Conventional
Arrangement	Papillary, cribriform	Papillary, follicular
	Nuclear palisading	
Morules	Occasionally present	Absent
Cell shape	Tall columnar, cuboidal spindle	Round, cuboidal, columnar
Cytoplasm	Moderately abundant	Variable
	Tail-like elongation	
Nuclei		
Peculiar nuclear clearing	Present	Absent
Ground glass appearance	Obscure	Present
Cytoplasmic inclusion	Present	Present
Background		
Colloid	Absent	Ropy strands
Lymphocytes	Absent	Occasionally present
Foam cells	Present	Occasionally present
Hyaline materials	Present	Absent

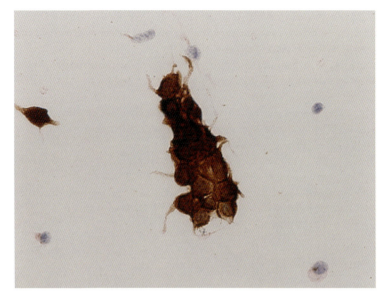

Figure 14. The carcinoma cells show nuclear and cytoplasmic positivity for beta-catenin. (Beta-catenin immunostaining, LBC, x400)

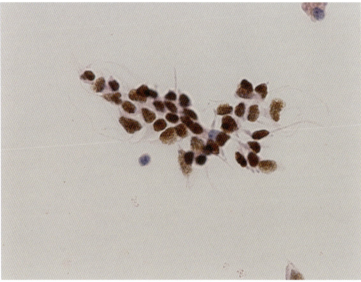

Figure 15. The carcinoma cells are positive for the estrogen receptor. (Immunostaining, LBC, x400)

References

1. Nikiforov YE. Diagnostic Pathology and Molecular Genetics of the Thyroid; A comprehensive guide for practicing thyroid pathology. Philadelphia: Lippincott Williams & Wilkins; 2009, p191-2.
2. Harach HR, Williams GT, Williams ED. Familial adenomatous polyposis associated thyroid carcinoma: a distinct type of follicular cell neoplasm. Histopathol 1994; 25:549-61.
3. Cetta F, Toti P, Petracci M, et al. Thyroid carcinoma associated with familial adenomatous polyposis. Histopathol 1997; 31:231-6.
4. Kini SR. Thyroid Cytopathology; An Atlas and Text. Philadelphia: Lippincott Williams & Wilkins; 2008, p163-9.
5. Hirokawa M, Maekawa M, Kuma S, et al. Cribriform-morular variant of papillary thyroid carcinoma - cytological and immunocytochemical findings of 18 cases. Diagn Cytopathol 2010; 38:890-6.
6. Koo JS, Jung W, Hong SW. Cytologic characteristics and β-catenin immunocytochemistry on smear slide of

cribriform-morular variant of papillary thyroid carcinoma. Acta Cytol 2011; 55:13-8.
7. Kuma S, Hirokawa M, Xu B, et al. Cribriform-morular variant of papillary thyroid carcinoma. Report of a case showing morules with peculiar nuclear clearing. Acta Cytol 2004; 48:431-6.
8. Hirokawa M, Kuma S, Miyauchi A, et al. Morules in cribriform-morular variant of papillary thyroid carcinoma: Immunohistochemical characteristics and distinction from squamous metaplasia. APMIS 2004; 112:275-82.
9. Jung CK, Choi YJ, Lee KY, et al. The cytological, clinical, and pathological features of the cribriform-morular variant of papillary thyroid carcinoma and mutation analysis of *CTNNB1* and *BRAF* genes. Thyroid 2009; 19:905-13.
10. Boonyaarunnate T, Olson MT, Bishop JA, et al. Cribriform morular variant of papillary thyroid carcinoma: clinical and cytomorphological features on fine-needle aspiration. Acta Cytol 2013; 57:127-33.
11. Cameselle TJ, Chan JK. Cribriform-morular variant of papillary carcinoma: a distinctive variant representing the sporadic counterpart of familial adenomatous polyposis-associated thyroid carcinoma? Mod Pathol 1999; 12:400-11.

Chapter 10

Papillary Carcinoma, Columnar Cell Variant - Diagnostic Pitfalls and Differential Diagnoses

Chiung-Ru Lai

Case Report

A 32-year-old woman was healthy and denied any systemic diseases. Multiple thyroid nodules were found incidentally during a routine health examination. Ultrasound examination revealed multiple nodules in both lobes of thyroid, with one showing hypoechoic and being 0.8 cm in diameter in the left lobe. The thyroid function tests were within the normal limits. No other lesions were identified in the head and neck area. Fine needle aspiration (FNA) of the nodule was performed (Figure 1) and the aspirate was submitted to the cytology laboratory as one ethanol-fixed smear for Papanicolaou stain, one air-dried smear for Liu's stain, and one SurePath BD CytoRich™ vial for liquid-based preparation (Becton, Dickinson and Company, Franklin Lakes, NJ).

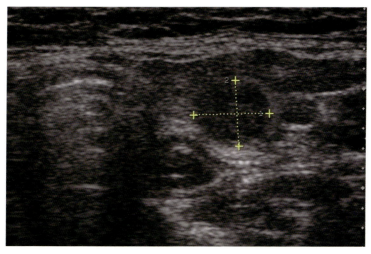

Figure 1. A hypoechoic nodule (7.8 mm x 6.6 mm) in the left lobe of the thyroid was aspirated.

Cytology/Pathology Findings

The smears showed moderate cellularity in a clean background devoid of colloid and blood, and consisted of loosely cohesive three-dimensional and monolayer clusters of cells (Figure 2). Occasional papillary fragments with vascular cores were present (Figure 3). Pseudostratified epithelium composed of cigar-shaped, elongated hyperchromatic nuclei in a picket-fence-like arrangement was apparent (Figures 4, 5, and 6). Nuclear grooves and intranuclear pseudoinclusions (NCIs) were found in very limited area (Figure 7). Immunocytochemical stains for CDX2 and BRAF were performed using the residual materials of liquid-based preparation, which revealed negative results for both CDX2 and BRAF. Then, FNA reported as papillary thyroid carcinoma (PTC), in favor of the columnar cell variant. The patient received total thyroidectomy and pathology confirmed a columnar cell variant papillary thyroid microcarcinoma (Figures 8 and 9) without the $BRAF^{V600E}$ mutation.

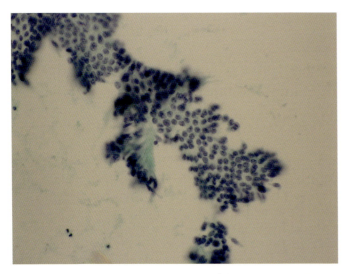

Figure 2. Moderately cellular smear showing loosely cohesive three-dimensional and monolayer clusters of cells. (Papanicolaou stain, x200)

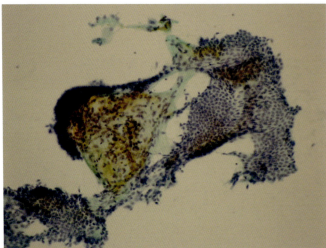

Figure 3. Vague papillary fragment with vascular cores. (Papanicolaou stain, x200)

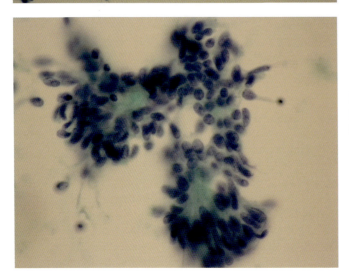

Figure 4. Tight cluster of cells with pseudostratified nuclei in a radiating pattern. (Papanicolaou stain, x400).

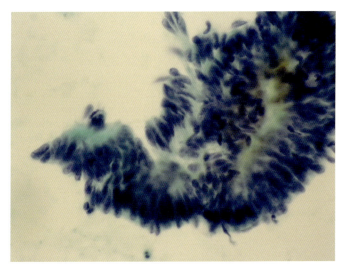

Figure 5. Pseudostratified columnar epithelium composed of cigar-shaped, elongated hyperchromatic nuclei in picket-fence-like arrangement. (Papanicolaou stain, x400)

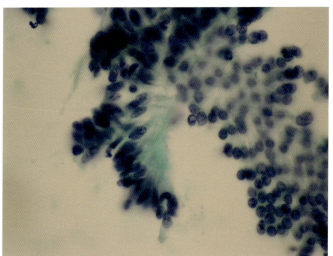

Figure 6. Note the columnar cells with pseudostratification in the left half of the cluster of cells. (Papanicolaou stain, x400)

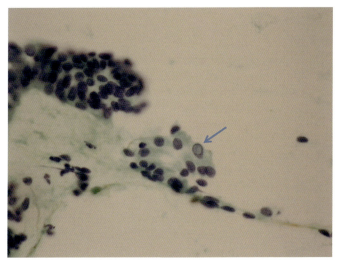

Figure 7. Intranuclear pseudoinclusion can be found in limited numbers. (Papanicolaou stain, x400)

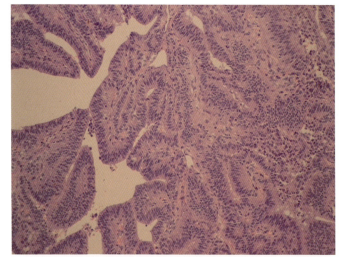

Figure 8. Histology sections of total thyroidectomy sample show papillary growth with fibrovascular cores and lined by pseudostratified tall columnar epithelial cells that were positive for TTF-1 and negative for CDX2. (H&E stain, x100)

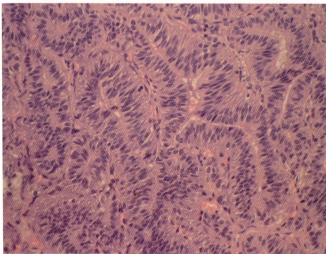

Figure 9. Characteristic pseudostratified columnar epithelium with elongated hyperchromatic nuclei and occasional subnuclear vacuolization. (H&E stain, x200)

Differential diagnosis
1. Malignant: PTC, tall cell variant
2. Malignant: PTC, columnar cell variant
3. Malignant: Metastatic endometrioid or colorectal adenocarcinoma
4. Benign: Hyperplastic nodule (papillary hyperplastic nodule)
5. Benign: Upper respiratory epithelial cells contamination from the aspiration procedure

The criteria of tall cell variant PTC have been recently lowered to more than 50% of cancer cells with a 2-3:1 height/width ratio (please refer to Chapter 8) (1). The nuclei frequently have the characteristic features of classic PTC showing oval and optically clear nuclei with nuclear grooves and NCIs (2). Therefore, it is easy to interpret the lesion as a PTC. However, you will find loosely cohesive clusters of cells with rows or parallel cords of tall cells, which raise the possibility of the tall cell variant (Figure 10) (please refer to Chapter 8). On the contrary, the characteristic PTC nuclear features are not apparent in the columnar cell variant (3). Although both subtypes have tall or columnar cell features, the differential diagnosis between them is not very difficult. The comparison of columnar and tall cell variant

PTC is summarized in Table 1.

The elongated overlapping and stratified nuclei with occasional supranuclear and/or subnuclear cytoplasmic vacuoles of columnar cell variant PTC may resemble those of metastatic endometrioid or colorectal adenocarcinoma. However, the latter types of cancer seldom metastasize to the thyroid. If it is a metastatic lesion in the thyroid, it usually happens for a disease at an advanced stage. Thus, the differential diagnosis could be easily made by the clinical presentation and history. The immunocytochemical stains for ER and CDX2 are not useful because they have been found to be positive in up to two thirds and 55% of columnar cell variant PTCs, respectively (4, 5).

The pseudostratification pattern of columnar cell variant PTC may resemble the upper respiratory epithelial cells that are sometimes inadvertently aspirated during the thyroid aspiration procedure (6). However, no cilia could be identified in any of these cells. In addition, the presence of vague PTC nuclear features or background colloid material would help a lot in the differential diagnosis. To rule our benign papillary proliferation in hyperplastic adenomatous nodule, please refer to Chapters 3 and 4.

Table 1. Differential diagnoses between columnar and tall cell variants of PTC

	Columnar cell variant	Tall cell variant
Incidence	0.2% (extremely rare)	3.2-19%
Age	Any age	Rare among pediatric and young patients
Height/width ratio	4-5:1	2-3:1
Cell-to-cell arrangement	Picket-fence-like pseudostratification	Parallel simple columnar
Nuclear grooves or intranuclear pseudoinclusions	Absence or paucity	Frequent
Locations of nucleus	Stratified	Central or basal

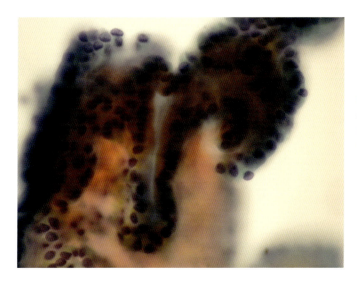

Figure 10. Characteristic parallel simple columnar tall cells (2~3:1 height/width ratio) with central nuclei. (Papanicolaou stain, x400)

Discussion

Columnar cell variant PTC is a rare thyroid cancer (accounting for 0.2% of all PTCs) and is characterized by columnar cells with hyperchromatic elongated nuclei in a pseudostratified arrangement (4). The classic nuclear features of conventional PTC are not frequently observed. The differential diagnoses among tall cell variant PTC, metastatic endometrioid or colorectal cancers, and contaminated respiratory epithelial cells, are not problematic with consideration of clinical presentation, past history, and overall cytomorphology.

The columnar cell variant was previously thought to be more aggressive than conventional PTC (7). However, recent studies have shown that the behavior of columnar cell variant is more related to its tumor size and extra-thyroid involvement rather than its histological subtype. A better prognosis is found in small-sized, circumscribed or encapsulated tumor in young female patients (4, 8). The $BRAF^{V600E}$ mutation has been identified in approximately one third of this variant, which is similar to that in conventional PTC (4). More studies are needed for further evaluation of the prognosis and behavior of this tumor in the future.

References

1. Ghossein R, LiVolsi VA. Papillary thyroid carcinoma tall cell variant. Thyroid 2008; 18:1179-81.
2. Sak S D. Variants of papillary thyroid carcinoma: multiple faces of a familiar tumor turk Patholoji Derg 2015; 31(Suppl):34-47.
3. Lloyd RV, Buehler D, Khanafshar E. Papillary thyroid carcinoma variants. Head Neck Pathol 2011; 5:51-6.
4. Chen JH, Faquin WC, Lloyd RV, et al. Clinicopathological and molecular characterization of the nine cases of columnar cell variant of papillary thyroid carcinoma. Mod Pathol 2011, 24: 739-49.
5. Enriquez ML, Baloch ZW, Montone KT, et al. CDX2 expression in columnar cell variant of papillary thyroid carcinoma. Am J Clin Pathol 2012; 137:722-6.
6. Jayaram G. Respiratory epithelial cells in fine needle aspirates of thyroid. Acta Cytol 1995; 39:834.
7. Sobrinho-Simoes M, Nesland J, Johnannessen J. Columnar cell carcinoma. Another variant of poorly differentiated carcinoma of the thyroid. Am J Clin Pathol 1986; 85:77.
8. Wenig BM, Thompson LDR, Adair CF, et al. Thyroid papillary carcinoma of columnar cell type: a clinicopathologic study of 16 cases. Cancer 1998; 82:740-53.

Chapter 11

Subacute Thyroiditis or Papillary Carcinoma

Tiesheng Wang

Subacute thyroiditis is a benign inflammatory condition. On the contrary, papillary thyroid carcinoma (PTC) belongs to a malignant neoplasm. The two diseases are distinct entities in clinicopathology, which are usually readily distinguished from each other. However, there are still some rare atypical cases encountered in clinical practice, which could be confused sonographically and/or cytopathologically, resulting in misdiagnosis (1-3). In this chapter, three illustrative clinical cases are presented and discussed.

1. Case A: Atypical "painless" subacute thyroiditis

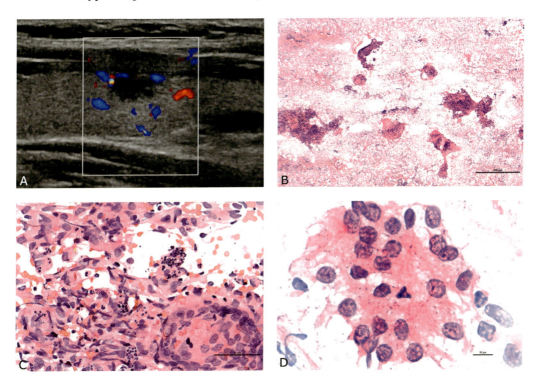

Figure 1. Subacute thyroiditis. 1A: An irregularly-shaped, hypoechoic solid nodule with ill-defined margin and decreased vascularity in the transverse image of the right thyroid lobe. 1B shows numerous multinucleated histiocytic-type giant cells in the background of cellular debris and inflammation on the low power view. 1C: Epithelioid histiocytes with curved nuclei and abundant granular to foamy cytoplasm, as well as multinucleated giant cells in the granuloma-like arrangement, admixed with neutrophils, lymphocytes, macrophages and follicular cells on the high magnification. 1D: Degenerative changes of the follicular cells with reactive atypia, but lacking the characteristic nuclear features of papillary thyroid carcinoma. 1B-1C are HE-stained smears.

1.1. Vignette

The patient was a 38-year-old woman who underwent a health check. Neck ultrasound scan incidentally revealed a solitary hypoechoic nodule of 0.4×0.4×0.5 cm in size with an irregular blurred margin in the right lobe of the thyroid gland (Figure 1A). Papillary thyroid microcarcinoma (PTMC) was suspected sonographically. Therefore, ultrasound-guided fine needle aspiration (FNA) biopsy was performed and cytopathology showed characteristic features of subacute thyroiditis. No nuclear features of PTC were observed for the follicular cells (Figure 1B-1D) (4). Consequently, PTMC was ruled out and a diagnosis of subacute thyroiditis was rendered.

1.2. Discussion

As a distinct clinicopathologic entity, subacute thyroiditis has its own characteristic manifestations in the clinical and laboratory tests, and rarely requires FNA biopsy. However, some patients with subacute thyroiditis do not experience pain or tenderness, and the nodule presents as painless, non-tender, and solitary with sonographic appearance of being closely similar to that of PTMC. It is important to realize that such atypical "painless" subacute thyroiditis does exist and can be misdiagnosed as PTMC based on clinical and sonographic evaluation only (1-3). For these cases, cytopathologic examination of the FNA sample is necessary to reach a reliable diagnosis.

2. Case B: PTMC with numerous multinucleated giant cells on FNA

2.1. Vignette

The patient was a 34-year-old female. Thyroid ultrasound scan detected a 0.5 cm solitary and hypoechoic nodule with an irregular contour and ill-defined margin in the left lobe of thyroid (Figures 2A and 2B). On sonography, PTMC was suggested and ultrasound-guided FNA was followed. The FNA specimen showed numerous multinucleated giant cells on the low power view (Figure 2C), raising the possibility of subacute thyroiditis. However, after careful examination, some tissue fragments of follicular cells were found in the clean background, almost without admixed inflammatory cells. The nuclei of the follicular cells were enlarged, variable in size, and irregular in contour, with finely granular chromatin, micronucleoli, nuclear grooves, and intranuclear pseudoinclusions (Figures 2D-2H). The diagnosis of PTMC was confirmed with FNA evaluation. On gross examination of the specimen of left lobectomy, a 0.5 cm solitary and grey-white nodule with an ill-defined and irregular border was noted (Figures 3A and 3B). Histopathological examination revealed a typical papillary growth pattern of the tumor cells with characteristic nuclear features of PTC (Figures 3C and 3D). Two types of multinucleated giant cells, i.e. histiocytic type and follicular cell type, were noticed. The latter was immunohistochemically positive for TG and TTF-1, and differed greatly from the osteoclast-like multinucleated giant cells as seen in undifferentiated carcinoma (Figures 3E-3H). No histopathological features of subacute thyroiditis were identified, except that a few of multinucleated histiocytic-type giant cells presented in the spaces between papillae but without other inflammatory cells (Figures 3E and 3F). The diagnosis of PTMC was reconfirmed.

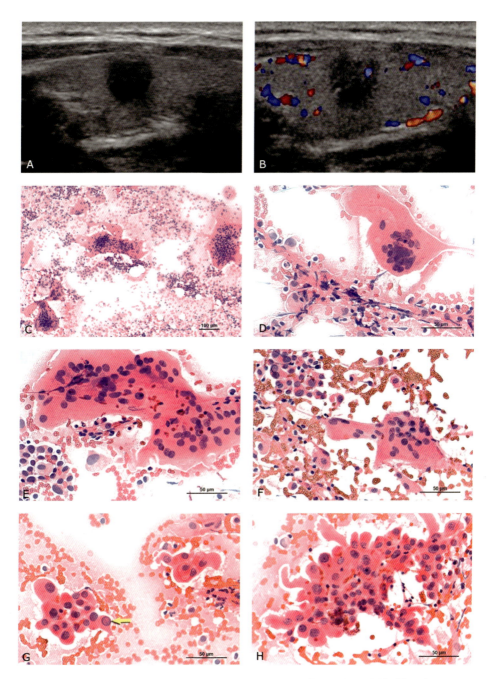

Figure 2. PTMC with numerous multinucleated giant cells on FNA. 2A and 2B: Thyroid sonograms show a 0.5 cm solitary and hypoechoic nodule with an irregular contour, ill-defined margin and decreased vascularity in the left lobe of thyroid. 2C: Numerous multinucleated giant cells on the low power view. 2D-2F: Notice tissue fragments of follicular cells in the clean background, almost without inflammatory cells admixed. 2G and 2H: High magnification to highlight that the nuclei of follicular cells are enlarged, variable in size, and irregular in contour, with finely granular chromatin, micronucleoli, nuclear grooves, and intranuclear pseudoinclusions (yellow arrow). 2C-2H are HE-stained smears.

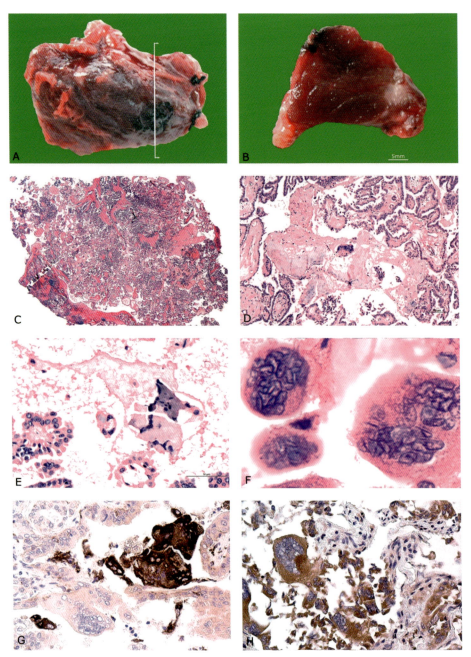

Figure 3. PTMC with numerous multinucleated giant cells on FNA. 3A and 3B: Fresh specimen of left lobectomy showing a grey-white nodule of 0.5 cm in diameter with an ill-defined and irregular margin. 3C and 3D: Typical papillary architectures with well-developed fibrovascular cores. 3E: Multinucleated histiocytic-type giant cells with pyknotic nuclei in the spaces between papillae. 3F: Several multinucleated giant cells with characteristic nuclear features of PTC are multinucleated follicular cell type giant cells. 3G: Multinucleated histiocytic type giant cells with strong immunostaining for CD68. 3H: Multinucleated follicular cell type giant cells with immunohistochemical positivity for TG. 3C-3F are tissue sections with HE stain. 3G and 3H demonstrate the immunohistochemical stain for CD68 and TGB, respectively.

2.2. Discussion

From the view of fluid mechanics, materials with low fluid resistance flow more easily into the capillary cavity. In FNA samples of thyroid, materials with the least resistance to flow are tissue fluid, blood, suspended exfoliated cells, and inflammatory cell populations if present, followed by follicular epithelial elements, the latter appears to be even more readily separated from the surface of papillary bodies, as well as slender papillary structures damaged by needle stroke. However, stromal elements are much more difficult to dislodge and this in part explains why stromal elements are less well represented in FNA specimens than in histological sections. For this reason, the proportions of various cellular and stromal components in thyroid FNA smears may significantly differ from those in thyroid tissue sections.

When numerous multinucleated giant cells are shown on low magnification, an initial impression of subacute thyroiditis may be given and may lead to misinterpretation of the FNA sample (4, 5). However, a clean background, almost without inflammatory cells admixed, and "bubble gum" colloid as well as the presence of two types of multinucleated giant cells are not in favor of the diagnosis of subacute thyroiditis (Table 1) (4). It is important to realize that the presence of numerous multinucleated giant cells does not rule out the diagnosis of PTC. In this instance, the key for differential diagnosis is not to miss the rarely existed tissue fragment of follicular cells with characteristic nuclear features of PTC. Careful study of the whole smear is necessary to achieve a proper cytopathological diagnosis.

Table 1. Clues for differential diagnosis of multinucleated giant cell in SAT* and PTC

Type of Giant Cells	Present in	IHC** Positive Markers	Pathological Characteristics
Histiocytic type	SAT, PTC	CD68, MAC387	Fusion of histiocytic cells involved in phagocytosis
Follicular cell type	PTC, occasional	TG, TTF-1	Proliferation and fusion of thyroid follicular epithelial cells
Striated muscle cell type	PTC, extremely rare	MSA, Myoglobin	Regeneration of striated muscle cells violated by extrathyroidal extension of PTC

*SAT: Subacute thyroiditis; **IHC: Immunohistochemical.

3. Case C: PTMC coexisting with subacute thyroiditis

3.1 Vignette

The patient was a 42-year-old female who have had recurrent subacute thyroiditis for more than three years. Ultrasound images showed multiple hypoechogenic areas varying in size in both lobes of thyroid, and among them were a 15×6 mm focal hypoechogenic lesion with an ill-defined margin in the left lobe, and a 7.1×7.6×6.4 mm hypoechogenic, partially circumscribed, nodule in the right lobe. The left thyroid lesion was strongly suspected as subacute thyroiditis and the right thyroid nodule exhibited suspicious ultrasound features of PTMC (Figure 4). Therefore, FNA was performed. At first, the palpable painful nodule in the left lobe was sampled, and its cytopathological features were consistent with subacute thyroiditis. Ultrasound-guided FNA of the right thyroid nodule was then performed and its cytopathology demonstrated a mixture of epithelioid cells, multinucleated giant cells, neutrophils, lymphocytes, macrophages, fragments of stromal tissue, and several fragments of follicular cells with full PTC nuclear features (Figure 5A-5D). Based on the cytopathological findings and unbearable severe neck pain for the patient, a total thyroidectomy was carried out. The histopathological examination of the surgical specimen revealed a PTMC lesion in the background of subacute thyroiditis (Figures 5E-5H).

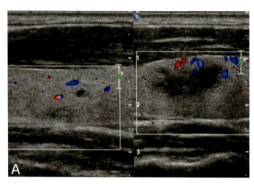 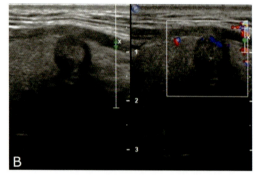

Figure 4. PTMC coexisting with subacute thyroiditis. On ultrasound, both lobe measurements are normal in size; but a 15×6 mm and a 7.1×7.6×6.4 mm focal hypoechogenic lesions were detected in the left lobe and in the lower pole of right lobe, respectively; the former was oval in shape and ill-defined for its margin, while the latter was avascular, and partially circumscribed.

3.2. Discussion

This is a rare case of subacute thyroiditis coexisting with PTMC, which may obscure the coexistence of PTMC (7). The clinical manifestations, ultrasound features and cytological evaluation revealed the presence of diffuse multiple lesions of subacute thyroiditis in both lobes of thyroid. During FNA of the target nodule that was suspected of PTC, the needle was inevitable to pass through inflammatory peripheral region, and the FNA cytology was therefore presented as a mixture of inflammatory and neoplastic components. The key for differential diagnosis is to search for syncytial tissue fragments of follicular cells with characteristic nuclear features of PTC.

It is usually easy to choose a palpable large nodule for FNA biopsy, and the critical small lesions may be missed. We thus propose ultrasound-guided FNA biopsy since it will not only be able to ensure that samples are taken from the critical lesions, but also help to choose the most suspicious parts based on the ultrasound characteristics of the lesions, thereby increasing the possibility of collecting essential diagnostic samples. As noted in this case, the first biopsy sample was taken from a palpable painful nodule in the left lobe and its cytological findings showed only the changes of subacute thyroiditis. Under ultrasound guidance, the small nodule suspected of PTC in the right lobe was sampled, and co-existence of PTMC with subcuate thyroiditis was revealed, providing the evidence for proper treatment of the patient.

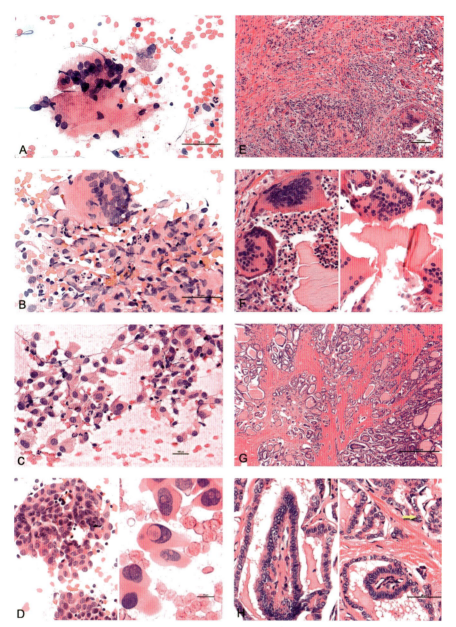

Figure 5. PTMC coexisting with subacute thyroiditis. 5A and 5B: Medium power view shows aggregates of epithelioid cells, multinucleated histiocytic type giant cells, and inflammatory cells. 5C: Aggregates of follicular cells mingled with neutrophils, lymphocytes and macrophages. 5D: Tissue fragments of follicular cells are syncytial (left) and several intranuclear pseudoinclusions could be observed (right). 5E: Low power view shows granulomatous inflammation in the fibrotic background. 5F: Medium power view shows encirclement of follicles by multinucleated histiocytic type giant cells and a mixture of acute and chronic inflammatory cells with abundant neutrophils within an effaced follicle. 5G: Papillae and irregularly shaped follicles were isolated and surrounded by proliferative fibrous tissue. 5H: Medium power view shows typical papillary structures with fibrovascular cores and covered with follicular cells with important nuclear features of PTC. Note the yellow arrow points to an intranuclear pseudoinclusion (5A-5D: FNA Smears; and 5E-5H: HE-stained tissue sections).

References

1. Woolf PD, Daly R. Thyrotoxicosis with painless thyroiditis. Am J Med 1976; 60(1):73-9.
2. Bartels PC, Boer RO. Subacute thyroiditis (de Quervain) presenting as a painless "cold" nodule. J Nucl Med 1987; 28:1488.
3. Daniels GH. Atypical subacute thyroiditis: preliminary observations. Thyroid 2001; 11:691-5.
4. García Solano J, Giménez Bascuñana A, Sola Pérez J, et al. Fine-needle aspiration of subacute granulomatous thyroiditis (De Quervain's thyroiditis): a clinico-cytologic review of 36 cases. Diagn Cytopathol 1997; 16(3):214-20.
5. Shabb NS, Tawil A, Gergeos F, et al. Multinucleated giant cells in fine needle aspiration of thyroid nodules: their diagnostic significance. Diagn Cytopathol 1999; 21(5):307-12.
6. Zeppa P, Benincasa G, Lucariello A, et al. Association of different pathologic processes of the thyroid gland in fine needle aspiration samples. Acta Cytol 2001; 45(3):347-52.
7. Nishihara, Hirokawa M, Ohye H, et al. Papillary carcinoma obscured by complication with subacute thyroiditis: sequential ultrasonographic and histopathological findings in five cases. Thyroid 2008; 18(11):1221-5.

Chapter 12

Hyalinizing Trabecular Tumor vs. Papillary Thyroid Carcinoma

Mitsuyoshi Hirokawa and Ayana Suzuki

Case

The patient was a 48-year-old female who was pointed out to have dyslipidemia in a medical checkup, and visited another hospital, where a nodule was demonstrated in the left lobe of the thyroid. She was referred to our hospital for close inspection. Ultrasonographic examination revealed two nodules in the thyroid. One nodule was located in the left lobe, measuring 26 mm x 17 mm x 24 mm. This nodule was slightly hypoechoic and homogeneous in its internal echogenicity. Its shape was slightly irregular, but its border was well-defined. The nodule was associated with multiple punctate hyperechogenic foci (Figure 1). Color Doppler ultrasound showed intra- and peri-tumoral hypervascular flow, called "tumor inferno" (Figure 2). Ultrasonographic interpretation was either papillary thyroid carcinoma (PTC) or hyalinizing trabecular tumor (HTT). Another nodule was located in the right lobe, measuring 10 mm x 6 mm x 6 mm, which was interpreted as a benign nodule. Aspiration cytology report for the left and right nodules was hyalinizing trabecular tumor and oxyphilic cell variant of follicular neoplasm, respectively. The patient underwent a total thyroidectomy.

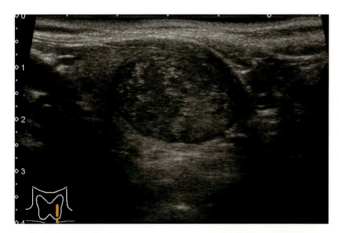

Figure 1. A slightly hypoechoic and homogeneous mass is seen in the left lobe of the thyroid. The mass contains with multiple punctate hyperechogenic foci. (Ultrasound B-mode image)

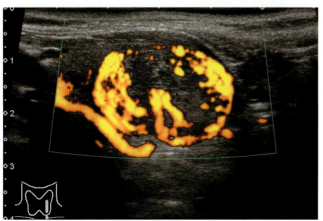

Figure 2. Intra- and peri-tumoral hypervascular flow called "tumor inferno" is seen. (Ultrasound color Doppler image)

Cytological Findings

The tumor cells appeared surrounding hyaline materials, which looked like papillary structure (Figure 3). The hyaline materials were located at the center of the clusters and radially elongated (Figure 4). Some clusters showed curved nuclear palisading. There were no papillary, follicular, or sheet-like arrangements. The cytoplasm was faintly stained and somewhat filamentous (Figure 5). The cell border was indistinct. The nuclei exhibited intranuclear cytoplasmic inclusions (NCIs) and nuclear grooves (Figure 6). Yellow bodies were not observed.

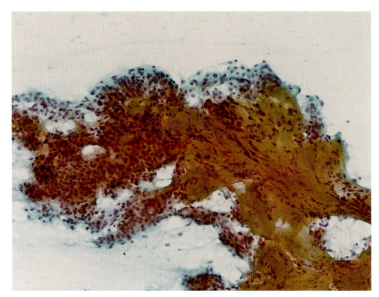

Figure 3. The tumor cells surround hyaline material. (Pap, x20)

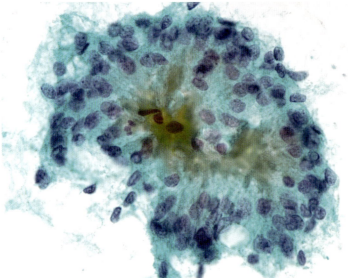

Figure 4. The hyaline materials are radially elongated. Curved nuclear palisading is seen. (Papanicolaou, x400)

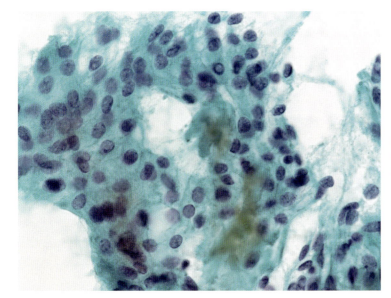

Figure 5. The cytoplasm is faintly stained and somewhat filamentous. (Pap, x40)

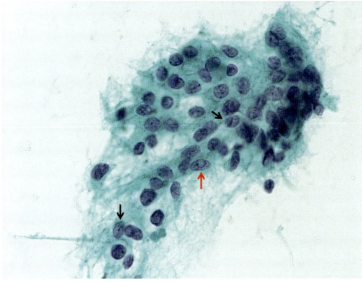

Figure 6. Intranuclear cytoplasmic inclusion (red arrow) and nuclear grooves are seen (black arrows).

(Papanicolaou, x400)

Pathological Findings

A solid tumor measuring 2.3 x 2.2 cm was located at the lower portion of the left thyroid. On the cut surface, the tumor was solid, whitish-yellow in color, and partially encapsulated by thin fibrous connective tissue (Figure 7). Microscopically, the tumor cells mainly exhibited a trabecular pattern (Figure 8). Follicular pattern with colloid and/ or microcalcification were also observed. The tumor cells showed NCIs, nuclear grooves, and yellow bodies (Figure 9). Hyaline materials were present not only at the periphery of trabecular tumor nests, but also between the tumor cells. The stroma was highly vascular. Immunohistochemically, the tumor cells displayed cell membranous positivity for Ki-67 (MIB-1) (Figure 10).

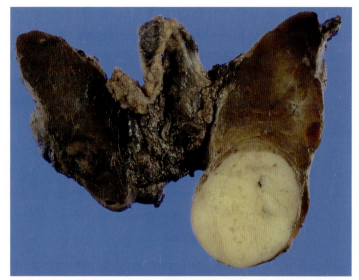

Figure 7. The tumor is solid, whitish-yellow in color, and partially encapsulated by the thin fibrous connective tissue.

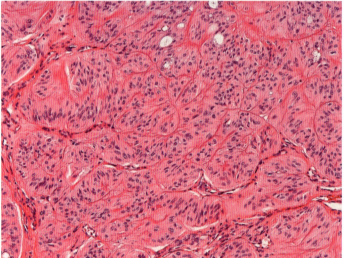

Figure 8. The tumor cells show trabecular pattern. Follicular pattern is seen in the upper portion. (HE, x200)

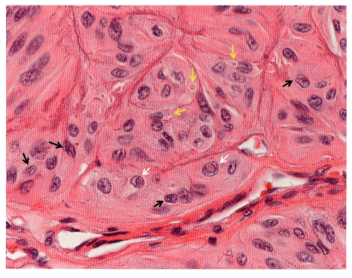

Figure 9. Intra- and inter-trabecular hyaline materials are present. The tumor cells show intranuclear cytoplasmic inclusions (white arrows), nuclear grooves (black arrows), and yellow bodies (yellow arrows). (HE, x400)

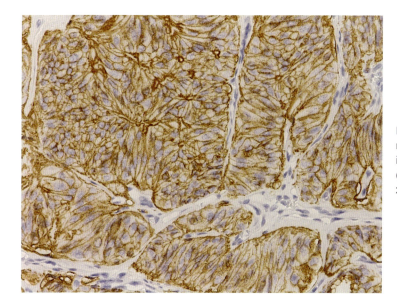

Figure 10. The cell membrane of the tumor cells is immunoreactive for Ki-67 (MIB-1). (Immunostaining, x200)

Discussion

Hyalinizing trabecular tumor (HTT) was identified by Carney *et al.* in 1987 as a type of benign follicular neoplasm of the thyroid (1). This tumor shares several histological features with PTC, including NCIs, nuclear grooves, and psammoma bodies. These and other findings such as lymph node metastasis and molecular biological evidence are similar to those of PTC, which have led to the suggestion that HTT and PTC are two tumors with a close relationship (2), but later micro-RNA profile did not support the proposed link of HTT with PTC (3).

HTT is a rare follicular cell-derived thyroid tumor characterized by a trabecular growth pattern and marked intra- and inter-trabecular hyalinization (4). The hyalinization denotes excessively produced basement membrane materials and constitutes an important diagnostic clue (5). Rothenberg *et al.* reported that intracytoplasmic, eosinophilic spheres (so-called yellow bodies) were observed in all of the 75 HTT cases they reviewed histologically, but not identified in PTC (6). Yellow bodies are consistent with giant lysosome and most probably represent a universal feature of this tumor. Microcalcification is occasionally seen, which is morphologically similar to the psammoma bodies seen in PTC (7). However, it appears within follicles composed of the tumor cells, and should be differentiated from true psammoma bodies. Psammoma bodies seen in PTC are formed in the stroma with papillary growth or within the lymph vessels.

Immunohistochemically, HTT exhibits the property of thyroid follicular cells: positive thyroglobulin and negative calcitonin. To distinguish HTT from PTC, immunostaining against cytokeratin 19 and Ki-67 (MIB-1) is useful (8-10). PTC is positive for cytokeratin 19, but HTT is negative. Ki-67 is a proliferation-related antigen that is present during all active phases of the cell cycle and is expressed in the nucleus. In PTC cases, the nuclei of carcinoma cells show a low labeling index. HTT however shows a strong cell membranous immunoreactivity for Ki-67 (MIB-1). The unique staining pattern for Ki-67 (MIB-1) (Figure 10) is useful to differentiate HTT from PTC.

On fine needle aspiration smears, HTT is easily confused with PTC because both show nuclear grooves and NCIs. NCIs are identified in all HTT cases, but PTC does not always exhibit them. Differential diagnoses of HTT and PTC are shown in Table 1. The smears aspirated from HTT are slightly cellular. The tumor cell clusters show pseudopapillary pattern with the hyaline materials in the center or periphery of the clusters (Figure 4). Hyaline materials are radially elongated (11). The border between the tumor cells and hyaline materials is extremely irregular or vague. They never exhibit the papillary, follicular or sheet-like arrangements that are seen in PTC (7). Vague and curved nuclear palisading may be seen. The tumor cells are mainly spindled; and elongated, polygonal and stellate cells are also observed (12). Cytoplasmic processes may be observed (7). The cytoplasm is faintly stained and somewhat filamentous (Figure 5). The cell border is indistinct. In contrast, the cytoplasm of PTC is densely stained and the cell border is distinct (Figure 11). Yellow bodies that are seen as hyaline-like materials with halo are frequently observed in HTT (Figure 12), but not in PTC. Therefore, the presence of yellow bodies is a reliable clue to make a diagnosis of HTT. Immunocytochemical staining for Ki-67 (MIB-1) is also useful (Figure 13) (13).

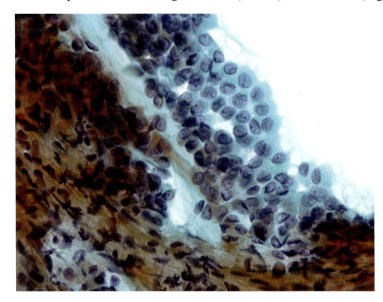

Figure 11. In papillary thyroid carcinoma, the carcinoma cell cluster and stroma are clearly separated. The cytoplasm is densely stained. (Papanicolaou, x400)

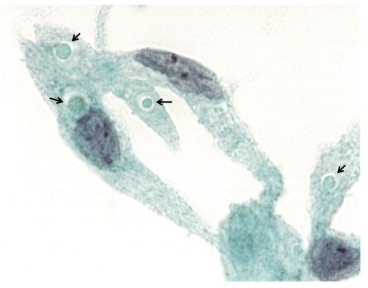

Figure 12. Yellow bodies (arrows) are seen as hyaline-like materials with halo. (Papanicolaou, LBC, x1000)

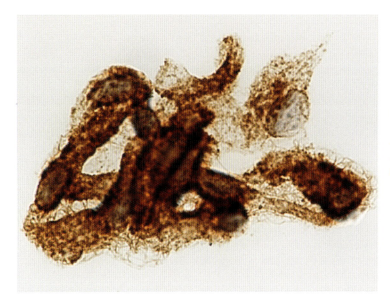

Figure 13. The tumor cells show cell membranous and cytoplasmic positivity for Ki-67 (MIB-1). (Immunostaining, LBC, x1000)

Table 1. Differential diagnoses of hyalinizing trabecular tumor and papillary thyroid carcinoma

	Hyalinizing trabecular tumor	Papillary thyroid carcinoma
Background	Hyaline material	Ropy colloid, psammoma body
	(basement membrane)	Foamy cells, lymphocytes
		Multinucleated giant cell
Arrangement	Radiating	Sheet-like, papillary, follicular
Nuclear palisading	Vague, curved	Distinct, straight
	(surrounding hyaline materials)	
Cell border	Indistinct	Distinct
Cell shape	Spindled, elongated,	Round, oval
	Cytoplasmic process	
Cytoplasm	Faintly stained	Densely stained
	Filamentous	Homogeneous
	Yellow bodies	Septate intracytoplasmic vacuoles
Nucleus	Intracytoplasmic inclusions (all cases),	Intracytoplasmic inclusions (not always),
	Grooves, perinucleolar halo	Grooves, perinucleolar halo
		Powdery chromatin
Immunostaining		
Cytokeratin 19	Negative	Positive
Ki-67 (MIB-1)	Cell membrane	Nuclei

References

1. Carney JA, Hirokawa M, Lloyd RV, et al. Hyalinizing trabecular tumors of the thyroid gland are almost all

benign. Am J Surg Pathol 2008; 32:1877-89.
2. Li J, Yang GZ, Gao LX, et al. Hyalinizing trabecular tumor of the thyroid: Case report and review of the literature. Exp Ther Med 2012; 3:1015-7.
3. Shue SY, Vogel E, Worm K, et al. Hyalinizing trabecular tumour of the thyroid. – differential expression of distinct miRNAs compared with papillary thyroid carcinoma. Histopathol 2010; 56: 632-40.
4. Nose V, Volante M, Papotti M. Hyalinizing trabecular tumor of the thyroid: an update. Endocr Pathol 2008; 19:1-8.
5. Katoh R, Kakudo K, Kawaoi A. Accumulated basement membrane material in hyalinizing trabecular tumors of the thyroid. Mod Pathol 1999; 12:1057-61.
6. Rothenberg HJ, Goellner JR, Carney JA. Hyalinizing trabecular adenoma of the thyroid gland. Am J Surg Pathol 1999; 23:118-25.
7. Kuma S, Hirokawa M, Miyauchi A, et al. Cytologic features of hyalinizing trabecular adenoma of the thyroid. Acta Cytol 2003; 47:399-404.
8. Hirokawa M, Carney JA, Ohtsuki Y. Hyalinizing trabecular adenoma and papillary thyroid carcinoma of the thyroid gland express different cytokeratin patterns. Am J Surg Pathol 2000; 24:877-81.
9. Hirokawa M, Carney JA. Cell membrane and cytoplasmic staining for MIB-1 in hyalinizing trabecular adenoma of the thyroid gland. Am J Surg Pathol 2000; 24:575-8.
10. Gupta S, Modi S, Gupta V, et al. Hyalinizing trabecular tumor of the thyroid gland. J Cytol 2010; 27:63-5.
11. Casey MB, Sebo TJ, Carney JA. Hyalinizing trabecular adenoma of the thyroid gland: Cytologic features in 29 cases. Am J Surg Pathol 2004; 28:859-67.
12. Goellner JR, Carney JA. Cytologic features of fine-needle aspirates of hyalinizing trabecular adenoma of the thyroid. Am J Clin Pathol 1989; 91:115-9.
13. Hirokawa M, Shimizu M, Manabe T, et al. Hyalinizing trabecular adenoma of the thyroid: its unusual cytoplasmic immunopositivity for MIB1. Pathol Int 1995; 45.399-401.

Chapter 13

Hashimoto's Thyroiditis or Papillary Carcinoma

Yun Zhu and Tiesheng Wang

Follicular epithelium in Hashimoto's thyroiditis may display a range of nuclear changes that mimic those encountered in papillary thyroid carcinoma (PTC), constituting important diagnostic pitfalls. Suspecting PTC on fine needle aspiration (FNA) of the thyroid with only Hashimoto's thyroiditis is not unusual in our practice. In this chapter, we discuss three cases that were misinterpreted, aiming to identify the cytologic features leading to misinterpretation in Hashimoto's thyroiditis, and explore how to avoid an over diagnosis of malignancy.

1. **Case 1: Follicular carcinoma, minimally invasive type**

    Clinical History
    A 23-year old woman with a family history of PTC was admitted to our hospital for a physical examination. Ultrasound detected an 8×8×9 mm, regularly shaped, partially circumscribed, and heterogeneous isoechoic thyroid nodule with a thin halo in the isthmus. Ultrasound-guided FNA (US-FNA) was performed as the patient strongly requested for.
    Cytological examination revealed an extremely cellular aspirate showing large numbers of tissue fragments with papillary-like architecture (Figure 1) in a background of sparsely scattered lymphocytes (Figures 1 and 2) and some multinucleated giant cells (Figure 3). The cell nuclei were enlarged, slightly crowded with granular chromatin and inconspicuous nucleoli (Figure 2), showing some equivocal features of conventional PTC. Overwhelmingly papillary-like fragments of follicular cells, a paucity of background lymphocytes, and a few cells exhibiting worrisome nuclear features of PTC as well as the family history led to the diagnosis of "indeterminate - not exclude PTC".
    On gross examination of the isthmus, a 0.8 cm, solitary reddish-brown, well-circumscribed nodule with a thick capsule was identified. Histopathological examination showed that the tumor cells split the thick and fibrotic capsule with complete transgression, which led to a diagnosis of follicular carcinoma minimally invasive type (Figure 4). Most follicular cells in this follicular carcinoma exhibited slightly crowded and overlapped nuclei with compact or coarsely granular chromatin and did not show worrisome nuclear features of PTC. Please refer to Chapters 3 and 4 for true-positive PTC for comparison in which several large branching tissue fragments of follicular cells with central fibrovascular cores (Figure 2 of Chapter 4) and typical nuclear features of PTC such as pale powdery chromatin, nucleoli, nuclear grooves and intranuclear cytoplasmic inclusions in a clean background (Figures 5 and 6 of Chapter 3, Figure 3 of Chapter 4, and cover page illustration).

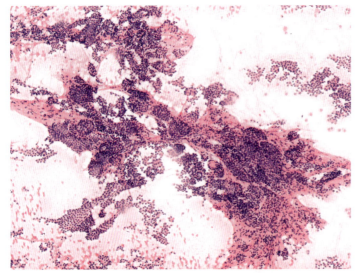

Figure 1. Medium power view of the papillary-like architecture. The component cells are minimally enlarged, and round with granular chromatin. Nuclear characteristics of papillary carcinoma are rarely observed besides the architecture. (HE stain, ×40)

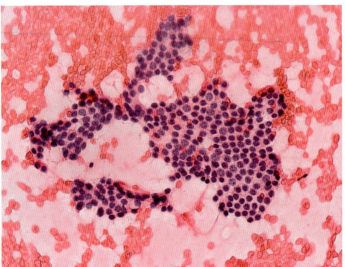

Figure 2. High magnification showing anastomosing trabeculae of follicular cells with syncytial arrangement. The nuclei are enlarged, slightly crowded and altered in polarity with granular chromatin and nucleoli. The background is clean and lacks colloid. (HE stain, ×200)

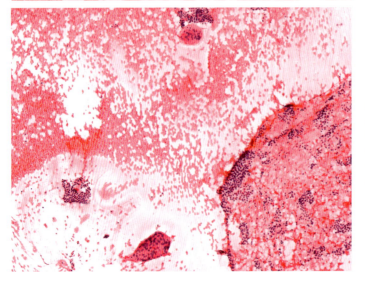

Figure 3. Note two isolated multinucleated giant cells in the aspirate. This aspirate is interpreted as "indeterminate-not exclude papillary carcinoma". (HE stain, ×40)

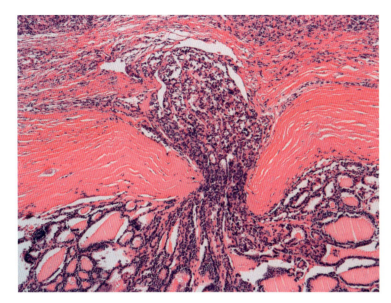

Figure 4. The invasion is seen as involving the entire and going beyond the capsule. Follicular cells in this follicular carcinoma have slightly crowed and overlapped nuclei with compact or coarsely granular chromatin, but do not exhibit worrisome nuclear features of PTC.
(HE stain, ×100)

2. **Case 2: Hashimoto's thyroiditis with marked Hürthle cell metaplasia**

   Clinical History

   This was a 49-year-old woman who underwent a health examination. Neck ultrasound scan discovered a diffusely enlarged gland with developing fibrosis. A hypoechoic focus of 3×3×4 mm in size with irregularly blurred margins in the right lobe of the thyroid gland was noticed. Papillary thyroid microcarcinoma (PTMC) was suspected sonographically. Therefore, US-FNA was performed.

   Cytological examination revealed extremely cellular aspirates with follicular cells, Hürthle cells, and inflammatory cells in varying proportions (Figures 5 and 6). Mildly enlarged and overlapped cells arranged in syncytial fashion (Figure 7), and they exhibited poorly defined cell borders. The atypical nuclei showed finely granular chromatin, micronucleoli and occasional nuclear grooves (Figure 8). A probably psammoma body (Figure 6), multinucleated giant cells (Figure 7) and extremely crowded cells with a three-dimensional arrangement (Figure 8) were also noticed, thus, a diagnosis of suspicious for PTC was rendered. Histological sections revealed Hashimoto's thyroiditis with marked Hürthle cell metaplasia and nuclear atypia (Figures 9 and 10), but neoplastic cells were not found.

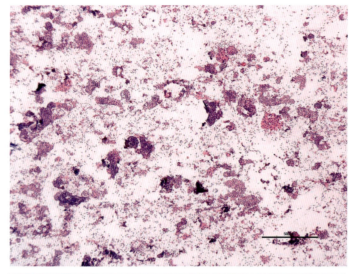

Figure 5. Extremely cellular aspirate in a background of Hashimoto's thyroiditis on the low power view. Note the follicular cells, Hürthle cells and inflammatory cells in varying proportions on the medium power view.
(HE stain, ×40)

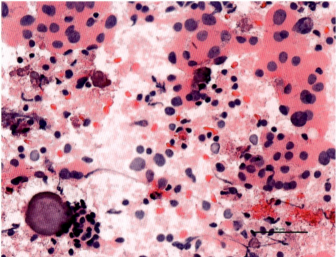

Figure 6. High magnification shows tissue fragments of markedly pleomorphic Hürthle cells with bizarre nuclei. This arrangement is not consistent with that of Hürthle cell neoplasm. The low left field contains a probably psammoma body.
(HE stain, ×400)

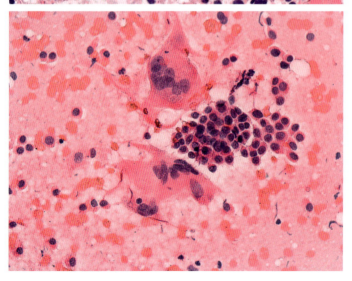

Figure 7. One group of mildly enlarged and overlapped cells arranged in a syncytial fashion with poorly defined cell borders and atypical nuclei. The nuclei exhibit finely granular chromatin, micronucleoli, and occasional nuclear grooves. Multinucleated giant cells are also noticed.
(HE stain, ×400)

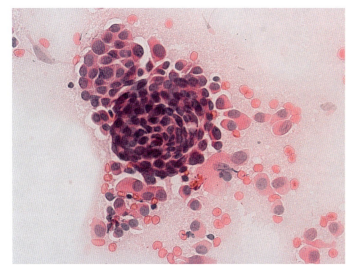

Figure 8. A syncytial fragment with extremely crowded nuclei, a smooth external contour, and a three-dimensional appearance. Scattered follicular cells in the peripheral area exhibit finely granular chromatin and occasional nuclear grooves. This aspirate is interpreted as suspicious for papillary carcinoma.
(HE stain, ×400)

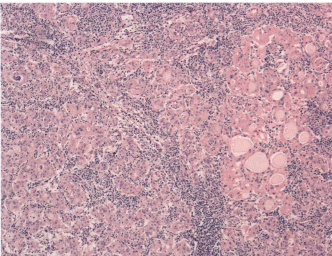

Figure 9. Subsequent thyroidectomy revealed Hashimoto's thyroiditis, but not a neoplastic nodule.
(HE stain, ×100)

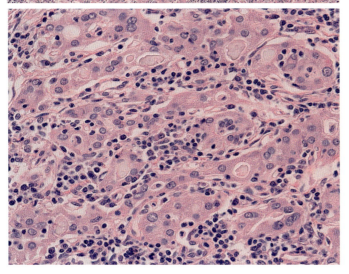

Figure 10. High magnification showing mildly crowded Hürthle cell metaplasia with mild nuclear atypia. Note the interfollicular lymphoid cell infiltration
(HE stain, ×200)

3. Case 3: Hashimoto's thyroiditis with an atypical hyperplastic nodule

   Clinical History
   This was a 45-year-old woman who was suffering from Hashimoto's thyroiditis for more than ten years. Ultrasound images showed multiple hypoechogenic areas varying in size in both lobes. Among them, a 13×11×10 mm focal hypoechogenic lesion was detected in the right lobe with ill-defined margins and microcalcification (Figure 11), raising a possibility of PTC. Consequently, FNA was performed. Cytological examination showed a few of syncytial or monolayered tissue fragments of follicular epithelium with markedly crowded and overlapped nuclei with nuclear contour irregularity (Figures 12 and 13). The chromatin was finely granular to powdery. Nucleoli and nuclear grooves were present (Figure 14). A diagnosis of PTC was rendered. Histological sections revealed a well-circumscribed follicular pattern tumor in a background of Hashimoto's thyroiditis (Figure 15). Some areas of this tumor presented mildly enlarged nuclei with nuclear contour irregularity and pale chromatin, reminiscent of PTC (Figure 16), which might include a differential diagnosis of follicular variant papillary thyroid carcinoma (FVPTC). However, there are debates on diagnostic criteria of this variant and observer variation between benign follicular adenoma and malignant FVPTC was reported to be significant (1). Chinese pathologists apply stricter criteria to non-invasive follicular pattern tumors with questionable PTC type nuclei. Finally, a diagnosis of Hashimoto's thyroiditis with an atypical hyperplastic nodule was rendered, which was probably equivalent to FVPTC in the Western practice or NIFTP (non-invasive follicular thyroid neoplasm with papillary-like nuclear features) proposed recently by Nikiforov *et al.* (2) (please refer to Chapter 6).

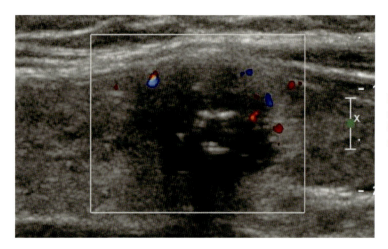

Figure 11. Ultrasound image shows a focal hypoechogenic lesion with an ill-defined margin and microcalcification.

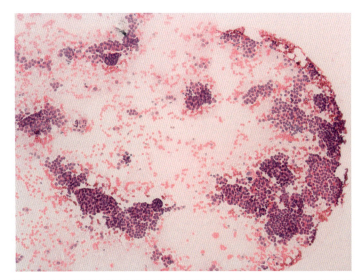

Figure 12. Showing syncytial or monolayered tissue fragments of follicular cells in neither follicular nor papillary pattern.
(HE stain, ×100)

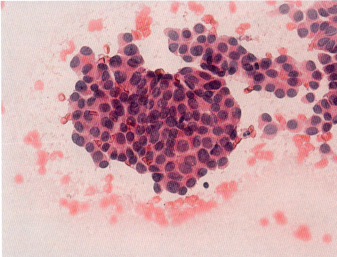

Figure 13. Markedly crowded and overlapped nuclei with an irregular nuclear contour.
(HE stain, ×400)

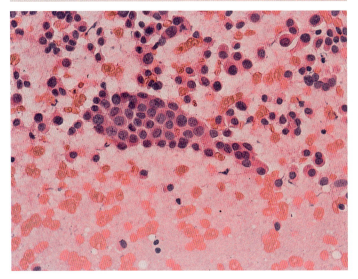

Figure 14. The chromatin is finely granular. Nucleoli and grooves are present.
(HE stain, ×400)

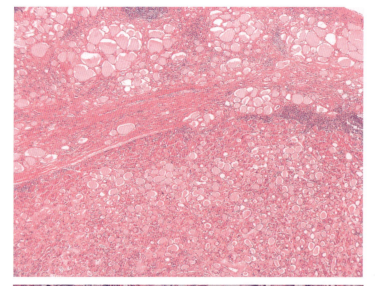

Figure 15. Low power view shows a partly encapsulated tumor with a follicular growth pattern coexisted with Hashimoto's thyroiditis. (HE stain, ×40)

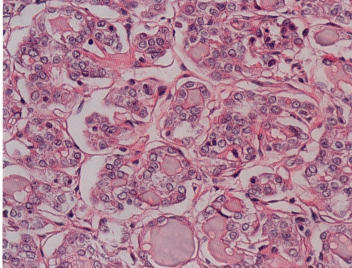

Figure 16. Mildly enlarged nuclei with finely dispersed chromatin, empty appearance, and a prominent nuclear membrane. (HE stain, ×200)

Discussion

Hashimoto's thyroiditis is a main pitfall of overdiagnosis of PTC in thyroid cytology as reported in many literatures (3-9). There are various cytologic features simulating PTC in Hashimoto thyroiditis (please refer to Chapters 3, 4, and 6). In adequate specimens, it would not make us confused too much for diagnosis of Hashimoto's thyroiditis. However, the nuclei of the oxyphilic or non-oxyphilic follicular epithelium in Hashimoto thyroiditis often exhibit considerable nuclear atypia, and there may have aggregates of a few of follicles containing cells that are indistinguishable from those seen in PTC as shown in Figures 6, 7 and 8 (8-10). It is one of the most significant pitfalls especially when the aspirate is strikingly cellular such as in Case 1 (6, 7). Useful cytological features to differentiate Hashimoto's thyroiditis from PTC are also listed in the Table 1 of Chapter 3. Kini et al. suggested that the minimal criteria for the diagnosis of PTC should include a syncytial-type tissue fragment of follicular epithelium, regardless of its architectural pattern, displaying a typical nuclear morphology, i.e., pale appearing enlarged nuclei with fine, dusty, or powdery chromatin, and a chromatin bar or ridge; single or multiple micro and/or macronucleoli; and intranuclear cytoplasmic inclusions (Table 1) (6). These criteria have been proven extremely effective in our experience.

Table 1. Minimal criteria for the cytological diagnosis of PTC

1. Syncytial tissue fragments with or without any architectural configurations
2. Enlarged nuclei with finely granular, powdery or watery chromatin and nuclear contour irregularity
3. Nuclear pseudoinclusions
4. Nuclear grooves
5. Multiple micro-and/or macronucleoli

Harvey et al. reviewed thyroid FNA cases whose diagnoses were suspicious or positive for a thyroid neoplasm but the subsequent thyroidectomy specimen revealed Hashimoto's thyroiditis only, and have concluded lymphocyte-infiltrating epithelial cell group is a significant feature that would help differentiate between thyroid neoplasm and Hashimoto's thyroiditis (7). The tissue fragments of follicular cells intimately permeated by lymphoid cells occur much more frequently in thyroiditis alone than in PTC coexisting with Hashimoto's thyroiditis in cytologic specimens. However, the cytologic evaluation greatly depends on the area sampled by the biopsy needle. When the nodule is discrete and encapsulated or non-capsulated but enlarged with few lymphoplasmacytic infiltrate, coexisted thyroiditis can be overlooked since the lymphocytes are extremely sparse or not sampled. Conversely, Hashimoto's thyroiditis with nonneoplastic follicular or Hürthle cell nodules usually has a lymphocytic infiltrate. Therefore, aspiration biopsy will exhibit follicular cells, Hürthle cells and inflammatory cells in varying proportions as shown in Case 2 (Figures 6 and 10), indicating a non-neoplastic process.

In case that the cellularity is marginal, sparsely scattered follicular cells exhibiting several features may seem to accord with the minimal criteria for the diagnosis of PTC, which may render a definite diagnosis really difficult (6). Fortunately, a repeated FNA or a core needle tissue biopsy often solves the problem, and such a circumstance occurs rarely in our experience.

Conclusion

It is essential to retain a conservative diagnosis until the minimal criteria of PTC are fulfilled. One single cytological feature of PTC proves to be meaningless to conclude malignancy in Hashimoto's thyroiditis since Hashimoto thyroiditis has several overlapping features with PTC. Extreme caution should also be taken when there are focal features suggestive of PTC, and the authors recommend to apply AUS category of the Bethesda, Thy 3a of the British system, TIR3A of the Italian system, or Indeterminate B (others) of the Japanese system instead of definite malignancy or suspicious for malignancy to these samples.

References

1. Kakudo K, Katoh R, Sakamoto A Asa S, DeLellis RA, Carney JA, Naganuma H, Kameyama K, Takami H. Thyroid gland: international case conference. Endocr Pathol 2002; 13:131-4.
2. Nikiforov Y, Seethala RR, Tallini G, et al: Revision of the normenclature for encapsulated follicular variant of papillary thyroid carcinoma: Terminology shift as paradigm for reducing overtreatment of indolent tumors. JAMA Oncol, 2016 Apr 14. doi: 10.1001/jamaoncol.2016.0386. [Epub ahead of print]
3. Nguyen GK, Ginsberg J, Crockford PM, et al. Hashimoto's thyroiditis: cytodiagnostic accuracy and pitfalls. Diagn Cytopathol 1997; 16;531-6.
4. Berho M, Suster S. Clear nuclear changes in Hashimoto's thyroiditis. A clinicopathologic study of 12 cases. Ann Clin Lab Sci 1995; 25:513-21.
5. Lee J, Hasteh F. Oncocytic variant of papillary thyroid carcinoma associated with Hashimoto's thyroiditis: a case report and review of the literature. Diagn Cytopathol 2009; 37:600-6.
6. Kini SR. Thyroid cytopathology: an atlas and text. 2nd edition, 2015, p212-213.
7. Harvey AM, Truong LD, Mody DR. Diagnostic pitfalls of Hashimoto's/Lymphocytic thyroiditis on fine-needle aspirations and strategies to avoid overdiagnosis. Acta Cytologica 2012; 56: 352-360.
8. Haberal AN, Toru S, Ozen O, et al. Diagnostic pitfalls in the evaluation of fine needle aspiration cytology of the thyroid: correlation with histopathology in 260 cases. Cytopathology 2009; 20:103-8.
9. Anand A, Singh KR, Kushwaha JK, et al. Papillary thyroid cancer and Hashimoto's thyroiditis: an association less understood. Indian J Surg Oncol 2014; 5:199-204.
10. Rosai J, Kuhn E, Carcangiu ML. Pitfalls in thyroid tumour pathology. Histopathology 2006; 49:107-20.

Chapter 14

MALT Lymphoma vs. Hashimoto Thyroiditis

Mitsuyoshi Hirokawa and Ayana Suzuki

Case

The case was a 21-year-old female who noticed anterior neck swelling one year ago. She visited another hospital for medical check-up, and ultrasonographic examination revealed multiple nodules in her thyroid. Her serum TSH was increased (8.14 µIU/ml). She was referred to our hospital for close inspection. Her serum TSH, thyroglobulin, and thyroglobulin antibody were 5.155 µIU/mL, 880.00 ng/mL, and 40.6 IU/mL, respectively. Serum thyroperoxidase antibody was negative. Ultrasonography revealed multiple nodules in both lobes of the thyroid (Figure 1). The largest nodule was measured 28 mm x 10 mm x 22 mm. The nodules were hypoechoic and heterogeneous. The borders were irregular and indistinct. Both ultrasonographic examination and aspiration cytology were suspicious of malignant lymphoma. Flow cytometry CD45 gating using aspirated materials revealed light chain restriction (κ/λ ratio, 10.9) (Figure 2). To confirm the diagnosis of malignant lymphoma, a total thyroidectomy was performed.

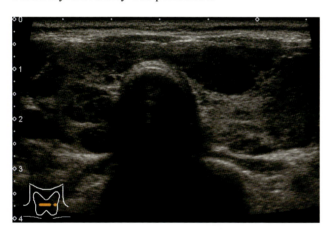

Figure 1. Multiple hypoechoic and heterogeneous nodules are seen in both lobes of the thyroid. (Ultrasound B-mode image)

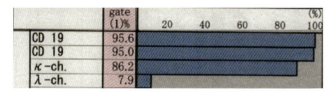

Figure 2. Report of flow cytometry CD45 gating shows light chain restriction.

Cytological Findings

The aspirated materials were highly cellular, and composed of lymphoid cells (Figure 3). A few follicular cells with oncocytic features were present (Figure 4). Most of the lymphoid cells were small to moderate-sized, but a small number of large-sized lymphoid cells were intermingled. The chromatin pattern of lymphoid cells was similar regardless of the difference in size (Figure 5). Micronucleoli were observed, even in small-sized lymphoid cells. Lymphoglandular bodies were not apparent.

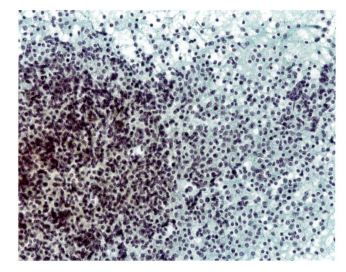

Figure 3. A large number of lymphoid cells are smeared. (Pap, x200)

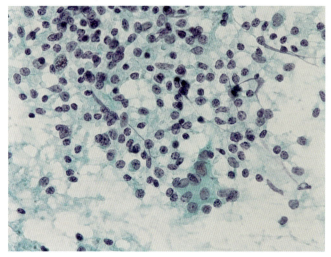

Figure 4. A small cluster of follicular cells with oncocytic features. (Papanicolaou, x400)

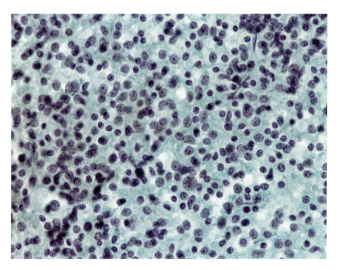

Figure 5. Lymphoid cells have similar chromatin pattern regardless of the difference in size. (Papanicolaou, x400)

Pathological Findings

The resected thyroid was enlarged due to multiple nodular lesions (Figure 6). The nodules were tan to whitish-yellow in color. The borders were indistinct and tended to merge each other. The nodules were composed of various-sized lymphoid cells (Figure 7). Most of them were small to medium in size. Proliferative follicular cells and lymphoid cells were intimately intermingled (lymphoepithelial lesions) (Figure 8) and an aggregation of lymphoid cells within thyroid follicles (packing) (Figure 9) was observed. Lymphoid cells did not invade extrathyroidal tissue. The nonneoplastic thyroid tissue was consistent with Hashimoto thyroiditis.

Immunohistochemically, most of lymphoid cells were positive for CD20. Monoclonality (κ/λ-light chain restriction) was not confirmed. CD23 immunostaining manifested disrupted follicular dendritic cell meshwork (follicular colonization) within a large and irregular shaped germinal center (Figure 10). Cytokeratin AE1/AE3 immunostaining highlighted lymphoepithelial lesions and packing (Figure 11). In flow cytometry with CD45 gating, the κ/λ ratio was 15.3. G-banding analysis revealed chromosomal abnormality, 46, XX, der (2) add (2) (p11.2) del (2) (q?). Clonal rearrangements of the IgH gene were not identified.

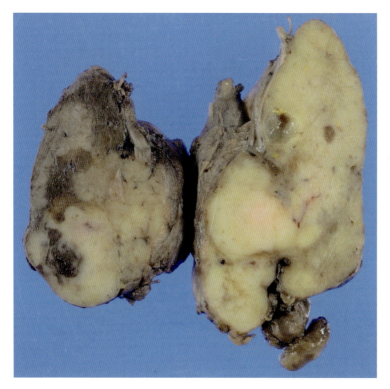

Figure 6. Enlarged thyroid contains multiple nodules.

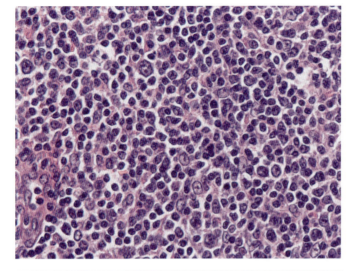

Figure 7. The nodule is composed of mainly small to medium-sized lymphoid cells. (HE, x400)

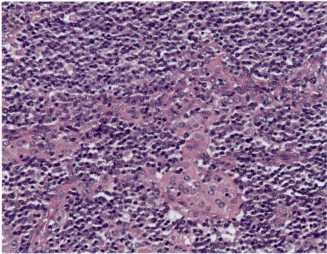

Figure 8. A lymphoepithelial lesion composed of proliferative follicular cells and lymphoid cells. (HE, x200)

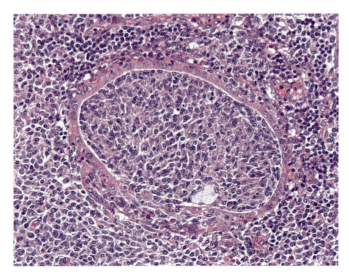

Figure 9. An aggregation of lymphoid cells within thyroid follicles (packing). (HE, x200)

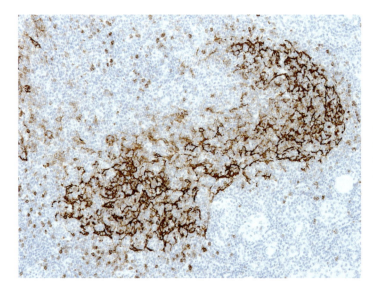

Figure 10. CD23 immunostaining manifests disrupted follicular dendritic cell meshwork within enlarged germinal center. (Immunostaining, x100)

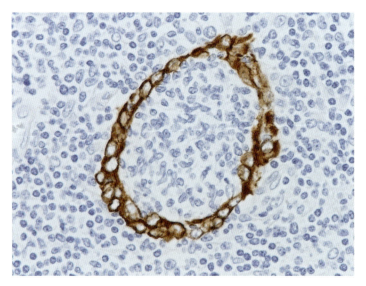

Figure 11. Cytokeratin AE1/AE3 immunostaining highlights packing. (Immunostaining, x400)

Discussion

Primary thyroid lymphoma is defined as lymphoma that arises within the thyroid gland. This excludes the lymphoma invaded by metastasis or direct extension. Primary thyroid lymphomas are uncommon, and estimated to be 5% of all thyroid malignant neoplasms (1). They tend to occur in middle-aged to older women, and are usually associated with Hashimoto thyroiditis. Almost all of them are B cell origin, including diffuse large B-cell lymphoma (DLBCL), extranodal marginal zone B-cell lymphoma (EMZBCL), and follicular lymphoma (2).

Macroscopically, the tumors involve either one lobe or both lobes. The tumors are soft to firm, solid, and lobulated. They are solitary, multinodular, or diffuse. The cut surface is bulging, and it displays a fish fresh appearance. The margin of the lesions is frequently indistinct because they merge Hashimoto thyroiditis with aggregation of lymph follicles. DLBCL may show hemorrhage, necrosis, and extrathyroidal invasion. The lesions of

EMZBCL are usually limited within the thyroid.

DLBCL is a predominant type of primary thyroid lymphoma, and it exhibits the diffuse involvement of large, atypical lymphoid cells (Figure 12). DLBCL may or may not be associated with the area of EMZBCL, the former is thought to be EMZBCL with large cell transformation.

Almost all of EMZBCLs, so-called MALT lymphomas, arise in the setting of acquired mucosa-associated lymphoid tissue (MALT). This type shows a vaguely nodular or follicular pattern, and the boundary between the lymphoma and Hashimoto disease is indistinct. The lesion is heterogeneous, and composed of small atypical lymphoid cells, centrocyte-like cells, monocytoid B-cells, large atypical lymphoid cells, and plasma cells (3). Some cases exhibit excessive plasma cell differentiation. Such cases had been referred to as extramedullary plasmacytoma, but they are currently considered a form of EMZBCL. A case of EMZBCL associated with amyloid deposition has been reported (4). Follicular colonization (infiltration into germinal center of the lymph follicles, packing (infiltration into the lumen of preserved thyroid follicular structure) (Figure 10), and lymphoepithelial lesion (proliferative nests composed of both follicular epithelia and lymphoma cells) (Figures 9 and 11) are features of EMZBCLs. EMZBCL generally shows good prognosis.

Aspiration cytology is a widely accepted technique for the diagnosis of the thyroid lesions, and it is not difficult cytologically to diagnose DLBCL. The smear from DLBCL is highly cellular, and it is mainly composed of a large number of atypical lymphoid cells (Figure 12). They are large-sized and monotonous. Mitosis, large nucleoli, and nuclear irregularity are frequently observed. There are lymphoglandular bodies in the background. Two-cell pattern may be seen because of an association with non-neoplastic small-sized lymphocytes.

MALT lymphoma shows a mixture of small to medium-sized atypical lymphocytes, monocytoid B-cells, immunoblasts, and plasma cells (2). Thus, it is frequently difficult to distinguish MALT lymphoma from Hashimoto thyroiditis (5). We believe that it is important to pay attention to the chromatin pattern. The chromatin patterns of lymphocytes seen in non-neoplastic lymphoid proliferations vary depending on their sizes. The heterochromatin is rich and granular in small lymphocytes, compared to diminished and fine in large lymphocytes. In contrast, lymphoid cells seen in MALT lymphoma show similar chromatin pattern regardless of the difference in size. An additional clue is the presence of the nucleoli in small-sized lymphoid cells. Kaba et al. have described that small to medium-sized cells displaying irregularly shaped nuclei with prominent nucleoli are neoplastic cells, and lymphoepithelial clusters and mountain range-like clusters are clues of MALT lymphoma (6). Follicular cells seen in lymphoepithelial clusters are not oncocytic, but in Hashimoto thyroiditis, they are oncocytic (please refer to Chapters 13 and 15).

It is difficult to distinguish between MALT lymphoma and Hashimoto thyroiditis by cytomorphology alone (7). Core needle biopsy, though not considered as the first choice for the diagnosis of lymphomas, has been reported to have a higher diagnostic accuracy (8). We recommend κ/λ light chain restriction analysis using flow cytometry (5, 9). When thyroid lymphoma is ultrasonographically suspected, we routinely examine flow cytometry CD45 gating using aspirated materials. We consider that more than 3.0 of the κ/λ ratio suspects lymphoma. In the present case, the κ/λ light chain restriction was confirmed in both aspirated materials and resected thyroid.

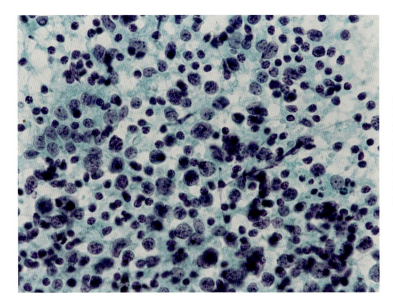

Figure 12. Diffuse large B-cell lymphoma, showing a two-cell pattern composed of the large-sized atypical lymphoid cells and non-neoplastic small-sized lymphocytes. (Papanicolaou, x400)

References

1. Pedersen RK, Pedersen NT. Primary non-Hodgkin's lymphoma of the thyroid gland: a population based study. Histopathol 1996; 28:25-32.
2. Kini SR. Color Atlas of Differential Diagnosis in Exfoliative and Aspiration Cytopathology. Philadelphia: Lippincott Williams & Wilkins; 1999. p249.
3. Lee SC, Hong SW, Lee YS, et al. Primary thyroid mucosa-associated lymphoid tissue lymphoma; a clinicopathological study of seven cases. J Korean Surg Soc 2011; 81:374-9.
4. Nobuoka Y, Hirokawa M, Kuma S, et al. Cytologic findings and differential diagnoses of primary thyroid MALT lymphoma with striking plasma cell differentiation and amyloid deposition. Diagn Cytopathol 2014; 42:73-7.
5. Adamczewski Z, Stasiołek M, Dedecjus M, et al. Flow cytometry in the differential diagnostics of Hashimoto's thyroiditis and MALT lymphoma of the thyroid. Endokrynol Pol 2015; 66:73-8.
6. Kaba S, Hirokawa M, Higuchi M, et al. Cytological findings for the diagnosis of primary thyroid mucosa-associated lymphoid tissue lymphoma by fine needle aspiration. Acta Cytol 2015; 59:26-6.
7. Sangalli G, Serio G, Zampatti C, et al. Fine needle aspiration cytology of primary lymphoma of the thyroid: a report of 17 cases. Cytopathol 2001; 12:257-63.
8. Screaton NJ, Berman LH, Grant JW. Head and neck lymphadenopathy: evaluation with US-guided cutting-needle biopsy. Radiol 2002; 224:75-81.
9. Stacchini A, Pacchioni D, Demurtas A, et al. Utility of flow cytometry as ancillary study to improve the cytologic diagnosis of thyroid lymphomas. Cytometry B Clin Cytom 2015; 88:320-9.

Chapter 15

Medullary (C Cell) Thyroid Carcinoma or Oxyphilic Follicular Neoplasms

Yun Zhu and Tiesheng Wang

Brief Clinical Summary
   A 56-year-old woman was admitted to our hospital for a physical examination.

Ultrasound Findings
   Neck ultrasound detected a 13 × 11 × 10 mm, regularly shaped, hypoechoic thyroid nodule with rich vascularity in the right lobe of the thyroid. The nodule was solid with minor cystic changes and blurred margins. Ultrasound-guided fine needle aspiration (US-FNA) was performed as malignancy was suspected.

Cytological Findings
   Cytological examination revealed a cellular aspirate with the neoplastic cells in a dispersed pattern (Figure 1A). The neoplastic cells were predominately plasmacytoid with extremely marginal location of the nuclei. The nuclei contained coarsely granular chromatin with occasional macronucleoli (Figures 1B-1D). Dense acellular materials resembling the amyloid were also noticed (Figure 1E). The amyloid displayed green birefringence with Congo red stain under crossed polarized light. Although the amyloid sometimes strongly resembles the colloid, it is virtually not very difficult to recognize and distinguish them on hematoxylin-eosin-stained slide. Amyloid always has an ambiguous margin with an uneven distribution of amorphously fibrillar-like materials in the inside, whereas colloid often has a sharp margin with smooth flat surface, usually with a few cracks that are not presented in the amyloid. Figure 1F shows a giant cell with coarsely granular chromatin, and the macronucleolus is not appreciated.

List of differential Diagnoses
   1. Malignant: Medullary (C cell) thyroid carcinoma
   2. Malignant: Hürthle cell carcinoma
   3. Malignant: Plasmacytoma
   4. Malignant: Oxyphilic variant of papillary thyroid carcinoma
   5. Malignant: Mixed medullary and follicular cell carcinomas
   6. Indeterminate (follicular neoplasm): Hürthle cell adenoma
   7. Benign: Nonneoplastic Hürthle cell nodules

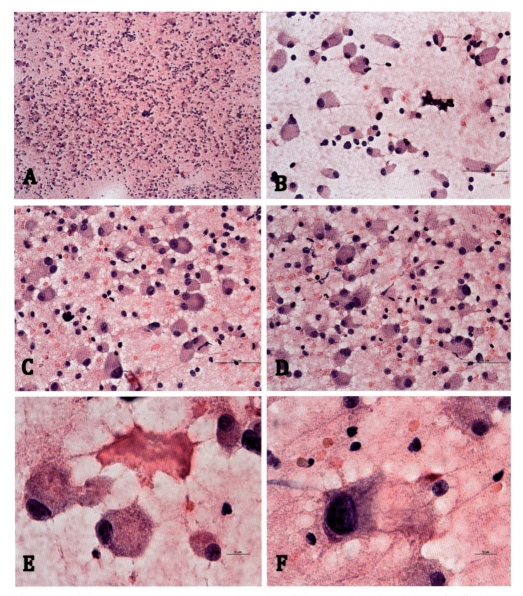

Figure 1. 1A: Low-power view shows an adequate cellular aspirate with a dispersed cell pattern. 1B-1D: The cells are monomorphic with eccentric nuclei and abundant eosinophilic cytoplasm. Note the extremely marginal location of the nucleus. Bi-nucleation occurs frequently. Both Hürthle cell neoplasm and medullary carcinoma were considered for differential diagnoses. 1E: High magnification shows the plasmacytoid cells with occasional macronucleoli. Dense acellular material is noticed, probably representing amyloid. 1F: A giant cell with a bizarre nucleus that contains coarse chromatin. (HE stain)

Immunostaining and Histological Diagnosis

Smear staining showed positive reactivity for calcitonin and negativity for thyroglobulin (Figures 2A and 2B), strongly suggesting a diagnosis of medullary carcinoma that was confirmed by the subsequent thyroidectomy. A monomorphic cell pattern, composed of exclusively uniform, cuboidal cells with appreciable eosinophilic cytoplasm, is encountered in histologic sections, bearing a morphologic resemblance to oncocytes (Figures 2C and D). Papillary growth pattern with fibrovascular core is one of the characteristic features of this case, which was daiagnosed as papillary type medullary carcinoma (Figures 2C and D) (1)

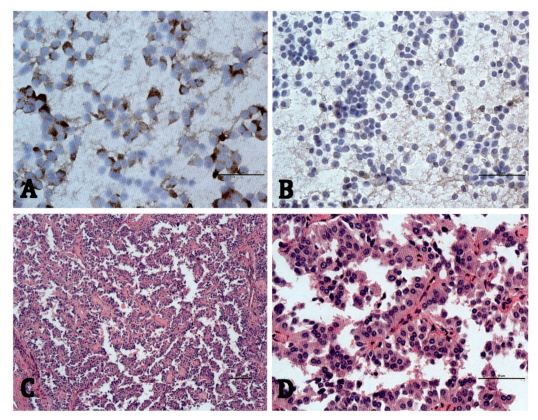

Figure 2. 2A and 2B: The calcitonin (A) stain is positive, whereas the thyroglobulin (B) stain is negative in the dispersed tumor cells. 2C: A medullary carcinoma papillary type confirmed by the thyroidectomy specimen. 2D: Histologic section showing an exclusively uniform, cuboidal cell pattern. The neoplastic cells exhibit appreciable eosinophilic cytoplasm with eccentric nuclei. (A, B: immunostain, C, D: HE stain)

Differential Diagnosis

Figures 3A-3C exhibits an aspirate of medullary carcinoma with a monomorphic cell pattern. The neoplastic cells were dispersed with abundant eosinophilic cytoplasm. Binucleation occurred frequently. The extremely marginal location of the nuclei with coarsely granular to salt-pepper type chromatin was the most important feature (3-5). Please refer to the Take Home Message (summary of cytological findings of C cell carcinoma) in Chapter 16. Figures 3D-3F shows the aspirate of a Hürthle cell carcinoma for comparison. The neoplastic cells were dispersed or arranged in a pseudo-follicular pattern, which is rarely seen in medullary carcinoma (5, 7-10). The nuclei are mostly eccentric, occasionally central, whereas the nuclei of plasmacytoid cells in medullary carcinoma always present at extremely marginal location (3-6). The cytological presentations of medullary carcinomas differ with different fixations and stains used (Table 1 and please refer to Chapter 16 for Papanicolaou stain). With wet-fixation Hematoxylin-eosin-stained preparations, the characteristic macronucleoli of Hürthle neoplasm cells are appreciable, and the granular cytoplasm is also different from that of the cells of medullary carcinoma. The granularity of Hürthle cells is more apparent and to some extent deeply stained than that of medullary carcinoma. The medullary carcinoma cells are comparable to those seen in tissues and the nuclei show delicate chromatin details. The salt-pepper chromatin pattern is obvious, which is very important for the differential diagnosis from Hürthle cell neoplasms (Table 2). In fact, a very cellular aspirate with a dispersed cell pattern formed by monomorphic small to medium-sized Hürthle cells with prominent macronucleoli makes the diagnostic features of Hürthle cell neoplasm (5, 7-10).

Most papillary carcinomas are easily recognized by the typical cytomorphology. Occasionally, papillary carcinoma presents a dispersed or loosely cohesive cell pattern with appreciable eosinophilic cytoplasm and eccentric nuclei, reminiscent of medullary carcinoma (2, 3). The differentiating features are listed in the Table 2 in Chapter 3. Figures 4A-4C from oncocytic variant papillary carcinoma exhibit a cellular aspirate composed of large polygonal cells with abundant eosinophilic cytoplasm and mildly eccentric nuclei. Cytoplasmic inclusions are apparent but not helpful for diagnosis as they are frequently presented in both medullary carcinoma and papillary carcinoma (2, 3). Finely granular chromatin and nuclear grooves were clues to the diagnosis of papillary carcinoma, which were identified in the subsequent thyroidectomy. Figure 4D-4F from medullary carcinoma shows a cellular aspirate composed of dispersed cells with similar eosinophilic cytoplasm but extremely eccentric nuclei that contain pseudoinclusions. Unfortunately, the cytological preparations failed to exhibit coarse or salt-pepper chromatin due to the air-dried fixation. A differential diagnosis between papillary carcinoma and medullary carcinoma is considered. The histologic sections revealed a medullary carcinoma.

Table 1. Comparison of medullary carcinoma cells with wet-fixation hematoxylin-eosin staining, wet-fixation Papanicolaou staining and air-dried Romanowsky type staining

	Wet-fixation hematoxylin-eosin staining	Air-dried Romanowsky type staining	Wet-fixation Papanicolaou staining
Cell and nuclear size	Comparable to that seen in histological sections; smaller than that seen in air-dried smears	Larger than cells seen in tissues	Comparable to that seen in histological sections; smaller than that seen in air-dried smears
Nuclear morphology	Delicate chromatin detail; coarsely granular to salt and pepper type chromatin	Loss of chromatin detail; coarse chromatin usually not apparent	Delicate chromatin detail; coarsely granular to salt and pepper type chromatin
Cytoplasm	Variable; eosinophilc with fibrillar cytoplasm	Azurophilic cytoplasmic granules	Variable; usually cyanophilic with fibrillar cytoplasm
Amyloid	Eosinophilic; acelluar substance in the background showing ambiguous margin with uneven distribution of amorphous fibrillar-like materials	Amyloid seen within and outside of cells, stained blue-grey or violet	Cyanophilic; fluffy, finely granular or dense acellular material in the background, sometimes indistinguishable from the colloid
Architecture of the tissue fragments	Well visualized	Poor details with thick tissue fragments; visualized if the smear is thin	Well visualized

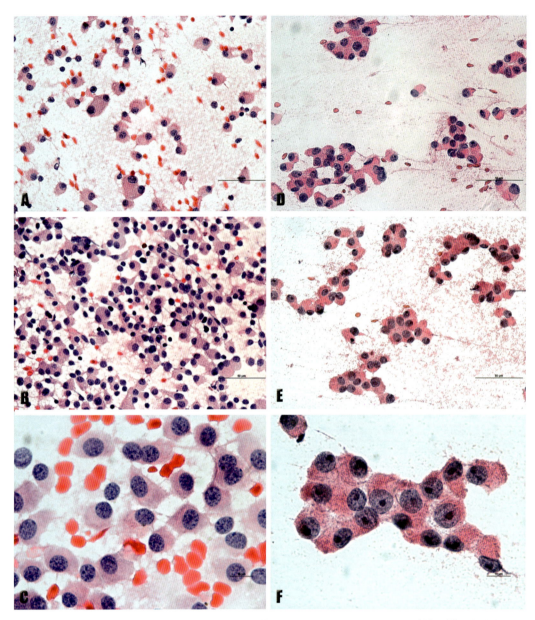

Figure 3. Medullary thyroid carcinoma (3A-3C) vs. Hürthle cell carcinoma (3D-3F). Medullary carcinoma shares a similar cytomorphology with Hürthle cell carcinoma, and they may be mistaken for each other. 3A and 3B: Medium-power view shows dispersed cells with abundant eosinophilic cytoplasm and extremely eccentric nuclei. Binucleation is frequently noticed. 3C: High magnification shows coarsely granular to salt-pepper type chromatin. The macronucleoli are not seen. 3D-3F: FNA of Hürthle cell carcinoma for comparison. 3D and 3E: The cells are discrete or arranged in a pseudo-follicular pattern. The nuclei are mostly eccentric and occasionally central. 3F: The characteristic macronucleoli are appreciable. Note coarse granularity in the cytoplasm, which is different from that of medullary carcinoma in wet-fixation hematoxylin-eosin staining (3C). The granularity is the result of abundant mitochondria. (HE stain)

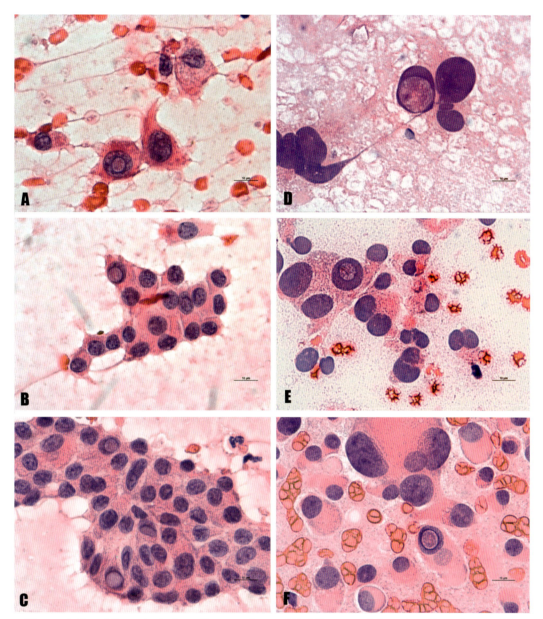

Figure 4. Oxyphilic variant of papillary carcinoma (4A-4C) vs. medullary thyroid carcinoma (4D-4F). 4A-4C: Cellular aspirate that is composed of large polygonal cells with abundant eosinophilic cytoplasm and mildly eccentric nuclei. Finely granular chromatin, nuclear grooves and cytoplasmic inclusions suggest a diagnosis of papillary carcinoma, which was confirmed on the subsequent thyroidectomy. 4D-4F: The aspirate shows dispersed cells with eosinophilic cytoplasm, eccentric nuclei, and obvious pseudoinclusions. A differential diagnosis between papillary carcinoma and medullary carcinoma was considered. The surgical tissue confirmed the diagnosis of medullary carcinoma. Please note epithelial sheet arrangements with tight cohesion in 4B and 4C, whereas no tight epithelial arrangements are appreciated in 4D to 4F. (HE stain)

Explanatory Notes

The diagnostic accuracy of medullary carcinoma is very high because it commonly presents characteristic features, including a dispersed cell pattern formed by pleomorphic cells with extremely eccentric nuclei that contain coarsely granular to salt-pepper type chromatin (3-6). However, medullary carcinoma cells sometimes demonstrate a monomorphic cell pattern, comprised exclusively of plasmacytoid cells with abundant eosinophilic cytoplasm, and sharing strong similarity with oxyphilic cell neoplasms, thus constituting the important diagnostic pitfalls (3-6). Unfamiliarity with the varied cytopathologic features and inappropriate cytologic preparations are the main reasons for typing errors in our initial experience, and only more than half have been reported to be classified accurately in literature (11). Measurements of calcitonin levels in the needle washout has been reported to improve diagnostic accuracy and make the cytological diagnosis confidently (please refer to Chapter 23 for more details) (11). Dispersed neoplastic cells from an adequate aspirate with ideal cytologic preparation constantly show fibrillar cytoplasm and typical nuclear morphology of coarsely granular to salt-pepper type chromatin. It is also the most important characteristic feature to distinguish medullary carcinoma cells from cells of Hürthle cell neoplasm (Table 2). Diagnosis of Hürthle cell lesion is a challenge in thyroid cytology as nonneoplastic Hürthle cell nodules in Hashimoto's thyroiditis and in multinodular goiter and Hürthle cell neoplasm display similar cytological findings (7-10). In our experience, although the cytological criteria for differentiating Hürthle cell neoplasm from metaplastic Hürthle cell nodules are subtle, the differentiation could still achieve a high degree of accuracy with ideal cytologic preparation. Figure 5 shows an aspirate of a Hürthle cell nodule from a multinodular goiter. Hürthle cells present as sheets of epithelium in a honeycomb or follicular pattern, with well-defined cell borders and abundant cytoplasm in the background of watery colloid (Figures 5A and 5B). The nuclei are always centrally located with compact chromatin, and they do not possess macronucleoli (Figures 5C and 5D). Figures 6A-6C depict an aspirate from Hashimoto's thyroiditis, showing dispersed or cohesive cells with pleomorphic nuclei, containing finely granular chromatin, in a background of inflammatory cells. Figures 6D-6F exhibit an aspirate of Hürthle cell adenoma for comparison. Predominant Hürthle cells occur singly, in loosely cohesive groups, or in syncytial tissue fragments. The nuclei are eccentric with finely granular chromatin, but the macronucleoli are not present. The background is clean without any colloid or lymphocytes. Although the macronucleolus has been suggested as the most important characteristic feature in distinguishing Hürthle cell neoplasms from nonneoplastic Hürthle cell nodules, it is not present in every case of Hürthle cell neoplasms (5). An admixture of regular follicular cells, oncocytes with highly pleomorphic in size, transition forms, degenerative changes with histiocytes, lymphocytes or colloid in the background, absent macronucleus could serve as the clues to the diagnosis of nonneoplastic Hürthle cell nodules. We do not have much experience in distinguishing Hürthle cell adenoma with Hürthle cell carcinoma. Kini *et al.* suggested that small cell size, syncytial-type tissue fragments, high nucleus/cytoplasm ratios, infrequent intranuclear cytoplasmic inclusions and psammoma bodies might be useful diagnostic clues (5).

A distinction between Hürthle cell neoplasm and medullary carcinoma can be made on the basis of the extremely marginal location of the nuclei with coarsely granular to salt-pepper type chromatin for the medullary carcinoma cells and prominent macronucleoli for the Hürthle cells. Sometimes apparent cytoplasmic granularity could be observed in Hürthle cells, which is different from the fibrillar cytoplasm of medullary carcinoma cells with ideal cytological preparation. Calcitonin immunostaining, and serum calcitonin and carcinoembryonic antigen levels as well as a family history of multiple endocrine neoplasia type 2 are very helpful for the cytological interpretations.

Table 2. Features differentiating medullary carcinoma from monomorphic plasmacytoid cells and Hürthle cell neoplasm

	Medullary carcinoma	Hürthle cell neoplasm
Cellularity	Variable	Variable
Presentation	Cells mostly isolated, or in loosely cohesive groups with a typical dispersed pattern	Cells dispersed, in cohesive groups or in syncytial tissue fragments
Cells	Monomorphic to markedly pleomorphic; well to poorly defined cell borders	Tending to be uniform in a given case; well to poorly defined cell borders
Cytoplasm	Variable, scant to abundant fibrillar-like cytoplasm	Usually abundant, apparent granularity with wet-fixation hematoxylin-eosin stain
Nucleus	Extremely marginal location; frequently binucleated or multinucleated; coarsely granular to salt and pepper type chromatin; common intranuclear pseudoinclusion; not apparent nucleoli	Central or eccentric location; frequently seen binucleation; finely granular chromatin; prominent single macronucleolus
Immunostain	Calcitonin +; thyroglobulin -	Calcitonin -; thyroglobulin +
Background	Clean; amorphous, acellular material resembling the amyloid	Colloid variable; usually clean, sometimes bloody

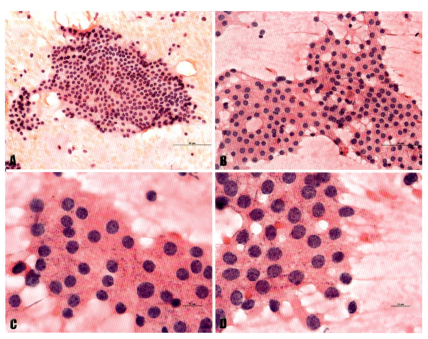

Figure 5. An aspirate of a Hürthle cell nodule from multinodular goiter. 5A and 5B: Hürthle cells present as sheets in a honeycomb or follicular pattern and have well-defined cell borders and appreciable eosinophilic cytoplasm in a background of watery colloid. 5C and 5D: The nuclei are mostly central-placed with compact chromatin and do not contain macronucleoli. (HE stain)

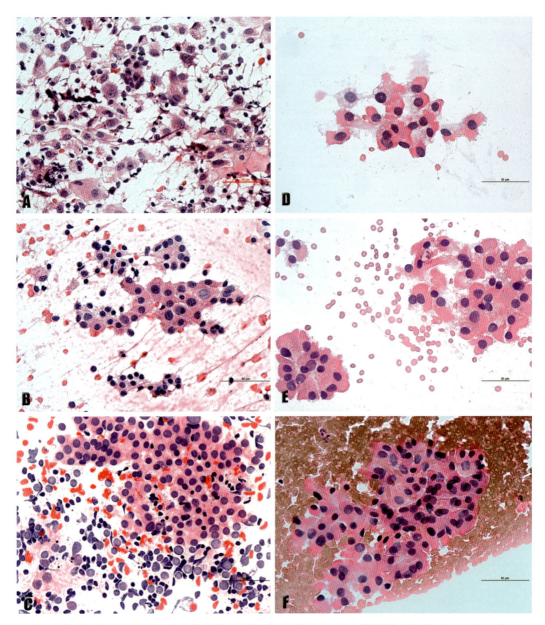

Figure 6. Hashimoto's thyroiditis (6A-6C) vs. Hürthle cell adenoma (6D-6F). 6A-6C: An aspirate from Hashimoto's thyroiditis showing dispersed or cohesive cells with abundant eosinophilic cytoplasm and pleomorphic nuclei, containing finely granular chromatin, in a background of inflammatory cells. 6D-6F: An aspirate of Hürthle cell adenoma for comparison. Hürthle cells occur singularly in loosely cohesive groups, or in syncytial tissue fragments in a clean background. The nuclei are eccentric with finely granular chromatin, but they lack prominent macronucleoli. (HE stain)

References
1. Kakudo K, Miyauchi A, Takai S, et al. C-cell carcinoma of the thyroid -papillary type-. Acta Pathol Jpn 1979; 29:653-9.

2. Lee J, Hasteh F. Oncocytic variant of papillary thyroid carcinoma associated with Hashimoto's thyroiditis: a case report and review of the literature. Diagn Cytopathol 2009; 37:600-6.
3. Kakudo K, Miyauchi A, Ogihara T, et al: Medullary carcinoma of the thyroid. Giant cell type. Arch Pathol Lab Med 1978; 102:445-7.
4. Kaushal S, Iyer VK, Mathur SR. Fine needle aspiration cytology of medullary carcinoma of the thyroid with a focus on rare variants: a review of 78 cases. Cytopathol 2011; 22:95-105.
5. Kini SR et al. Thyroid cytopathology: an atlas and text, 2nd edition, 2015.
6. Forrest CH, Frost FA, de Boer WB, et al. Medullary carcinoma of the thyroid: accuracy of diagnosis of fine-needle aspiration cytology. Cancer 1998; 25:295-302.
7. Nguyen GK, Ginsberg J, Crockford PM, et al: Hashimoto's thyroiditis: cytodiagnostic accuracy and pitfalls. Diagn Cytopathol 1997; 16:531-6.
8. Alaedeen DI, Khiyami A, McHenry CR. Fine-needle aspiration biopsy specimen with a predominance of Hürthle cells: a dilemma in the management of nodular thyroid disease. Surgery 2005; 138:650-6.
9. Elliott DD, Pitman MB, Bloom L, et al: Fine-needle aspiration biopsy of Hürthle cell leions of the thyroid gland: a cytomorphologic study of 139 cases with statistical analysis. Cancer 2006; 108:102-9.
10. Auger M. Hürthle cells in fine-needle aspirates of the thyroid: a review of their diagnostic criteria and significance. Cancer Cytopathol 2014; 122:241-9.
11. Trimboli P, Cremonini N, Ceriani L, et al: Calcitonin measurement in aspiration needle washout fluids has higher sensitivity than cytology in detecting medullary thyroid cancer: a retrospective multicenter study. Clin Endocrinol (Oxf) 2014; 80:135-40.

Chapter 16

Medullary (C Cell) Carcinoma or Metastatic Carcinoma to Thyroid

Junko Maruta

Brief Clinical Summary

An 80-year-old female was found having a high level of serum CEA level at general checkup. A tumor lesion in the left lobe of the thyroid gland was detected by computed tomography, but no other mass lesions were identified in the organs of the chest and abdomen. She was referred to the Noguchi Thyroid Clinic and Hospital Foundation, a specialized institute for thyroid disease, for further evaluation of the thyroid nodule.

Ultrasound Findings

Ultrasound revealed a solid tumor with an irregular shape, unclear border, and homogeneous echo with coarse high echo (Figure 1). Elastography gave an impression of a hard tumor mass (Figure 2). A diagnosis of adenomatous nodule was made based on the basis of the ultrasound findings.

Cytological Illustrations

Ultrasound-guided fine needle aspiration (US-FNA) smear demonstrated weakly cohesive aggregations of cells. Neither follicle formation nor sheet-like clusters were found. The tumor cells were round or polygonal with eccentric nuclei (Figures 3 and 4). The cytoplasm was oxyphilic and the nuclei were atypical with an irregular contour. Mononuclear and multinucleated cells were present with significant variation in nuclear size. The nuclear morphology of the giant cells and multinucleated cells was similar to that of the surrounding small mononuclear cells. Nucleoli were indiscernible in finely granular chromatin. Nuclear inclusions in the cytoplasm could be observed occasionally (Figure 5). No mitosis was found. Mucous substance, tumor necrosis, granulocytes, lymphocytes or amyloid deposits were not found in the smear background.

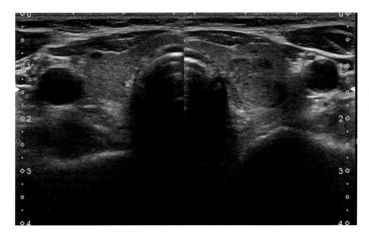

Figure 1. Ultrasound examination demonstrates a left thyroid nodule.

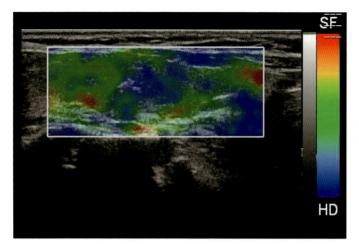

Figure 2. Elastography demonstrates blue color indicating hard consistency of the nodule.

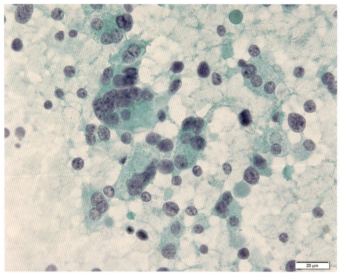

Figure 3. Conventional smear demonstrates numerous isolated cells with variously shaped nuclei and wide cyanophilic cytoplasm. (Papanicolaou stain, x400)

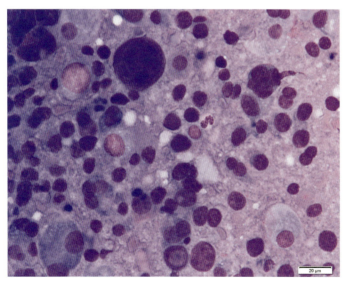

Figure 4. Conventional smear shows variously sized nuclei with basophilic wide cytoplasm. (Diff-Quik stain, x400)

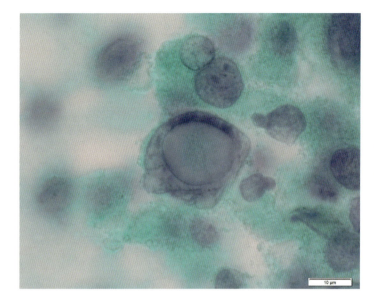

Figure 5. Cytoplasmic nuclear inclusions are found in few tumor cells. (Papanicolaou stain, x1000)

List of Differential Diagnoses
1. Benign: atypical adenoma
2. Indeterminate: follicular neoplasm
3. Malignant: undifferentiated carcinoma
4. Malignant: poorly differentiated carcinoma
5. Malignant: papillary carcinoma, poorly differentiated or aggressive variant
6. Malignant: medullary (C cell) carcinoma, giant cell type
7. Malignant: metastatic carcinoma from the other primary site

Differential Diagnosis in Cytology

Follicular neoplasm and atypical adenoma were excluded because there were no follicular structures observed in the smear and the chromatin findings were different from those of follicular neoplasm or atypical adenoma. Many isolated cells, increased irregular piles of cell clumps, and a high nuclear grade with increased chromatin were in favor of malignant diagnosis and less likely to be a follicular neoplasm of low malignant potential.

Undifferentiated carcinoma (Figure 6) was excluded because there were no inflammatory cells and necrosis in the background. Although there were giant cells, typical small round nuclei of neuroendocrine (C cell) carcinoma type were evident; this observation did not fit the undifferentiated carcinoma (1, 2).

Poorly differentiated thyroid carcinoma was excluded because there were no cellular patterns such as trabecular, solid, or insular structure. The chromatin patterns of the tumor cells were also different from those of poorly differentiated carcinoma or follicular neoplasm (Please refer to Chapter 21).

Papillary carcinoma was excluded because there was no ground-glass nuclear appearance or nuclear grooves. Although cytoplasmic nuclear inclusions were observed, they are reported to be present in both papillary carcinoma and medullary carcinoma (2).

Metastatic renal or breast cancer or invasion from esophageal cancer can possibly form the secondary (metastatic) carcinoma in the thyroid gland. When cytology is combined with immunocytochemistry for calcitonin (Figure 7) and/or measurement of calcitonin levels in the needle washout fluids after aspiration (FNA-calcitonin), an accurate diagnosis of medullary

(C cell) carcinoma can be made (please refer to Chapters 15, 18, 22 and 23) (3). Neither glandular structures suggesting adenocarcinoma nor keratinization indicating squamous cell carcinoma was found in this case, which helps to rule out metastatic adenocarcinoma or squamous cell carcinoma.

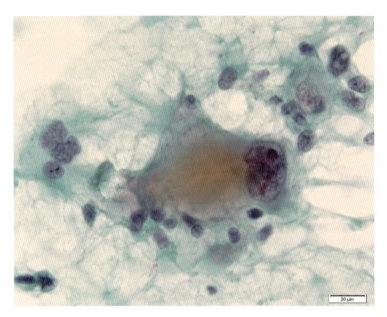

Figure 6. For your comparison, an example from a case of undifferentiated carcinoma is shown. Note the giant nuclei with prominent nucleoli. (Papanicolaou stain, x400)

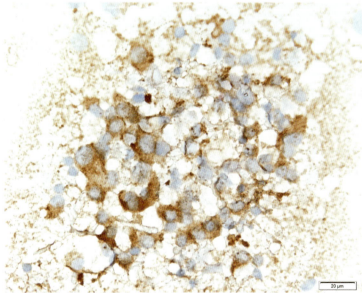

Figure 7. Most of the tumor cytoplasm is positively stained for calcitonin (Immunoperoxidase stain for calcitonin, x400).

Histological Diagnosis: Medullary (C cell) carcinoma, giant cell type

The primary tumor was 1.3 x 1.2 cm in size with partial calcification, but without apparent tumor capsule. There were multiple intrathyroid spreads, less than 0.2 cm in size, in the thyroid parenchyma.

Solid medullary proliferation, multinucleated cells, salt and pepper chromatin, nuclear cytoplasmic inclusion were observed in this rare variant of medullary carcinoma (Figures 8 and 9) (2). Positive immunoreactivities for calcitonin (Figure 10) and CEA (Figure 11) confirmed the diagnosis. Negative immunoreactivity for thyroglobulin also supported the diagnosis. MIB-1 (Ki67 proliferation) index was low (Figure 12), less than 1%, indicating a low-risk medullary carcinoma and denied the high-risk undifferentiated carcinoma, poorly differentiated carcinoma, or metastatic carcinoma (4). Amyloid deposits have been reported in 50-70 % of the cases with medullary carcinoma, but it was not found in this case cytologically and histologically (5). Metastatic lesions were identified in two of the seven dissected paratracheal lymph nodes, whereas no metastatic lesions were found in the dissected lateral cervical lymph nodes. Extrathyroid invasion or distant metastasis was not found and the tumor stage was concluded as T1N1aM0.

In the preoperative tests, serum calcitonin was found to be elevated to 960 pg/ml and serum CEA to 28 pg/ml, and these values dropped significantly after total thyroidectomy (the serum calcitonin dropped to 37 pg/ml, and the CEA to 1.6 pg/ml). Medullary carcinoma is a thyroid carcinoma originating from C cells and calcitonin production is essential for this diagnosis, while CEA is not included in the diagnostic criteria. However, CEA is a useful marker for diagnosis of medullary carcinoma and about 86% of C cell tumors have been reported to be positive for CEA stain (6).

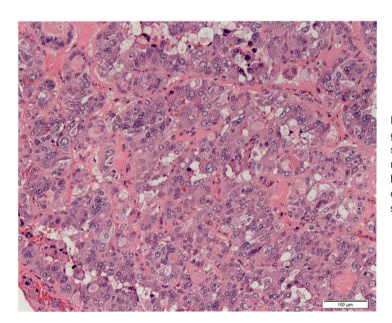

Figure 8. Solid medullary growth of C cell carcinoma is shown. The tumor cells have round nuclei and wide slightly basophilic cytoplasm. Amyloid deposits was not found in the stroma. (HE stain, x100)

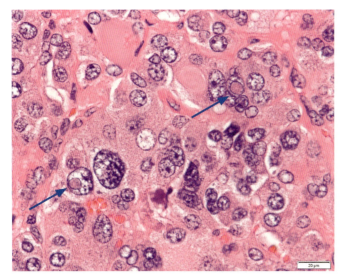

Figure 9. The tumor cells have giant nuclei and wide granular cytoplasm. A few cytoplasmic nuclear inclusions (arrow) are demonstrated in this high magnification. (HE stain, x400)

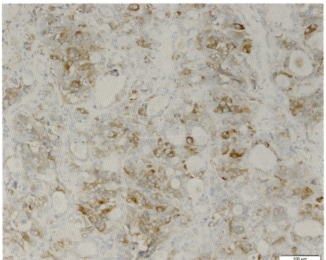

Figure 10. Immunohistochemistry for calcitonin confirmed positive reaction in tumor cell cytoplasm. (Immunoperoxidase stain for calcitonin, x100).

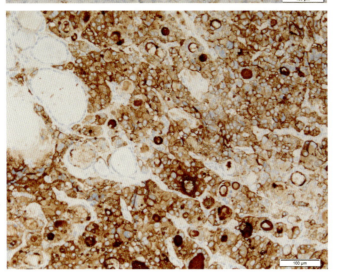

Figure 11. Positive immunostain for CEA confirmed the diagnosis, medullary (C cell) carcinoma of the thyroid. Note negative reaction in non-neoplastic follicular cells in the upper left field. (Immunoperoxidase stain for CEA, x100).

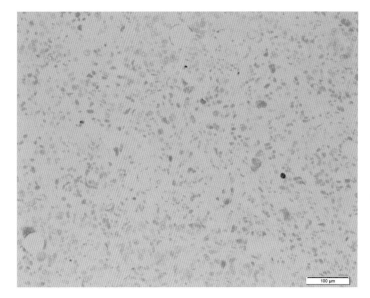

Figure 12. Although cellular atypia is significant in this case, proliferation index measured by Ki-67 immuno-stain is low, and only less than 1% if tumor cells are labelled. (Immunoperoxidase stain for Ki-67, x100).

Take Home Message (summary of the cytological findings of medullary carcinoma)
1. Neither papillary nor follicular structures were observed in the FNA smear
2. Isolated cells with varied shapes (round, polygonal, spindle (Figure 13), or a plasmacytoid appearance (Figure 14) (7)
3. Round nuclei with salt and pepper chromatin (neuroendocrine nuclear features) (Figure 15) (7)
4. Wide cytoplasm with granularity (azurophilic cytoplasmic granule in Romanowsky (Giemsa)-stained smear) (Figure 4) (please refer to Figure 23 of Supplemental Chapter 5)
5. Amyloid deposits in the smear background (Figure 16) (7) (please refer to Figure 1 of Chapter 15)
6. Demonstration of calcitonin in the FNA washout (3) (please refer to Figure 23)
7. Positive immunohistochemical markers include calcitonin, CEA, wide spectrum keratin, chromogranin A, synaptophysin, neuron specific enolase, and TTF1. An important negative marker is thyroglobulin (8) (please refer to Chapter 30)
8. Neuroendocrine granules at the electron microscopic level (9, 10, 11)

Diagnostic Clues
1. Clinical information on genetic tests and serum levels of markers are helpful.
2. Amyloid deposits are present in only half of the cases.
3. Cytoplasmic nuclear inclusion is reported in both medullary carcinoma and papillary carcinoma.
4. There are several histological variants (giant cell, melanotic, papillary, follicular and poorly differentiated), which may create a pitfall in the diagnosis of medullary carcinoma.
5. Necrosis and mitosis are rare
6. Psammoma body type calcification is rare.
7. Cystic change is rare.

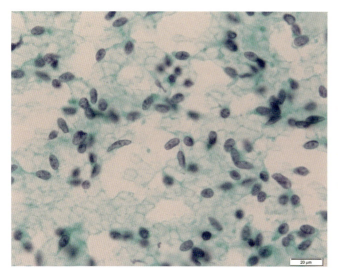

Figure 13. Predominant spindle cells are characteristics of this case of C cell carcinoma, which required a differential diagnosis from mesenchymal tumors and undifferentiated carcinoma. (Papanicolaou stain, x400)

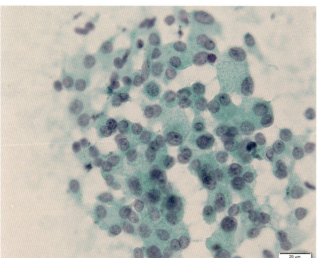

Figure 14. Plasmacytoid type C cell carcinoma. Please note round and regular size nuclei in contrast to Figures 3 ∼ 5 of giant cell type C cell carcinoma. (Papanicolaou stain, x400)

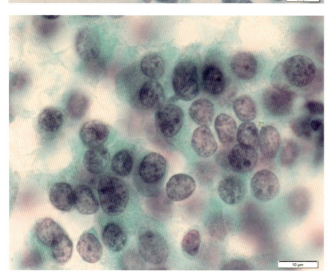

Figure 15. In this high magnification, the salt and pepper chromatin of neuroendocrine type nuclei of C cell carcinoma is apparent. (Papanicolaou stain, x1000)

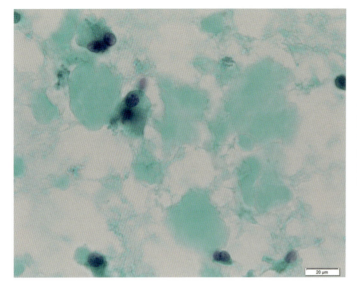

Figure 16. Amyloid deposits may be found in more than half of C cell carcinoma. It is acellular dense amorphous mass stained in blue with Papanicolaou stain. (Papanicolaou stain, x400)

References

1. Pusztaszeri MP, Bongiovanni M, Faquin WC. Update on the cytologic and molecular features of medullary thyroid carcinoma. Adv Anal Pathol 2014; 21(1):26-35.
2. Kakudo K, Miyauchi A, Ogihara T, et al. Medullary carcinoma of the thyroid. Giant cell type. Arch Pathol Lab Med 1978; 102(9):445-7.
3. Trimboli P, Treglia G, Guidobaldi L, et al. Detection rate of FNA cytology in medullary thyroid carcinoma: a meta-analysis. Clin Endocrinol (Oxf) 2015; 82(2):280-5.
4. Tisell LE, Oden A, Muth A, et al. The Ki67 index a prognostic marker in medullary thyroid carcinoma. Br J Cancer 2003; 89(11):2093-7.
5. DeLellis RA, Lioyd RV, Heitz PU, et al. Pathology and genetics of tumor of endocrine organs: WHO classification of tumors. Lyon; IARC Press; 2004; p86-91.
6. Kakudo K, Takami H, Katayama S, et al. Carcinoembryonic antigen and nonspecific cross-reacting antigen in medullary carcinoma of the thyroid. Acta Pathol Jpn 1990; 40(2):261-6.
7. Papaparaskeva K, Nagel H, Droese M. Cytological diagnosis of medullary carcinoma of the thyroid gland. Diagn Cytopathol 2000; 22(6):351-8.
8. Forrest CH, Frost FA, de Boer WB, et al. Medullary carcinoma of the thyroid: accuracy of diagnosis of fine-needle aspiration cytology. Cancer 1998; 84(5):295-302.
9. Kakudo K, Miyauchi A, Katayama S. Ultrastructural study of thyroid medullary carcinoma. Acta Pathol Jpn 1977; 27:605-22.
10. Kini SR, Miller JM, Hamburger JI, et al. Cytopathologic features of medullary carcinoma of the thyroid. Arch Pathol Lab Med 1984; 108(2):156-9.
11. Kakudo K, Miyauchi A, Katayama S, et al. Ultrastructural study of poorly differentiated medullary carcinoma of the thyroid. Virch Arch A Pathol Anat Histopathol 1987; 410:455-60.

Chapter 17

Intrathyroid Epithelial Thymoma/Carcinoma Showing Thymus-like Differentiation vs. Poorly Differentiated Carcinoma

Mitsuyoshi Hirokawa and Ayana Suzuki

Case

The patient was a 63-year-old male with a history of taking Levothyroxine 100 μg/day for eight years to treat Hashimoto thyroiditis. He underwent a clinical survey and enlargement of the thyroid was pointed out. Because fine needle aspiration cytology suspected poorly differentiated carcinoma, he was referred to our hospital. The levels of thyroglobulin and thyroperoxidase antibodies were 1867.0 IU/mL and >600.0 IU/mL, respectively. He had a family history of papillary thyroid carcinoma (PTC) and Grave's disease for his sister and Hashimoto thyroiditis for his parents. Ultrasonographic examination revealed a mass measuring 64 x 31 x 47 mm in the right lobe of thyroid (Figure 1). The mass was hypoechoic and heterogeneous, and contained cystic areas. The border was indistinct. The background of the thyroid was consistent with chronic thyroiditis. Aspiration cytology for the mass suspected poorly differentiated carcinoma, intrathyroid epithelial thymoma (ITET)/carcinoma showing thymus-like differentiation (CASTLE), or metastatic carcinoma. Because the other primary site was not detected, he underwent total thyroidectomy with central and right lateral neck lymph node resection.

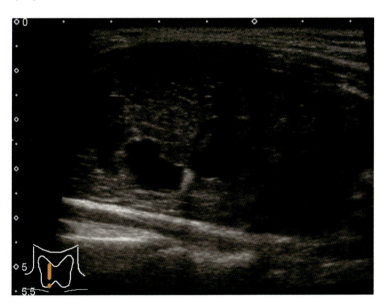

Figure 1. A hypoechoic and heterogeneous mass in the right thyroid lobe, containing cystic areas. (Ultrasound B-mode image)

Cytologic Findings

The aspirated materials were highly cellular, and there was no any colloid material in the background (Figure 2). Carcinoma cells formed solid, three-dimensional clusters (Figure 3). Papillary, follicular or sheet-like arrangements were not seen. Carcinoma cells were large in size and round to polygonal in shape. The cytoplasm was moderately to densely stained with lightgreen and the cell border was indistinct. Nuclear arrangement was crowded. The nuclei showed a variety of sizes and they had prominent nucleoli (Figure 4). Lymphocytes and plasma cells were observed not only in the background, but also within carcinoma cell clusters (Figure 5).

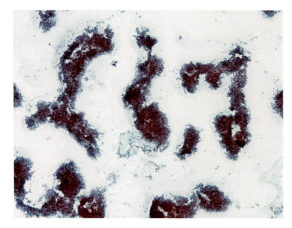

Figure 2. Cellular materials are smeared. There are no colloid materials in the background. (Pap, x4)

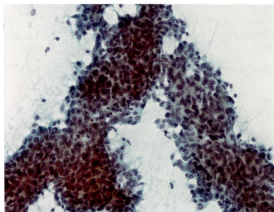

Figure 3. Carcinoma cells show solid three-dimensional clusters.(Papanicolaou, x200)

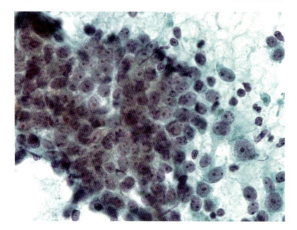

Figure 4. Lymphocytes are observed within and around the carcinoma cell clusters. (Papanicolaou, x400)

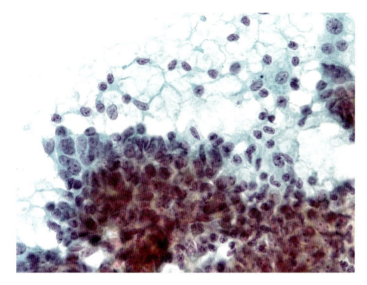

Figure 5. Lymphocytes are observed within and around the carcinoma cell clusters. (Pap, x40)

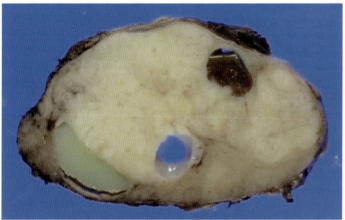

Figure 6. Carcinoma is tan to yellowish in color and slightly lobulated, and contains cystic spaces.

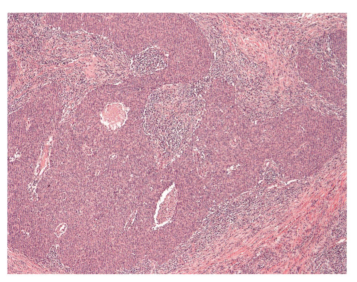

Figure 7. Carcinoma cells proliferate forming anastomosing large solid nests. Comedo-like necrosis is seen in two places. (HE, x40)

Pathologic Findings

A mass, measuring 6.3 x 4.0 cm, occupied the right lobe of the thyroid. On cut surface, the mass was tan to yellowish in color and slightly lobulated, and contained cystic spaces (Figure 6). Microscopically, carcinoma cells were round to oval and proliferated forming lobulated or anastomosing large solid nests (Figure 7). Comedo-like necrosis was seen. Carcinoma cells were large and showed prominent nucleoli (Figure 8). Tubular formation and squamous differentiation were focally observed. The stroma was abundant and associated with infiltration of lymphocytes and plasma cells. The lymphocytes and plasma cells were also observed within carcinoma cell nests. Carcinoma showed infiltrative growth, but it remained within the thyroid.

Immunohistochemically, the carcinoma cells were positive for p63, and focally positive for high molecular weight cytokeratin 34-beta E12 (HMWCK). CD5 (Figure 9), thyroglobulin, TTF-1, and PAX8 were all negative. The Ki-67 (MIB-1) labeling index was approximately 50%.

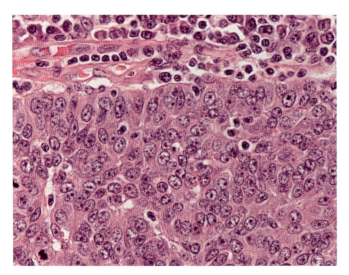

Figure 8. Carcinoma cells are large and their nucleoli are prominent. (HE, x400)

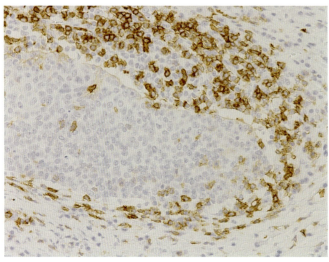

Figure 9. Carcinoma cells are negative for CD5. The positive cells are lymphocytes. (Immunostaining, x200)

Discussion:

CASTLE is a very rare malignant thyroid carcinoma showing architectural resemblance to thymic epithelial tumors (1). The carcinoma type was initially proposed by Miyauchi et al. in 1985 as intrathyroidal epithelial thymoma (2). The carcinoma affects middle-aged adults with a slight female predominance (M:F = 1:1.3), and it appears as a painless mass in the lower pole of the thyroid (3). About 30% of the cases have nodal metastasis at surgery, but the prognosis is not so poor.

Microscopically, the tumor consists of lobulated large nests of squamoid or syncytial-appearing cells and abundant lymphocytic infiltration (1, 3-5). Squamous differentiation in whorled clusters resembling Hassall's corpuscles may be present. There are a large number of lymphocytes in the tumor nests and stroma, similar in thymic carcinoma. CASTLE can have squamous, glandular, and neuroendocrine components, indicating that the carcinoma arises from a multipotential stem cell (6).

The immunohistochemical phenotype of CASTLE is also analogous to thymic carcinoma (3-8). Immunoreactivity for CD5 is characteristic (Figure 8) (7-9) (please refer to Chapter 28). Our case did not express the antigen, but the diagnosis of CASTLE cannot be denied completely. CASTLE is also strongly positive for both p63 and HMWCK (9-11), but negative for TTF-1 and thyroglobulin (12, 13).

Aspirated materials are usually cellular. Carcinoma cells appear as large cell clusters. The clusters are three-dimensional and they have no any internal structures, such as papillary or follicular structure. The clusters may contain a few lymphocytes. Nuclei are round, oval, or short spindled. Nuclear chromatin is vesicular or finely granular. Intranuclear cytoplasmic inclusions are not observed. Nucleoli are usually large and distinct. Cytoplasm varies from clear to dense. Naked nuclei may be prominent. The cell border is usually distinct. The tumor cells may show squamous differentiation or intracytoplasmic lumina with or without a magenta body (14). A small to moderate number of lymphocytes and plasma cells are seen in the background.

The differential diagnoses included poorly differentiated carcinoma, CASTLE, and metastatic carcinoma for this case. Medullary (C cell) carcinoma, anaplastic carcinoma, squamous cell carcinoma, and mucoepidermoid carcinoma may be also supposed (15). In our experience, the distinction between CASTLE and poorly differentiated carcinoma is mostly difficult (please refer to Chapter 21). The presence of follicular cell differentiation such as colloid, follicular structure, or trabecular structure indicates poorly differentiated carcinoma (16). Endothelial cells adhering to solid cluster are characteristic of insular type of poorly differentiated carcinoma (16, 17). Whereas, keratinization, intracytoplasmic lumina, and lymphocytes within cell clusters favor the diagnosis of CASTLE (14, 18). The location of the tumor may be useful because CASTLE usually arises at the lower pole of the thyroid (19). Unfortunately, the tumor in our case was too large to identify its precise location.

Mucoepidermoid carcinoma (MEC) exhibits characteristics of both squamous differentiation and mucin-producing cells (20). Two types of mucoepidermoid carcinoma occur in the thyroid; conventional MEC, and sclerosing MEC with eosinophilia. The latter may be suggested by the presence of eosinophils. The cytologic findings of conventional MEC and CASTLE are similar. It is not easy to make an accurate diagnosis of CASTLE preoperatively.

A panel of immunostaining for CD5 (Figures 10 and 11), TTF-1, and thyroglobulin with cytological preparations may be useful to confirm the diagnoses of CASTLE (please refer to Chapter 28).

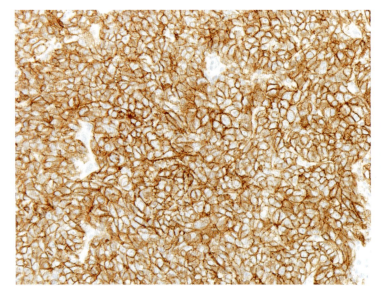

Figure 10. In a typical case, the cell membrane of carcinoma cells is positive for CD5. (Immunostaining, x200)

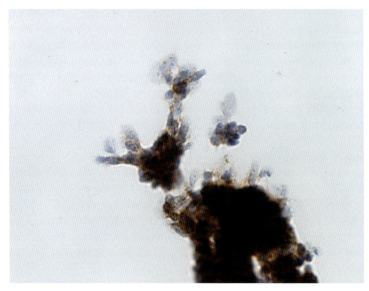

Figure 11. Carcinoma cells are positive for CD5. (Immunostaining, LBC, x400)

References
1. DeLellis RA, Lloid RV, Heitz PU, et al. WHO Classification of tumours, Pathology & Genetics, Tumours of endocrine organs. Lyon: IARC press; 2004, p96-97.
2. Miyauchi A, Kuma K, Matsuzuka F, et al. Intrathyroidal epithelial thymoma: an entity distinct from squamous cell carcinoma of the thyroid. World J Surg 1985; 9:128-35.
3. Ito Y, Miyauchi A, Nakamura Y, et al. Clinicopathologic significance of intrathyroidal epithelial thymoma/carcinoma showing thymus-like differentiation: a collaborative study with Member Institutes of The Japanese Society of Thyroid Surgery. Am J Clin Pathol 2007; 127:230-6.
4. Luo CM, Hsueh C, Chen TM. Extrathyroid carcinoma showing thymus-like differentiation (CASTLE) tumor-a new case report and review of literature. Head Neck 2005; 27:927-33.
5. Piacentini MG, Romano F, De Fina S, et al. Carcinoma of the neck showing thymic-like elements (CASTLE): report of a case and review of the literature. Int J Surg Pathol 2006; 14:171-5.

6. Hirokawa M, Miyauchi A, Minato H, et al. Intrathyroidal epithelial thymoma/carcinoma showing thymus-like differentiation; comparison with thymic lymphoepithelioma-like carcinoma and a possibility of development from a multipotential stem cell. APMIS 2013; 121:523-30.
7. Dorfman DM, Shahsafaei A, Miyauchi A. Intrathyroidal epithelial thymoma (ITET)/carcinoma showing thymus-like differentiation (CASTLE) exhibits CD5 immunoreactivity: new evidence for thymic differentiation. Histopathology 199832:104-9.
8. Berezowski K, Grimes MM, Gal A, et al. CD5 immunoreactivity of epithelial cells in thymic carcinoma and CASTLE using paraffin-embedded tissue. Am J Clin Pathol 1996; 106:483-6.
9. Reimann JD, Dorfman DM, Nosé V. Carcinoma showing thymus-like differentiation of the thyroid (CASTLE): a comparative study: evidence of thymic differentiation and solid cell nest origin. Am J Surg Pathol 2006; 30:994-1001.
10. Dotto J, Pelosi G, Rosai J. Expression of p63 in thymomas and normal thymus. Am J Clin Pathol 2007; 127:415-20.
11. Cîmpean AM, Raica M, Encica S. Overexpression of cytokeratin 34beta E12 in thymoma: could it be a poor prognosis factor? Rom J Morphol Embryol 1999-2004; 45:153-7.
12. Kakudo K, Bai Y, Ozaki T, et al. Intrathyroid epithelial thymoma (ITET) and carcinoma showing thymus-like differentiation (CASLE): CD5-positive neoplasms mimicking squamous cell carcinoma of the thyroid. Histol Histopathol 2013; 25:543-56.
13. Liu Z, Teng XY, Sun DX, et al. Clinical Analysis of Thyroid Carcinoma Showing Thymus-Like Differentiation: Report of 8 Cases. Int Surg 2013; 98:95-100.
14. Hirokawa M, Kuma S, Miyauchi A. Cytological findings of intrathyroidal epithelial thymoma/carcinoma showing thymus-like differentiation: a study of eight cases. Diagn Cytopathol 2012; 40 (Suppl 1):E16-20.
15. Kini SR. Thyroid Cytopathology; An Atlas and Text. Philadelphia: Lippincott Williams & Wilkins; 2008, p419.
16. Pukait S, Agarwal S, Mathur SR, et al. Fine needle aspiration cytology features of poorly differentiated thyroid carcinoma. Cytopathol 2015 (early view)
17. Kane SV, Sharma TP. Cytologic diagnostic approach to poorly differentiated thyroid carcinoma: a single-institution study. Cancer Cytopathol 2015; 123:82-91.
18. Chang S, Joo M, Kim H. Cytologic findings of thyroid carcinoma showing thymus-like differentiation: a case report. Korean J Pathol 2012; 46:302-5.
19. Liu X, Hadeti B, Zhang W, et al. Thyroid carcinoma showing thymus-like differentiation: a clinicopathologic study of 8 cases. Zhonghua Bing Li Xue Za Zhi. 2011; 40:89-93.
20. Baloch Z, Solomon AC, LiVolsi VA. Primary mucoepidermoid carcinoma and sclerosing mucoepidermoid carcinoma with eosinophilia of the thyroid gland: a report of nine cases. Mod Pathol 2000; 13:802-7.

Chapter 18

Parathyroid Adenoma and its Differential Diagnoses

Kayoko Higuchi and Nami Takada

Clinical Summary:

An 89 year-old male presented with hypercalcemia during a follow-up after colectomy for colon cancer. He had no symptoms, but primary hyperparathyroidism due to parathyroid adenoma was suspected based on the results of blood tests, computed tomography (CT), and ultrasound (US) scan. Resection of the right lower parathyroid gland and a partial thyroidectomy were performed.

Clinical Tests:

Blood tests revealed that the patient's levels of calcium and intact parathyroid hormone had increased to 14.6 (8.5~10.5) mg/dl and 365 (10~65) pg/ml, respectively.

Ultrasound and CT Findings:

With US, a hypoechoic mass measuring 1.5 cm in diameter was detected in the right lower portion of the thyroid gland (Figure 1A). Color Doppler demonstrated little vascularity in the periphery of the mass (Figure 1B). A low-density mass measuring about 1 cm in diameter was found in the back of the right thyroid lobe on CT (Figure 2), which had a clear margin and a heterogeneous interior.

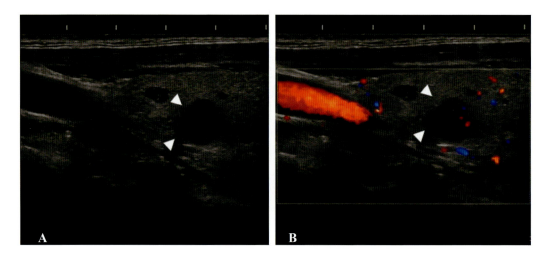

Figure 1. US images of the right side of the neck. A: A hypoechoic mass measuring 1.5 cm in diameter is detected in the right lower portion of the thyroid gland, which has a clear margin and a heterogeneous interior. B: Color Doppler shows little vascularity in the periphery of the lesion.

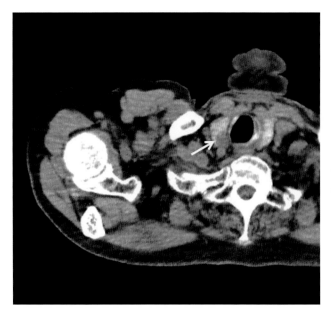

Figure 2. CT images of the right side of the neck. A low-density mass measuring about 1 cm in diameter is shown in the back of the right thyroid lobe.

Cytological Findings:

Papanicolaou-stained scrape smears of the nodule were made. On the low power view, cellular smears showed large 3-dimensional clusters and large branching tissue fragments with fibrovascular stroma (Figure 3). Epithelial cells were found along the border of the fibrovascular stroma (Figure 4). Tumor cells exhibiting trabecular or acinar patterns were also seen in loosely cohesive syncytial clusters. The tumor cells were cuboidal to polyhedral in shape and had clear to finely granular cytoplasm, small round nuclei with granular chromatin, and small or indistinct nucleoli (Figures 5 and 6). Some clusters consisted of small cells with a high nuclear to cytoplasmic ratio. In addition, the nuclei were uniformly round with granular chromatin, which displayed crowding and overlapping (Figure 7). A characteristic dispersed cell pattern was observed, and many naked nuclei appeared to have their cytoplasm stripped away (Figure 8).

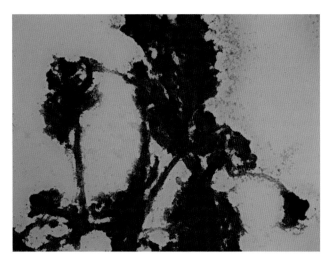

Figure 3. Scrape smear of the parathyroid adenoma demonstrating large branching tissue fragments with fibrovascular stroma. (Papanicolaou stain, x100)

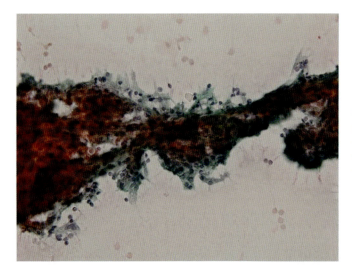

Figure 4. Scrape smear of the parathyroid adenoma showing epithelial cells along the borders of the fibrovascular stroma. (Papanicolaou stain, x400)

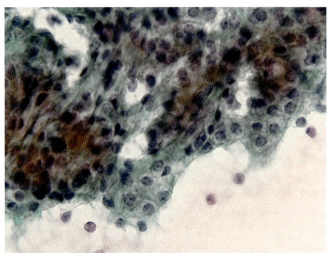

Figure 5. Scrape smear of the parathyroid adenoma. The tumor cells form trabecular patterns, and they have cuboidal clear to finely granular cytoplasm, small round nuclei with granular chromatin, and small or indistinct nucleoli. (Papanicolaou stain, x100)

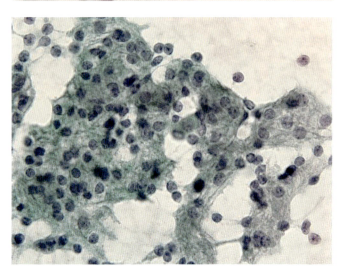

Figure 6. Scrape smear of the parathyroid adenoma. The tumor cells form syncytial clusters with small nuclei that exhibit vague acinar patterns. (Papanicolaou stain, x100)

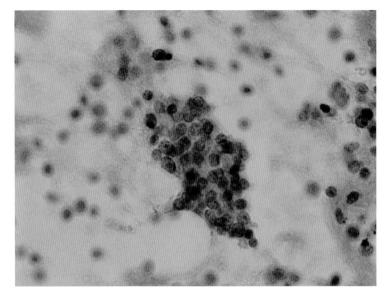

Figure 7. Scrape smear of the parathyroid adenoma. Some clusters consist of small cells with a high nuclear to cytoplasmic ratio. The cells have uniform round nuclei with granular chromatin that exhibits crowding and overlapping. (Papanicolaou stain, x100)

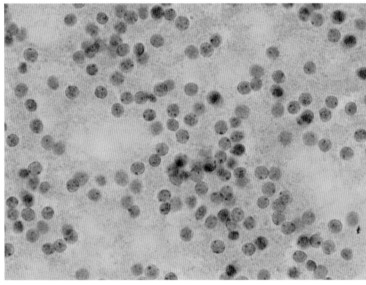

Figure 8. Scrape smear of the parathyroid adenoma showing many dispersed naked nuclei that appear to have had their cytoplasm stripped off. (Papanicolaou stain, x100)

Histological Diagnosis:

Right lower parathyroid glandectomy and a partial thyroidectomy were performed. Macroscopically, the lesion had a thin fibrous capsule and measured 15 mm in diameter, and its cut surface was white and solid. Histological sections demonstrated solid/acinar proliferation of clear/slightly granular chief cells with a rich sinusoidal network and compressed normal parathyroid tissue outside the capsule (Figures 9 and 10). A diagnosis of parathyroid adenoma was made.

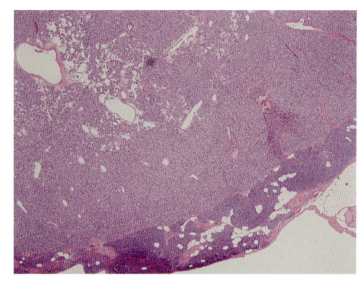

Figure 9. Histological section. Left to right: the parathyroid adenoma, compressed normal parathyroid tissue, and the thyroid gland. (H&E stain, x40)

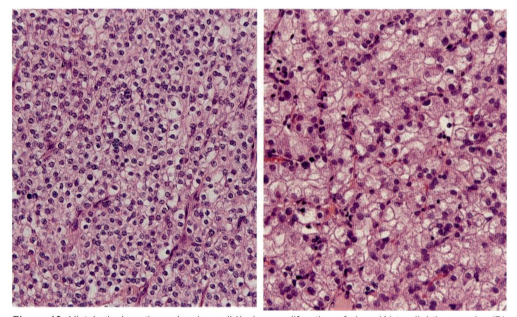

Figure 10. Histological sections showing solid/acinar proliferation of clear (A) to slightly granular (B) chief cells and a rich sinusoidal network. (H&E stain, x200)

List of Differential Diagnoses
1. Benign: Parathyroid adenoma/hyperplasia
2. Indeterminate: Follicular neoplasm
3. Malignant: Metastatic follicular carcinoma in lymph node
4. Malignant: Poorly differentiated carcinoma
5. Malignant: Medullary (C cell) carcinoma

Differential Diagnoses:

Parathyroid tumors are rarely identified within the thyroid, and they may be interpreted as thyroid nodules on US examination (1). Therefore, the increasing use of fine needle aspiration (FNA) cytology to evaluate the thyroid nodules raises the chance to encounter unsuspected parathyroid lesions. Parathyroid adenoma and thyroid follicular tumors are morphologically similar on cytological smears, and the differentiation between them is frequently difficult (2); however, the distinction between thyroid and parathyroid neoplasia is very important as it affects treatment strategies.

There is considerable cytomorphologic overlap between parathyroid adenoma and thyroid follicular tumor (Table 1). Both lesions represent bloody samples with follicular pattern composed of small round cells. Some huge nuclei associated with hyperchromasia are occasionally intermingled with small-sized tumor cells. Such atypical cells seen in parathyroid adenoma are referred to as endocrine atypia, liking those in medullary thyroid carcinoma (please refer to Figures 5 and 9 in Chapter 16). In the follicular tumor of thyroid, these findings lead to a diagnosis of atypical adenoma. The presence of hyaline colloid within follicular clusters indicates follicular tumor of the thyroid because the colloid is rarely observed in parathyroid adenoma.

There are two clues cytologically to differentiate between parathyroid adenoma and thyroid follicular tumors. One is the cellular arrangement. Parathyroid adenoma appears as predominantly trabecular pattern (Figure 11). The trabeculae are relatively flat and thick, and are not usually associated with colloid materials within the clusters. The trabeculae may show branching. Similar clusters are also seen in poorly differentiated carcinoma, but the carcinoma cells are more atypical (please refer to Chapter 21). In contrast, follicular neoplasm of the thyroid shows a typically microfollicular pattern, and the hyaline colloid is frequently observed (please refer to Chapter 20).

Another important clue is the chromatin pattern. Coarse granular chromatin pattern (salt and pepper chromatin) is a characteristic common for neuroendocrine tumors (please refer to Chapters 15 and 16). As parathyroid adenoma is one of neuroendocrine tumors, the chromatin pattern of the tumor is justifiably coarse granular (Figure 12). Coarse granular chromatin pattern is also characteristic of medullary (C cell) thyroid carcinoma (please refer to Figure 15 in Chapter 16), but the carcinoma cells are more discohesive and do not show the trabecular pattern. The chromatin pattern of follicular tumor of the thyroid is granular or fine granular (Figure 13).

When we encounter a case of intrathyroidal tumor showing thick trabecular pattern and coarse granular chromatin pattern, we should consider of the possibility of parathyroid adenoma. Currently, two methods are used to identify parathyroid lesions by FNA. One method is the parathyroid hormone (PTH) assay using the wash-out fluid of the aspiration needle (3) (please refer to Chapter 23); however, the method is limited to cases in which parathyroid cell proliferation was suspected before the aspiration. Another method is the immunocytochemical identification of parathyroid cells using specific antibodies (4, 5). It is well known that PTH is a specific marker for the parathyroid cells and their tumors (Figure 14). However, PTH immunostaining is frequently weak or focally positive (4, 5). Chromogranin A, one of the neuroendocrine markers, is positive for the parathyroid-derived cells (Figure 15) (4, 5), but also expresses in medullary (C cell) carcinoma of the thyroid. PTH and chromogranin A are both expressed in the cytoplasm. Therefore, the immunostaining using these antibodies is not helpful for the naked cells that are frequently present in the parathyroid lesions. Thyroid transcription factor-1 (TTF-1) and PAX8 antibodies react with the thyroid-derived cells (Figures 16 and 17) (6), and does not react with the parathyroid-derived cells. By contrast, GATA-3 antibody reacts with the parathyroid-derived cells (Figure 18), and does not react for the thyroid-derived cells (4, 7). As TTF-1, PAX8 and GATA-3 are expressed in the nuclei, the immunostaining can be adopted for the naked cells. In conclusion, we recommend a panel of GATA-3, TTF-1, and PAX8 immunostaining to differentiate between the parathyroid and thyroid lesions (Table 1) (please refer to Table 1 of Chapter 28).

Table 1. Differential diagnoses of parathyroid adenoma and non-oxyphilic thyroid follicular neoplasm

		Parathyroid adenoma	Non-oxyphilic thyroid follicular neoplasm
Cellularity		Hypo or hypercellular	Hypercellular
Background		Bloody or clean	Bloody or clean
		No colloid, rarely hyaline colloid	No watery colloid or proteinaceous material
		Occasionally proteinaceous material	Hyaline colloid
Arrangement		Predominantly trabecular (thick)	Predominantly mircofollicular
		Sheet-like, occasionally microfollicular	Occasionally trabecular (thin)
		Relatively flat cell cluster	Three-dimensional cell cluster
		Branching cell cluster	Tissue fragment with stroma
		Isolated and naked nuclei	Intertwined capillaries (LBC)
Cell shape		Small, round to cuboidal	Larger, round
Cytoplasm		Scant to moderate	Moderate
		Clear or indiscernible or granular	Indistinct cell border
		Occasionally oxyphilic	
		Distinct or indistinct cell border	
Nucleus		Round, small sized	Round, variably enlarged
		High N/C ratio,	Moderate to high N/C ratio
		Huge nuclei with hyperchromasia	Huge nuclei with hyperchromasia
		Smooth nuclear membrane	Smooth nuclear membrane
		Coarsely granular chromatin	Granular chromatin,
		(salt and pepper chromatin)	
		Micronucleoli	Micro to macronucleoli
Immunostaining			
	PTH	Positive	Negative
	GATA-3	Positive	Negative
	Thyroglobulin	Negative	Positive
	TTF-1	Negative	Positive
	PAX8	Negative	Positive

PTH: Parathyroid hormone, TTF-1: Thyroid transcription factor 1, LBC: Liquid-based cytology

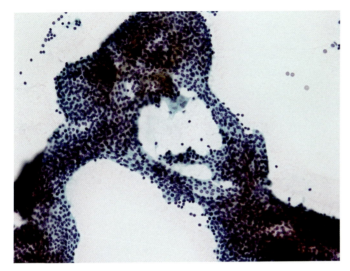

Figure 11. Parathyroid adenoma. Tumor cells display a trabecular pattern that is relatively flat and thick. (Papanicolaou stain, x100)

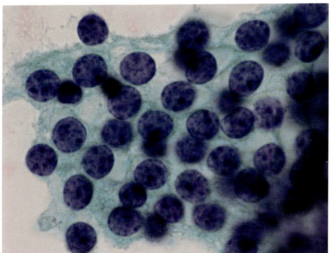

Figure 12. Parathyroid adenoma. The chromatin pattern is coarse granular (salt and pepper chromatin). (Papanicolaou stain, x1000)

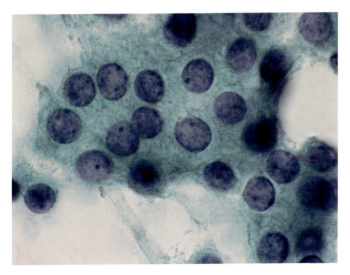

Figure 13. Follicular tumor of the thyroid. The chromatin pattern is fine granular. (Papanicolaou stain, x1000)

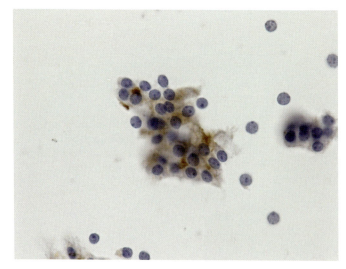

Figure 14. Parathyroid adenoma. PTH is weakly positive in the cytoplasm. (LBC, SurePath, PTH immunostaining, x400)

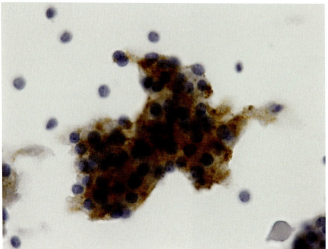

Figure 15. Parathyroid adenoma. Chromogranin A is strongly positive in the cytoplasm. (LBC, SurePath, Chromogranin A immunostaining, x400)

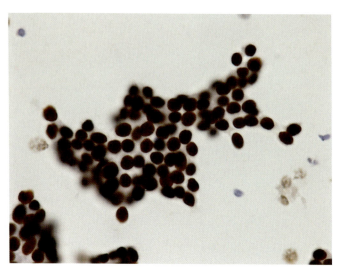

Figure 16. Follicular tumor of the thyroid. TTF-1 is strongly positive in the nuclei. (LBC, SurePath, TTF-1 immunostaining, x400)

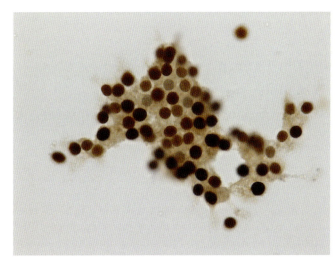

Figure 17. Thyroid benign follicular cells. PAX8 staining is strongly positive in the nuclei. (LBC, SurePath, PAX8 immunostaining, x400)

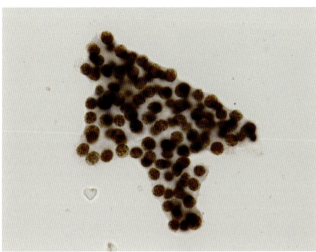

Figure 18. Parathyroid adenoma. GATA-3 staining is strongly positive in the nuclei. (LBC, SurePath, GATA-3 immunostaining, x400)

References

1. Tseleni-Balafouta S, Gakiopoulou H, Kavantzas N, et al. Parathyroid proliferations: a source of diagnostic pitfalls in FNA of thyroid. Cancer 2007; 111:130-6.
2. Kini SR. Chaptor 21. Lesions of the parathyroid glands. In Thyroid cytopathology: an atlas and text. 2nd ed. Philadelphia: Lippincott Williams & Wilkins. 2015; 12868-13262/15102 (e-book version).
3. Miyauchi A, Kakudo K, Fujimoto T, et al. Parathyroid cyst: analysis of the cyst fluid and ultrastructural observation. Arch Pathol Lab Med 1981; 105:497-9.
4. Takada N, Hirokawa M, Suzuki A, et al. Diagnostic value of GATA-3 in cytological identification of parathyroid tissues. Endocr J 2016; (in press).
5. Heo I, Park S, Jung CW, et al. Fine needle aspiration cytology of parathyroid lesions. Korean J Pathol 2013; 47:466-71.
6. Suzuki A, Hirokawa M, Takada N, et al. Diagnostic significance of PAX8 in thyroid squamous cell carcinoma. Endocr J 2015; 62:991-5.
7. Betts G, Beckett E, Nonaka D. GATA3 shows differential immunohistochemical expression across thyroid and parathyroid lesions. Histopathology 2014; 65:288-90.

Chapter 19

Risk-Classification of Follicular Pattern Lesions in Thyroid FNA Cytology
(Part 1: Benign Follicular Pattern Lesions or Follicular Neoplasms)

Kennichi Kakudo, Emiko Taniguchi, Shinya Satoh and Kaori Kameyama

Brief Clinical History

During a medical examination, nodular thyroid enlargement was found in a 36-year-old female, and she was referred to the Ito Hospital for further check-up. A dominant, 30.7 x 26.6 mm, nodule was found in the right lobe of thyroid on ultrasound examination (Figure 1). It was a well-circumscribed isoechoic nodule with cystic change, and FNA cytology was performed from the solid portion of the nodule.

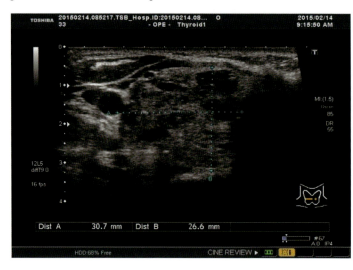

Figure 1. A well-circumscribed dominant nodule, 30.7 x 26.6 mm, is identified in the right lobe of the thyroid. It is an isoechoic nodule with cystic change. (Ultrasound)

Cytological Findings

Cellular lesions characterized predominantly by macro-follicle fragments or mono-layered flat sheets of follicular cells were observed with abundant colloid (Figure 2). These follicular cells had round to oval, evenly spaced monomorphic nuclei and cyanophilic pale cytoplasm (the so-called honeycomb-like arrangement). These follicular cells had fine, granular chromatin and inconspicuous nucleoli in the round nuclei (Figure 3). Only negligible nuclear overlapping and nuclear crowding were noted in the clusters.

Histological Diagnosis: Adenomatous goiter

Histological sections of the thyroid showed vague nodularity without capsulation (Figure 4). Central scar fibrosis was noted. These nodules showed colloid-filled macro-follicular or normo-follicular structures covered by flat to columnar follicular cells with pyknotic nuclei. Clusters of small follicles protruding into a large dilated colloid follicle (also known as Sanderson's polsters, a characteristic of hyperplastic nodules) were often observed (Figure 5).

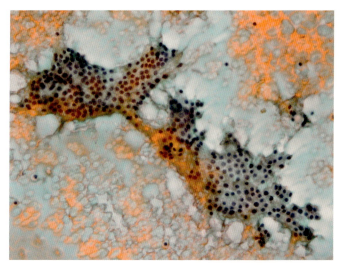

Figure 2. Monolayered flat sheets of follicular cells with abundant colloid. The follicular cells show round to oval evenly spaced monomorphic nuclei and cyanophilic pale cytoplasm (honeycomb-like arrangement). (Papanicolaou stain, x200)

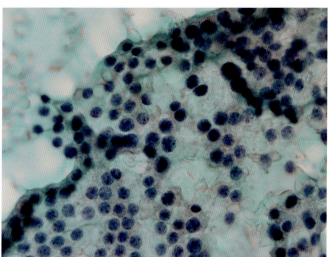

Figure 3. Monolayered flat sheets of follicular cells with round nuclei containing finely granular chromatin and inconspicuous small nucleoli. (Papanicolaou stain, x400)

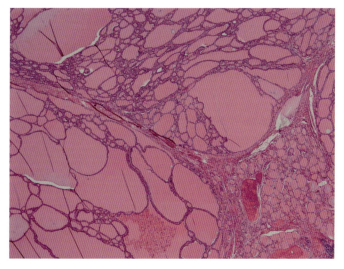

Figure 4. Multiple nodular hyperplastic lesions are separated by thin fibrous tissue and comprising macrofollicular architecture. These follicles are lined by flat or cuboidal follicular cells with abundant pinkish colloid. (HE stain, x40)

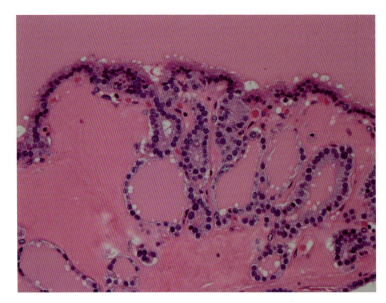

Figure 5. A cluster of small follicles protruding into a large dilated colloid follicle (Sanderson's polster) is shown. These follicles are covered with cuboidal cells containing small round pyknotic nuclei. (HE stain, x200)

Benign Follicular Pattern Lesions and Its Differential Diagnosis from Follicular Neoplasms (FN) of High-risk Indeterminate Category (Table 1)

The two important diagnostic criteria of benign cytological diagnosis are 1) normal appearance of follicular cell clusters and 2) various amounts of colloid substance in the smear background (Figures 6A and 6B) (1-4). Normal-appearing (benign) follicular cell clusters form large flat sheets of follicular cells with evenly distributed round nuclei are shown in the Figure 6. The difference in nuclear sizes is shown in Figure 7, with normal follicular cells on the left and neoplastic follicular cells on the right. Contrary to benign follicular cell clusters, characteristics of the FN (high-risk indeterminate) category usually include scant or no colloid in the smear background, and a cellular smear with 3-dimensional cell clusters with nuclear crowding and overlapping (Figures 7 and 8). Of note, nuclear crowding and overlapping are often accompanied by nuclear enlargement, irregular nuclear contour, hyperchromasia, and conspicuous nucleoli (Figure 8). Cases without these nuclear features should be classified into the benign category (Table 1) (1-4). Cases with nuclear atypia related to papillary thyroid carcinoma (PTC) type nuclear features, such as pale chromatin, nuclear grooves, and/or cytoplasmic nuclear inclusions, should be placed into the PTC lineage (indeterminate/PTC cannot be ruled out, suspicious for malignancy, or malignant) categories (5-6) (please refer to Chapters 1, 2 and 4). The chromatin pattern of parathyroid tumor is coarse granular and different from that of normal or neoplastic follicular cell tumors (please refer to Figures 12 and 13 in Chapter 18).

Table 1. Comparison between benign follicular cell clusters and neoplastic follicular cell clusters (high-risk indeterminate category)

Characteristics	Benign follicular cells	Follicular neoplasms
Colloid background	rich	scant or no colloid
Microfollicles	rare or artifact	variably present
Dispersed cells	rare or artifact	variably present
3-dimensional clusters	rare or artifact	variably present
Nuclear position	honeycomb sheets	syncytial sheets
Nuclear crowding	absent	present
Nuclear overlapping	absent	present
Nuclear enlargement	absent	present
Nuclear/cytoplasmic ratio	low	increased
Nucleoli	inconspicuous	conspicuous

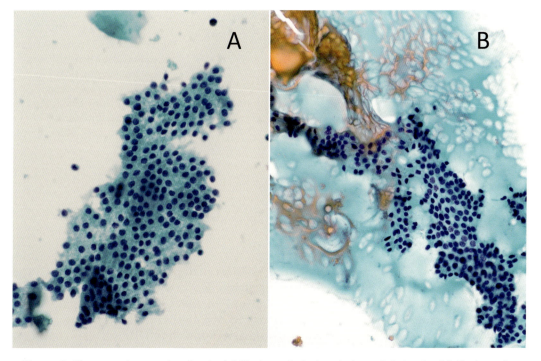

Figure 6. The normal appearing (benign) follicular cell clusters in large flat sheets of follicular cells. Note the small round pyknotic nuclei. These nuclei are distributed evenly in the so-called honeycomb-like arrangement. A fragment of thick colloid (top of panel A) in a liquid-based preparation (A) and watery thin colloid (blue-green in background) in a conventional smear (B). (A: liquid-based cytology and B: conventional smear, Papanicolaou stain, x200)

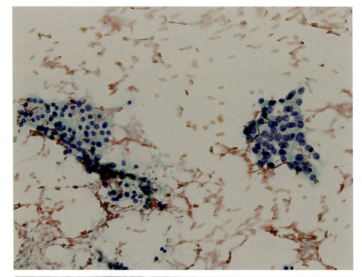

Figure 7. A normal looking follicular cell cluster (left) and a neoplastic follicular cell cluster (right) in the same field. Note the nuclear size difference between the two clusters. Nuclear crowding and overlapping are observed in the right neoplastic cluster. (Papanicolaou stain, x200)

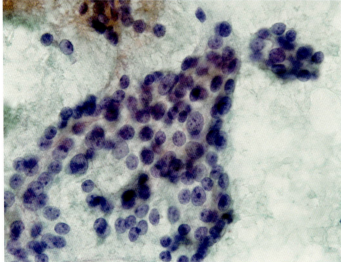

Figure 8. A loosely cohesive large trabecular cluster demonstrating nuclear overlapping. Note the large and variably-sized nuclei with granular chromatin and conspicuous nucleoli. (Papanicolaou stain, x400)

Benign Follicular Pattern Lesions and Its Differential Diagnosis from PTC and Indeterminate (PTC cannot be ruled out) Categories

When PTC type nuclear features are identified under high power magnification, reaching a correct diagnosis (malignant, PTC) may be easy (please refer to Chapters 3 and 4) (Figure 9D). However, a false positive diagnosis may occur with cellular aspirates containing papillary-like and monolayered tissue fragments (please refer to Figure 6 of Chapter 4). Use of higher magnification is necessary to confirm the uniform and small nuclei of benign-appearing follicular cells in the honeycomb pattern, which will allow a more confident diagnosis of benign disease (Figure 9C). Therefore, ruling out PTC type nuclear features in follicular pattern lesions is essential for achieving accurate benign diagnosis (Figure 9). This is the only method to avoid the possible pitfall of mistaking benign cases with PTC cases displaying worrisome nuclear features. Improper assessment of PTC type nuclear features in follicular pattern lesions may result in either high rate of PTCs in surgically treated patients of benign cytological diagnosis or high proportion of PTCs in surgically treated patients with indeterminate cytological diagnosis (follicular neoplasm).

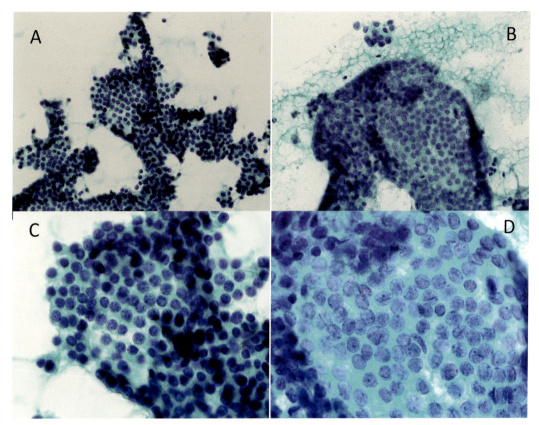

Figure 9. Comparison between benign follicular cell sheet (A and C) and malignant papillary carcinoma in sheet-like arrangements (B and D). The nuclei of the papillary carcinoma in B and D are larger, paler, more crowded, and more irregular in contour. Note the multiple nuclear grooves in D. Under low magnification, the difference between A and B may often be overlooked, and misinterpretation may occur. (Papanicolaou stain, A and B, x200 and C and D, x400)

Conclusions

Follicular pattern lesions are divided into benign, low-risk indeterminate, and high-risk indeterminate categories in the American (AUS/FLUS and FN/SFN) (2, 7), Italian (TIR3A and TIR3B) (8, 9), British (Thy 3a and Thy 3f) (10, 11) and Japanese (Indeterminate A1: favorable benign, A2: borderline and A3: favorable malignant) (5, 6) systems (please refer to Chapter 2). It is important for cytopathologists to identify benign lesions; the benign cytological diagnosis spares patients unnecessary diagnostic surgeries, and those patients can often be conservatively managed with periodic clinical examinations (12). How to reduce the number of patients classified into the indeterminate category has been discussed in several reports, and diagnostic surgery has been recommended for all patients with FNs (high-risk indeterminate category) traditionally (3, 4). However, it was changed to more conservative manner in the 2015 ATA guideline (12) (please refer to Chapters 1 and 2). The comparison between characteristics of benign follicular lesions and FNs (high-risk indeterminate category) is shown in Table 1.

Take Home Message

Important diagnostic features of benign follicular cells (exclusion criteria from the indeterminate category) are:
1. Abundant colloid in the background.
2. Follicular cells with minimally enlarged round nuclei (uniformly sized nuclei).
3. Follicular cells in a honeycomb sheet arrangement (no overlapping).

References

1. Kini SR. Thyroid cytopathology: an atlas and text. 1st ed. Philadelphia: Lippincott Williams & Wilkins; 2008.
2. Ali SZ and Cibas ES (ed). The Bethesda system for reporting thyroid cytopathology. Definitions, criteria and explanatory notes. Springer, New York, USA: 2010, p1-166.
3. Abele JS, Levine RA. Diagnostic criteria and risk-adapted approach to indeterminate thyroid cytodiagnosis. Cancer Cytopathol 2010; 118:415-22.
4. Renshaw AA, Gould EW. Reducing indeterminate thyroid FNAs. Cancer Cytopathol 2015; 123:237-43.
5. Kakudo K, Kameyama K, Miyauchi A, et al. Introducing the reporting system for thyroid fine-needle aspiration cytology according to the new guidelines of the Japan Thyroid Association. Endocr J 2014; 61:539-52.
6. Kameyama K, Sasaki E, Sugino K, et al. The Japanese Thyroid Association reporting system of thyroid aspiration cytology and experience from a high-volume center, especially in indeterminate category. J Basic Clin Med 2015; 4:70-4.
7. Baloch ZW, LiVolsi VA, Asa SL, et al. Diagnostic terminology and morphologic criteria for cytologic diagnosis of thyroid lesions: a synopsis of the National Cancer Institute Thyroid Fine-Needle Aspiration State of the Science Conference. Diagn Cytopathol 2008; 36:425-37.
8. Fadda G, Basolo F, Bondi A, et al. Cytological classification of thyroid nodules. Proposal of the SIAPEC-IAP Italian consensus working group. Pathologica 2010; 102:405-6.
9. Nardi F, Basolo F, Crescenzi A, et al. Italian consensus for the classification and reporting of thyroid cytology. J Endocrinol Invest 2014; 37:593-9.
10. Lobo C, McQueen A, Beale T, et al. The UK royal college of pathologists' thyroid fine-needle aspiration diagnostic classification: is a robust tool for the clinical management of abnormal thyroid nodules. Acta Cytol 2011; 55:499-506.
11. Perros P, Colley S, Boelaert K, et al. Guidelines for the management of thyroid cancer Third edition British Thyroid Association Chapter 5.1, p19-24; Clin Endocrinol 2014; 81 (Suppl S1).
12. Haugen BR, Alexander EK, Bible KC, et al. 2015 American Thyroid Association management guidelines for adult patients with thyroid nodules and differentiated thyroid cancer. Thyroid 2015; 26:1-134.

Chapter 20

Risk-Classification of Follicular Pattern Lesions in Thyroid FNA Cytology
(Part 2: Follicular Adenoma or Follicular Carcinoma)

Kennichi Kakudo, Kaori Kameyama, Keiko Inomata and Shinya Satoh

Clinical Findings

A 66-year-old female patient noticed a lump in her neck, and she was referred to Ito Hospital for further checkup. She had a well-circumscribed elastic soft nodule in the left side of her neck. An ultrasound examination revealed partially hypoechoic and isoechoic solid nodule with a size of 43 x 33 x 55 mm and irregular margins in the left lobe of thyroid. Fine needle aspiration (FNA) cytology of the thyroid nodule was then performed.

Cytological Findings

The cellular smear showed a clean background and predominant microfollicular clusters (Figures 1 and 2) with well-preserved cellular cohesiveness and colloid substance. Nuclear overlapping and crowding in these clusters were also noted (Figures 1-4). Significant nuclear enlargement and high nuclear pleomorphism were observed in the clusters, demonstrating disturbed cellular polarity (Figures 3 and 4). The nuclei of the follicular cells were predominantly round- to oval-shaped, and had finely granular chromatin with conspicuous small nucleoli (Figures 3 and 4). Although some showed irregular nuclear contours, papillary thyroid carcinoma (PTC)-type nuclear features (nuclear grooves or nuclear cytoplasmic inclusions) were not observed. Isolated cells were few, and no tumor necrosis was observed in the background.

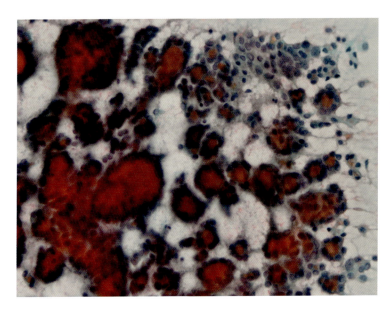

Figure 1. A cellular smear showing a predominantly microfollicular growth pattern. (Conventional smear, Papanicolaou stain, x100)

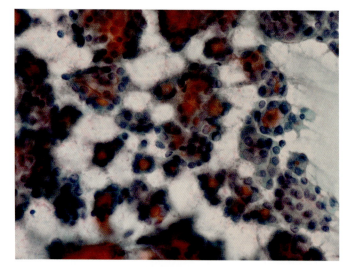

Figure 2. Microfollicles with central colloid substance are observed in the smear with clean background. (Conventional smear, Papanicolaou stain, x200)

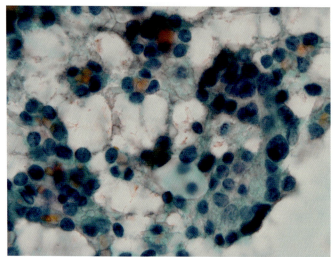

Figure 3. Nuclear pleomorphism and hyperchromasia with finely granular chromatin and conspicuous small nucleoli are observed in these clusters. (Conventional smear, Papanicolaou stain, x400)

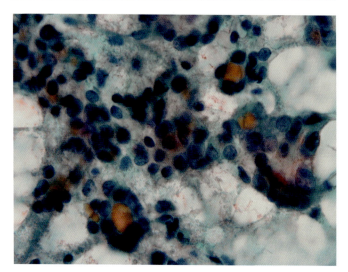

Figure 4. Nuclear crowding and overlapping are observed in the 3-dimensional clusters. (Conventional smear, Papanicolaou stain, x400)

List of Differential Diagnoses
1. Benign: adenomatous (hyperplastic) nodule
2. Low-risk indeterminate category (FLUS of the American system, TIR3A of the Italian system, and Thy 3a of the British system) or Indeterminate A1: follicular neoplasm (FN), favor benign of the Japanese system
3. High-risk indeterminate category (FN of the American system, TIR3B of the Italian system, and Thy 3f of the British system) or Indeterminate A3: FN, favor malignant of the Japanese system
4. Suspicious for malignancy, follicular variant PTC
5. Malignant: poorly differentiated carcinoma

Differential Diagnosis

Benign adenomatous nodule can be ruled out, because neither colloid-rich background nor benign-looking follicular cell clusters were observed (please refer to Chapter 19). The high-risk indeterminate category of the American (FN), Italian (TIR3B), British (Thy 3f), and Japanese (A3: FN, favor malignant) systems is the likely diagnostic category in this case. High grade nuclear atypia and disturbed cellular polarity, as well as nuclear crowding observed in Figures 1-4 do not fit the low-risk indeterminate category of the American (FLUS), Italian (TIR3A), British (Thy 3a), and Japanese (A1: FN, favor benign) systems (please refer to Chapters 2 and 5). Absence of PTC type nuclear features also rules out the indeterminate B category of the Japanese system, suspicious for malignancy, and follicular variant PTC (please refer to Chapter 4). Furthermore, absence of high-grade features (mitotic figures in the tumor cells and tumor necrosis in the smear background) did not favor poorly differentiated carcinoma type malignancy (please refer to Chapter 21). A total thyroidectomy was performed. The cut surface of the thyroid nodule in the left lobe demonstrated a solid nodule invading into the thyroid parenchyma.

Histological Diagnosis: Follicular carcinoma, widely invasive and angio-invasive type.

The nodule was a well-demarcated follicular tumor showing invasive growth into the thyroid parenchyma. A few vascular invasions were identified (Figures 5 and 6). The tumor cells formed follicular structure of various sizes with colloid, predominantly in a microfollicular growth pattern (Figure 7). Neither papillary growth nor PTC type nuclear features was identified.

Cytological Features of FN (High-risk Indeterminate Category) (Tables 1 and 2)

The characteristics of the high-risk indeterminate category (FN) include hypercellularity as well as arrangement of cells in predominantly follicular patterns (Figures 1 and 2) (1-3). Abundant cellular clusters showing nuclear crowding and overlap are always observed in the clusters. Furthermore, colloid is sparse or absent in the smear background. These tumor cells have larger nuclei than the normal follicular cells, and show significant nuclear size variation, irregular nuclear membrane, and hyperchromatic nuclear chromatin (Figures 3 and 4) (Tables 1 and 2). If the features mentioned above are lacking in a smear with more than 6 follicular cell clusters, the case should be classified into the benign category (please refer to Chapter 19). However, some cases may demonstrate characteristics between the two categories, such as cellular follicular lesions showing mild nuclear crowding, overlapping, and/or nuclear atypia (Figures 8 and 9). These cases are often classified into the low-risk indeterminate category in the American (FLUS) (1, 2), Italian (TIR3A) (3, 4), and British (Thy 3a) (5, 6) systems, regardless of the presence or absence of PTC type nuclear features. This category is further divided into the indeterminate A1: favor benign FN (without

PTC-N) category (Figure 8) and indeterminate B (with worrisome PTC-N) category (Figure 9) in the Japanese system (8), because the latter has a higher risk of malignancy (8-11) (please refer to Chapters 4-6).

Table 1. Cytological features suggestive for benign cellular follicular adenoma or low-risk (minimally invasive type) follicular carcinoma

1. Cellularity is variable but often highly cellular
2. Absent or scant colloid
3. Trabecular large tissue fragments
4. Syncytial type follicular cell clusters
5. Nuclear enlargement and irregularity
6. Microfollicular clusters
7. Nuclear crowding and overlapping (3-dimensional clusters)

Table 2. Cytological features observed more often in widely invasive type follicular carcinoma or poorly differentiated carcinoma

1. High grade nuclear crowding and overlapping (3-dimensional clusters) (Figures 1-4)
2. High nuclear grade (nuclear pleomorphism, hyperchromasia and prominent nucleoli) (Figure 10)
3. Occasional mitosis
4. Cellular aspirate with dispersed cells (loss of cellular cohesiveness) (Figure 11)
5. Necrosis in the background

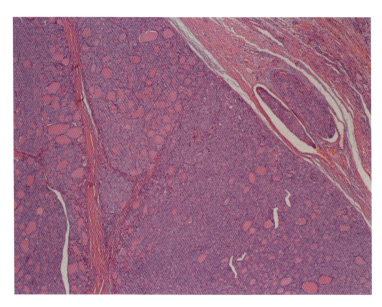

Figure 5. A follicular carcinoma with fibrous capsule is shown at low magnification. Note the vascular invasion by the tumor nest in the upper right field. (HE stain, x40)

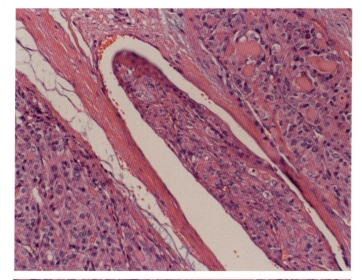

Figure 6. Higher magnification of the vascular invasion of Figure 7. Note the red blood cells in the vascular space and endothelial lining of the vessel. (HE stain, x200)

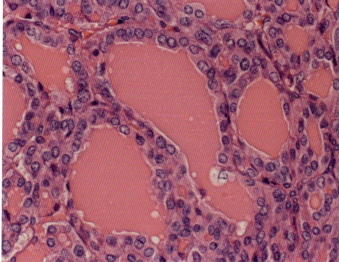

Figure 7. Follicular growth histology without papillary carcinoma nuclear features. Note the nuclear pleomorphism and hyperchromatic vesicular nuclei. (HE stain, x400)

Is Cytological Diagnosis of Follicular Adenoma and Follicular Carcinoma Valid?

For follicular pattern lesions, the cytological diagnosis of FN is considered to be a screening test, and a diagnostic lobectomy for histological confirmation is recommended for all patients with high-risk indeterminate cytology in most international clinical guidelines and diagnostic systems (1-4). This is because the diagnosis of follicular adenoma and follicular carcinoma (FTC) solely relies on the histological demonstration of invasiveness, and it is believed that it is not possible to detect invasiveness by cytological features. However, Kini emphasized that FNA cytology is able to accurately identify follicular adenoma, widely invasive FTC, and poorly differentiated carcinoma, while cellular follicular adenoma and minimally invasive FTC of low malignant potential have significant morphological overlap (7). This leaves a small proportion of cellular follicular adenomas and well-differentiated FTCs that cannot be differentiated cytologically from each other. These are interpreted as either cellular adenomas or suspicious for FTC, with an estimated risk of malignancy, in Kini's cytological practice (7). Similar to Dr. Kini's practice of thyroid cytology, risk stratification of the indeterminate category is traditionally carried out in high volume thyroid centers in Japan since 1992, initiated by Toriya *et al.* (12). This strategy is retained in the establishment of the Japanese system, and cases with overlapping morphology between benign follicular adenoma and low-risk FTC are subjectively placed in either A1: favor benign or A2: borderline in the Japanese system, depending on their cytological features (8).

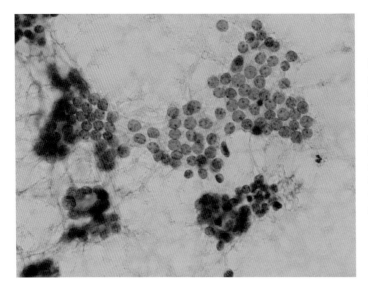

Figure 8. Cellular smear showing sheet-like clusters and microfollicles. Note the uniformly round nuclei and the well-preserved cellular polarity and cohesiveness. Benign category or low-risk indeterminate category may be recommended. Subsequent surgery showed follicular adenoma. (Conventional smear, Papanicolaou stain, x400)

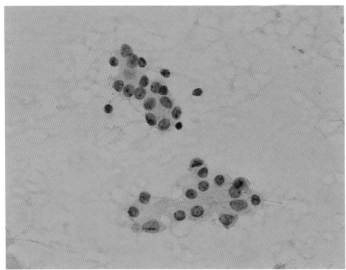

Figure 9. Mild irregularity of the nuclear contours and nuclear grooves are observed in a microfollicular pattern smear. Subsequent surgery revealed encapsulated non-invasive follicular variant papillary carcinoma (benign borderline tumor of NIFTP or WDT-UMP, please refer to Chapter 6). (Conventional smear, Papanicolaou stain, x400)

The Kameyama Scoring System for Subclassification of the FN Category into Benign, A1: Favor Benign, A2: Borderline, and A3: Favor Malignant Subcategories in the Japanese System

To develop a more objective evaluation method for follicular pattern lesions, Kameyama *et al.* developed a scoring system for subclassification of FN using three parameters (cellularity, nuclear overlapping, and nuclear atypia) (14). They scored the cellularity as 1 point when the cellular volume was small, 2 points when intermediate, and 3 points when high. The degree of nuclear overlapping (three dimensional clustering and loss of cellular polarity) was scored 1 point when mild, 2 points when moderate, and 3 points when high (Figure 4). Nuclear atypia was scored 1 point when mild, 2 points when moderate, and 3 points when high (Figures 4 and 10) (14). When the total score was 3, 4, or 5, the lesion was classified into category A1: favor benign, when 6 or 7, it was classified into category A2: borderline, and when 8 or 9, it was classified into category A3: favor malignant (Figures 3, 4, 10). The case illustrated in Figures 1-4 was scored with a cellularity of 3, nuclear crowding of 2, and nuclear atypia of 3 (total score: 8), and was classed into the A3: favor malignant category. Total scores below 3 and cases without nuclear overlapping and nuclear atypia are classed into the benign category, even if the sample is highly cellular. Cases with any (equivocal or unequivocal) PTC type nuclear features are excluded from category A and placed in the indeterminate B, suspicious for malignancy or malignancy categories depending on their nuclear features in the Japanese system (please refer to Chapters 2 and 4). The case in Figure 8 was scored with a cellularity of 2, nuclear crowding of 1, and nuclear atypia of 1 (total score 4), and was classified into A1: favor benign. The case in Figure 9 was categorized into the indeterminate B: others category because of the worrisome nuclear features of PTC.

Using this scoring system, Kameyama *et al.* reported the successful risk stratification of 400 cases of FN, with malignancy risks of 11.5% (A1), 53.8% (A2), and 81.8% (A3), respectively (14), which are significantly higher than the estimated risks of malignancy reported in the Japanese system (8). This difference may be due to further clinical triage of the patients recommended by the clinical guidelines by the Japanese Thyroid Association (15). Satoh *et al.* reported resection rates of patients with A1, A2, and A3 nodules of 53.5%, 87.5% and 100%, respectively (16). The risks of malignancy determined by histology in the three subcategories were 20.0% (3/15 nodules), 33.3% (3/9 nodules), and 45.5% (5/11 nodules), respectively (16), which were consistent with the proposed risks of malignancy (A1: 5-15%, A2:15-30%, and A3:40-60%) as shown in Table 1 and Figure 1 in Chapter 2 (8).

Renshaw *et al.* reported reductions of the overall rate of the indeterminate category by classifying some of the cases as either favor benign or suspicious for PTC (11). The favor benign diagnosis in the AUS/FLUS category by Renshaw *et al.* is almost equivalent to the indeterminate A1 favor benign subcategory in the Japanese system (11), and the PTC ruled out in the FN/SFN category may be equivalent to the indeterminate B category of the Japanese system (9-11).

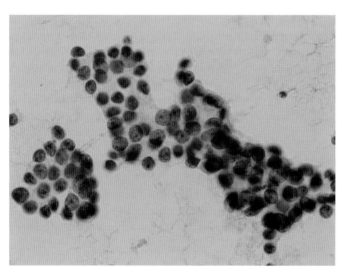

Figure 10. Nuclear crowding and overlapping in 3-dimensional clusters. Note the irregularly sized nuclei and marked nuclear hyperchromasia. Kameyama's total score was 8 (2+3+3), and the case was classified as indeterminate A3: favor malignant. Subsequent surgery revealed widely invasive type follicular carcinoma. (Conventional smear, Papanicolaou stain, x400)

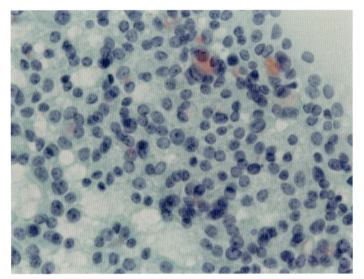

Figure 11. Cellular aspirate consisting of trabecular tissue fragments, numerous dispersed cells, and microfollicles with colloid substance. Note the loss of cellular polarity and cohesiveness, resulting in overlapped nuclei. Kameyama's total score was 7 (3+3+1), and the case was classified as indeterminate A2: borderline. Subsequent surgery demonstrated insular type follicular carcinoma. (Conventional smear, Papanicolaou stain, x400)

Exploratory Notes

There is a continuing debate among surgical pathologists on what constitutes the true invasion of follicular thyroid carcinoma (FTC) (17, 18). Interpretation of invasiveness and histopathologic diagnosis are subjective, and as a result, leading to marked interobserver variability (17, 18) as well as difficulty in or invalidation of cytological and histological correlation studies (7). We would like to emphasize that the poor reproducibility in histological diagnosis occurs almost exclusively between the benign cellular follicular adenoma and capsular invasion alone, minimally invasive FTCs of very low malignant potential (7, 18), in addition to between follicular adenoma and encapsulated PTC (18-21). These entities have been named FT-UMP (follicular tumor of uncertain malignant potential) and WDT-UMP (well-differentiated tumor of uncertain malignant potential) by Williams (22), and WDT-UB (well-differentiated tumor of uncertain behavior) by Liu *et al.* (23). Difficulty in cytological differentiation also occurs exclusively in cases between cellular follicular adenoma and minimally invasive FTC of very low grade malignant potential, similar to histological diagnosis (7). Goffredo *et al.* reported that only 2 of 1200 patients died of cancer in their study of patients with minimally invasive FTC, and these patients had a lifespan longer or comparable with the U.S. general population. Thus, the authors questioned the application of cancer terminology to this carcinoma of very low malignant potential (24). Our group proposed to classify this entity into the benign borderline category in 2012 because of its indolent biological behavior (25).

We have concluded that a conservative attitude is necessary for the diagnosis and clinical management of patients with follicular pattern lesions without nuclear atypia, nuclear crowding, and overlapping. Even if the histological diagnosis is malignant (minimally invasive FTC), a simple excision (lobectomy alone) is a curative treatment, and additional treatment such as a total thyroidectomy followed by radioactive iodine treatment is not necessary. Although diagnosis of malignancy for encapsulated follicular pattern lesions relies on histological identification of invasiveness, this judgement is subjective and poor in reproducibility in many studies (17, 18). A retrospective review of 66 cases of follicular carcinoma by Cipriani *et al.* showed significant observer variability, and nearly three-fourths of the cases were reclassified; surprisingly, 18 of the 66 (27%) cases were reclassified as a benign follicular adenoma (18).

It is essential to establish appropriate histological criteria to identify cancers that may develop recurrence or metastasis and result in cancer death at a significant rate, as well as to exclude indolent (borderline) lesions from true malignancy. Until this time comes, cytological examination is one of the most reliable methods to identify cases with a higher risk of malignancy to triage patients for surgical treatment or a lower risk of malignancy to close follow up. The authors of this chapter believe that the cytological FN category is no longer an indeterminate (vague, not established, uninformative or inconclusive) category and it is given a new role to accept borderline precursor tumors, both cellular follicular adenoma and minimally invasive FTC (low-risk FTC), in the future diagnosyic system for reporting thyroid cytopathology. The two tumors (benign follicular adenoma and malignant minimally invasive FTC) are in a same spectrum of tumors (clonal follicular cell neoplasms with very low grade malignant potential) and no distinction is necessary in clinical management.

Take Home Message

Subclassification of follicular pattern lesions will help establish stricter criteria of FN, regardless of the diagnostic system used. As a result, more cases with follicular pattern lesions can be placed into definite categories, as either benign or malignant. We believe that this training will ultimately reduce the rate of indeterminate categories (FN) in your cytology practice to possibly less than 10 % of the total samples. These stricter criteria should be particularly important to those systems that recommend diagnostic surgery unselectively to patients with FN nodule.

References

1. Baloch ZW, LiVolsi VA, Asa SL, et al. Diagnostic terminology and morphologic criteria for cytologic diagnosis of thyroid lesions: a synopsis of the National Cancer Institute Thyroid Fine-Needle Aspiration State of the Science Conference. Diagn Cytopathol 2008; 36:425-37.
2. Ali SZ, Cibas ES (ed). (2010) The Bethesda system for reporting thyroid cytopathology. Definitions, criteria and explanatory notes. Springer, New York, USA, p1-166.
3. Fadda G, Basolo F, Bondi A, et al. Cytological classification of thyroid nodules. Proposal of the SIAPEC-IAP Italian consensus working group. Pathologica 2010; 102:405-6.
4. Nardi F, Basolo F, Crescenzi A, et al. Italian consensus for the classification and reporting of thyroid cytology. J Endocrinol Invest 2014; 37:593-9.
5. Lobo C, McQueen A, Beale T, et al. The UK royal college of pathologists' thyroid fine-needle aspiration diagnostic classification: is a robust tool for the clinical management of abnormal thyroid nodules. Acta Cytol 2011; 55:499-506.
6. Perros P, Colley S, Boelaert K, et al. Guidelines for the management of thyroid cancer. Third Edition British Thyroid Association. Chapter 5.1 p19-24, Clin Endocrinol 2014;81(S1)
7. Kini SR. Thyroid Cytopathology: An Atlas and Text. 2nd ed. Philadelphia, Wolters Kluwer Health, 2015.
8. Kakudo K, Kameyama K, Miyauchi A, et al. Introducing the reporting system for thyroid fine-needle aspiration cytology according to the new guidelines of the Japan Thyroid Association. Endocr J 2014; 61: 539-52.
9. Renshaw AA. Focal features of papillary carcinoma of the thyroid in fine-needle aspiration material are strongly associated with papillary carcinoma at resection. Am J Clin Pathol 2002; 118:208-10.
10. Weber D, Brainard J, Chen L. Atypical epithelial cells, cannot exclude papillary carcinoma, in fine needle aspiration of the thyroid. Acta Cytol 2008; 52:320-4.
11. Renshaw AA, Gould EW. Reducing indeterminate thyroid FNAs. Cancer Cytopathol 2015; 123:237-43.
12. Kakudo K, Kameyama K, Miyauchi A. History of thyroid cytology in Japan and reporting system recommended by the Japan Thyroid Association. J Basic Clin Med 2013; 2:10-5.
13. Kakudo K, Kameyama K, Hirokawa M, et al. Subclassification of follicular neoplasms recommended by the

Japanese Thyroid Association reporting system of thyroid cytology. Int J Endocrinol 2015;2015:938305. doi: 10.1155/2015/938305.

14. Kameyama K, Sasaki E, Sugino K, et al. The Japanese Thyroid Association reporting system of thyroid aspiration cytology and experience from a high-volume center, especially in indeterminate category. J Basic Clin Med 2015; 4:70-4.
15. Japanese Thyroid Association. Guidelines for Clinical Practice for the Management of Thyroid Nodules in Japan. Nankodo Publishing Co, editor Nakamura H, Tokyo, 2013:1-277 (in Japanese).
16. Satoh S, Yamashita H, Kakudo K. Is the JTA reporting system for thyroid cytology useful for risk-classification of thyroid follicular neoplasm? Abstract Booklet of the 19th International Congress of Cytology (ICC2016) .
17. Mete O, Asa S. Pathological definition and clinical significance of vascular invasion in thyroid carcinomas of follicular epithelial derivation. Mod Pathol 2011; 24:1545-52.
18. Cipriani NA, Nagar S, Kaplan SP, et al. Follicular thyroid carcinoma: how have histologic diagnoses changed in the last half-century and what are the prognostic implications? Thyroid 2015; 25:1209-16.
19. Kakudo K, Katoh R, Sakamoto A, et al. Thyroid gland: international case conference. Endocr Pathol 2002; 13:131-4.
20. Hirokawa M, Carney JA, Goellner JR, et al. Observer variation of encapsulated follicular lesions of the thyroid gland. Am J Surg Pathol 2002; 26:1508-14.
21. Lloyd RV, Erickson LA, Casey MB, et al. Observer variation in the diagnosis of follicular variant of papillary thyroid carcinoma. Am J Surg Pathol 2004; 28:1336-40.
22. Williams ED. Guest editorial: Two proposals regarding the terminology of thyroid tumors. Int J Surg Pathol 2000; 8:181-3.
23. Liu Z, Zhou G, Nakamura M, et al. Encapsulated follicular thyroid tumor with equivocal nuclear changes, so-called well-differentiated tumor of uncertain malignant potential: a morphological, immunohistochemical, and molecular appraisal. Cancer Sci 2011; 102:288-94.
24. Goffredo P, Cheung K, Roman SA, et al. Can minimally invasive follicular thyroid cancer be approached as a benign lesion? a population-level analysis of survival among 1,200 patients. Ann Surg Oncol 2013; 20:767-72.
25. Kakudo K, Bai Y, Liu Z, et al. Classification of thyroid follicular cell tumors: with special reference to borderline lesions. Endocr J 2012; 59:1-12.

Chapter 21

Poorly Differentiated Carcinoma vs. Well Differentiated Carcinoma

Mitsuyoshi Hirokawa and Ayana Suzuki

Case Report

The patient was a 52-year-old female. She was pointed out to have enlargement of the thyroid by medical check-up. Thyroid function tests were within normal limits, and all of the thyroglobulin antibody, thyroperoxidase antibody, and thyroglobulin receptor antibody were negative. She was referred to our hospital for close inspection. Ultrasonographic examination revealed a nodule occupying the left lobe and isthmus of the thyroid. The nodule measured 51 mm x 24 mm x 47 mm. It was slightly hypoechoic, solid, homogeneous, irregular shaped, and not associated with microcalcification. The border of the nodule was indistinct. Color Doppler ultrasound revealed a hypervascular flow. Ultrasonographic interpretation was a malignancy. Cytological report was malignancy, and its differential diagnoses were poorly differentiated carcinoma (PDC), follicular carcinoma, metastatic carcinoma, or carcinoma showing thymus-like differentiation (CASTLE). As the other primary site was not detected, she underwent a total thyroidectomy with modified lymph node dissection on the left side.

Cytological Findings

The smear was highly cellular. Carcinoma cells appeared as three-dimensional clusters or individual cells (Figure 1). Microfollicle-like pattern was focally seen. Carcinoma cells were less cohesive and varied in size (Figure 2). The nuclei were large, and some of them showed grooves and indentation (Figure 2). Intranuclear cytoplasmic inclusions were not observed. Chromatin pattern was finely granular, and single large nucleolus was prominent (Figure 3). The cytoplasm was moderately abundant and densely stained. A few mitotic figures were scattered (Figure 4). Necrotic materials were not seen.

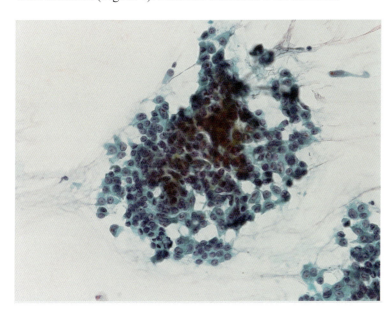

Figure 1. Three-dimensional and solid clusters are aggregated. (Pap, x20)

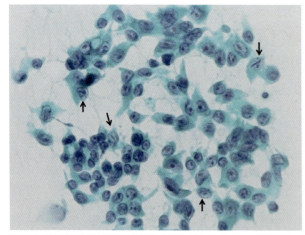

Figure 2. Carcinoma cells are less cohesive, and show large nuclei and moderately abundant cytoplasm. Some nuclei have grooves (arrow). (Papanicolaou, x400)

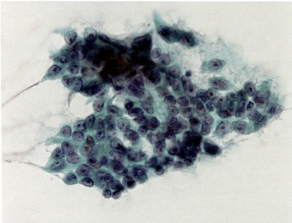

Fugure 3. The chromatin pattern is finely granular, and the nucleoli are large and prominent. (Pap, x40)

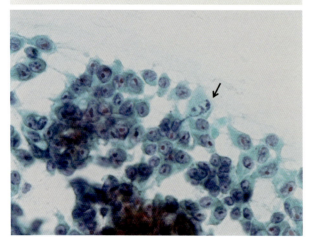

Figure 4. A mitotic figure is present (arrow). (Papanicolaou, x400)

List of Differential Diagnoses:
1. Benign: Hyperplastic nodule
2. Indeterminate: Follicular neoplasm

3. Malignant: Medullary (C cell) carcinoma
4. Malignant: Poorly differentiated carcinoma
5. Malignant: Metastatic carcinoma
6. Malignant: ITET/CASTLE

Pathologic Findings

The tumor occupied most of the left lobe and isthmus of the thyroid and measured 4.7 x 2.5 cm. On cut surface, it was solid, lobulated, whitish tan in color, invasive, and associated with multiple satellite nodules (Figure 5). Microscopically, carcinoma cells showed diffuse (Figure 6), alveolar (Figure 7), trabecular (Figure 8), and cribriform (Figure 9) growth patterns. There were no papillary or follicular patterns. The cytoplasm was moderately abundant and amphophilic. Some carcinoma cells revealed intracytoplasmic vacuoles in which mucous materials were not demonstrated. Carcinoma cells showed nuclear irregularity and a single prominent large nucleolus (Figure 10). Carcinoma cells invaded into the surrounding connective tissue. There were no metastatic lesions in dissected neck lymph nodes.

Immunohistochemically, the carcinoma cells were positive for cytokeratin 19 and galectin 3, and negative for HBME-1. Thyroglobulin was focally positive. Ectopic expression of beta-catenin was not observed. Estrogen receptor was negative, and p53 was positive (Figure 11). Ki-67 (MIB-1) labeling index was 5 to 10%. Pathological diagnosis was PDC.

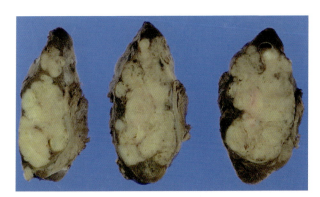

Figure 5. The thyroid is occupied with a solid, lobulated, invasive, whitish tan in color mass associated with multiple satellite nodules.

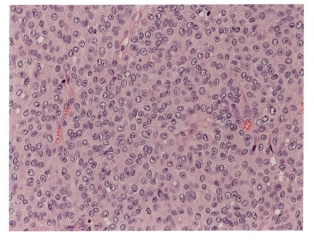

Figure 6. The carcinoma cells show diffuse growth pattern. (HE, x200)

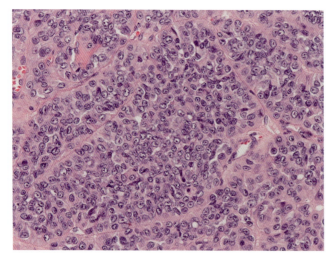

Figure 7. The carcinoma cells show alveolar growth pattern. (HE, x200)

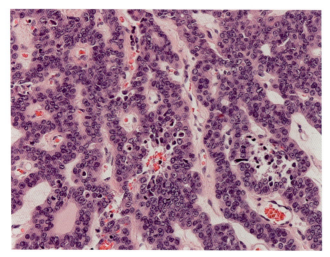

Figure 8. The carcinoma cells show trabecular growth pattern. (HE, x200)

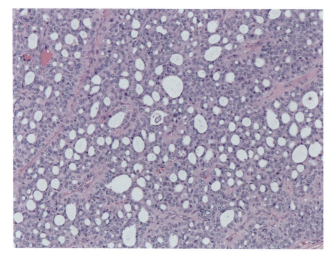

Figure 9. The carcinoma cells show cribriform growth pattern. (HE, x100)

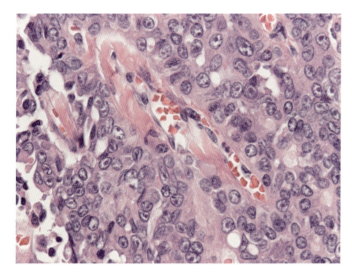

Figure 10. The nuclei of the carcinoma cells have irregularity and a single prominent large nucleolus. (HE, x400)

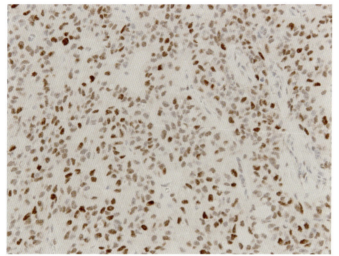

Figure 11. The carcinoma cells are positive for p53. (Immunostaining, x200)

Discussion

In 1983, Sakamoto *et al.* proposed PDC of the thyroid as a clinicopathologic entity for a high-risk group of papillary and follicular thyroid carcinomas (1). In 1984, Carcangiu *et al.* reported the poorly differentiated insular carcinoma, which presented solid clusters "insulae" of tumor cells containing a variable number of small follicles (2). Subsequently, various diagnostic criteria and terms concerning PDC have been employed. In 2004, World Health Organization (WHO) defined PDC as follicular cell neoplasm that shows limited evidence of structural follicular cell differentiation and occupies both morphologically and behaviorally an intermediated position between differentiated (follicular and papillary carcinomas) and undifferentiated (anaplastic) carcinomas (3). According to the classification, three different histologic patterns are recognized in PDC; insular, trabecular, and solid.

The cytological diagnosis of PDC is not easy because of the lack of well-established cytological features and a considerable degree of morphological overlap with other more common thyroid neoplasms. The architectural arrangement of carcinoma cells is the most important feature for rendering a diagnosis of PDC. Trabecular arrangement (Figures 1 and

12), large solid nests (Figure 3), and less-cohesive, singly dispersed cells (Figure 13) are characteristic of PDC, and they reflect histologically trabecular, insular, and solid growth patterns, respectively. Endothelial wrapping of cell clusters may be observed in the insular type (4-5). Purkait *et al.* have described that a peripheral orientation of the nuclei within cell clusters is characteristic of PDC, but the finding was not seen in the present case (5). Mitotic figures are occasionally observed (Figure 4), but necrotic materials are rarely demonstrated.

PDC is subdivided into papillary (please refer to mini-test case 1) and non-papillary types. As papillary arrangement and intranuclear cytoplasmic inclusions were not seen, the present case seemed to be non-papillary type. It is described that the cells of PDC are much smaller (please refer to Figure 11 in the Chapter 20) than the cells of differentiated thyroid cancers (follicular/papillary) and show scanty cytoplasm with a high N/C ratio (6, 7). However, in our experience, most of PDC are opposite, like the present case. We should keep in mind that PDC in Japan, where insular type (small cell type) PDC is rare, appears more atypical large cells than those of differentiated carcinoma. Typical papillary carcinoma cells with single cell pattern or solid clusters suggest the solid variant of papillary carcinoma (8, 9).

Non-papillary type PDC is frequently confused with follicular tumor; both can exhibit microfollicular pattern and inspissated colloid (7, 10). It is important to distinguish between an aggregation of microfollicles and multiple follicles within a large nest. The former is observed in follicular tumor, and the latter is present in PDC (7, 11). In addition, carcinoma cells in PDC are more atypical, except for the oxyphilic cell variant.

The distinction between PDC and CASTLE is problematic (please refer to Chapter 17). The presence of lymphocytes within cell clusters may indicate the latter (12, 13). The distinction between PDC and metastatic carcinoma is also difficult in the absence of colloid materials (please refer to Chapter 22). In such cases, clinical information and immunocytochemical examination are required. Conclusively, it is not difficult morphologically to recognize PDC as malignancy, but we have to differentiate it from other malignant tumors including well-differentiated carcinomas, CASTLEs, and metastatic carcinomas.

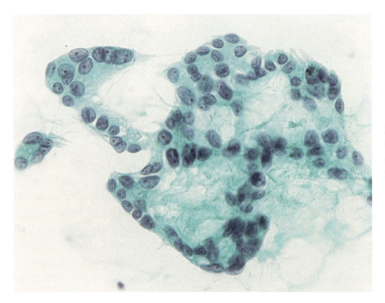

Figure 12. Poorly differentiated carcinoma showing trabecular arrangement. (Papanicolaou, x400)

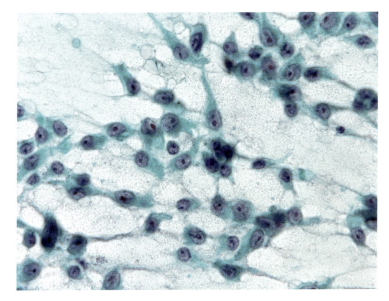

Figure 13. Poorly differentiated carcinoma showing less-cohesive, and singly dispersed arrangement. (Papanicolaou, x400)

References

1. Sakamoto A, Kasai N, Sugano H. Poorly differentiated carcinoma of the thyroid. A clinicopathologic entity for a high-risk group of papillary and follicular carcinomas. Cancer 1983; 52:1849-55.
2. Carcangiu ML, Zampi G, Rosai J. Poorly differentiated ("insular") thyroid carcinoma. A reinterpretation of Langhans' "wuchernde Struma". Am J Surg Pathol 1984; 8:655-68.
3. DeLellis RA, Lloyd RV, Heintz PU. Pathology and Genetics: Tumors of Endocrine Organs. WHO Classification of Tumors. Lyon: IARC Press, 2004, p73-76.
4. Kini H, Nirupama M, Rau AR, et al. Poorly differentiated (insular) thyroid carcinoma arising in a long-standing colloid goitre: A cytological dilemma. J Cytol 2012; 29:97-9.
5. Purkait S, Agarwal S, Mathur SR, et al. Fine needle aspiration cytology features of poorly differentiated thyroid carcinoma. Cytopathol 2015 (early view).
6. Kini SR. Thyroid Cytopathology: An Atlas and Text. Philadelphia, PA: Lippincott Williams & Wilkins; 2008, p220-32.
7. Kane SV, Sharma TP. Cytologic diagnostic approach to poorly differentiated thyroid carcinoma: a single-institution study. Cancer Cytopathol 2015; 123:82-91.
8. Giorgadze TA, Scognamiglio T, Yang GC. Fine-needle aspiration cytology of the solid variant of papillary thyroid carcinoma: a study of 13 cases with clinical, histologic, and ultrasound correlations. Cancer Cytopathol 2015; 123:71-81.
9. Damle N, Ramya S, Bal C, et al. Solid variant of papillary carcinoma thyroid in a child with no history of radiation exposure. Indian J Nucl Med 2011; 26:196-8.
10. Barwad A, Dey P, Nahar Saikia U, et al. Fine needle aspiration cytology of insular carcinoma of thyroid. Diagn Cytopathol 2012; 40 (Suppl 1):E43-47.
11. Patel KN, Shaha AR. Poorly differentiated and anaplastic thyroid cancer. Cancer Control 2006; 13:119-28.
12. Da J, Shi H, Lu J. Thyroid squamous-cell carcinoma showing thymus-like element (CASTLE): a report of eight cases. Zhonghua Zong Liu Za Zhi 1999; 21:303-4.
13. Liu Z, Teng XY, Sun DX, et al. Clinical analysis of thyroid carcinoma showing thymus-like differentiation: report of 8 cases. Int Surg 2013; 98:95-100.

Chapter 22

Metastatic Renal Cell Carcinoma vs. Follicular Neoplasm

Ayana Suzuki

Case Report
    The patient was a 67-year-old male who experienced pharyngeal discomfort for three months. He had a history of right nephrectomy for renal cell carcinoma (RCC) one year ago. He visited other hospital and a mass was detected in the right lobe of thyroid. As fine needle aspiration cytology was classified as "atypia of undetermined significance/follicular lesion of undetermined significance", he was referred to our hospital. Ultrasonographic examination showed a tumor, measuring 62 x 33 x 36 mm, in the right lobe of thyroid. It was multinodular, hypoechoic (Figure 1), and rich in blood flow. The left lobe was unremarkable. Aspiration cytology revealed malignant cells, and metastatic RCC was suspected by immunocytochemical analysis. He underwent right lobectomy with central and right lateral neck lymph node dissection.

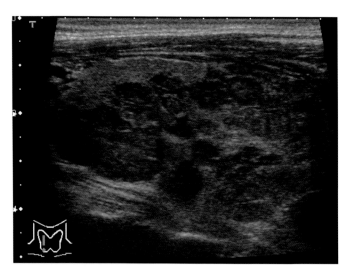

Figure 1. A multinodular and hypoechoic mass in the right lobe. (Ultrasound B-mode image)

Cytological Findings
    The aspirated materials were bloody and cellular. Colloid material was not observed. The atypical cells appeared as solid clusters or isolated naked cells (Figure 2). Apparent microfollicular pattern was not seen. They were large and round or spindle in shape. The cytoplasm was weakly stained and the cell border was indistinct (Figure 3). The nuclei were large and darkly stained, with a large and prominent nucleolus (Figure 4). As metastatic RCC was cytologically suspected, immunocytochemical examination using the liquid-based cytology sample was performed. The carcinoma cells were positive for CD10 (Figure 5), and negative for thyroglobulin and TTF-1.

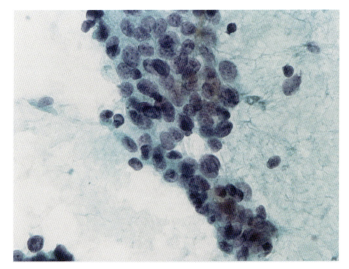

Figure 2: A solid cluster and a few isolated naked cells are seen. (Pap, x40)

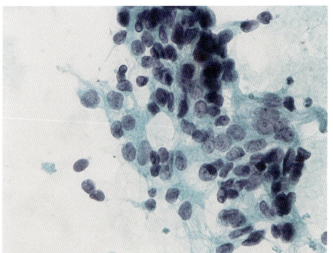

Figure 3. The cytoplasm is faintly stained and the cell border is indistinct. (Papanicolaou, x400)

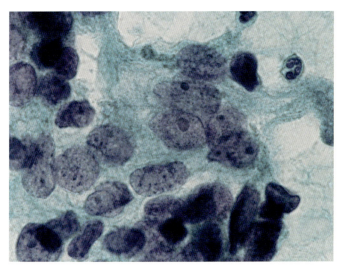

Figure 4. The nuclei are large and darkly stained. Some nuclei have a large prominent nucleolus. (Papanicolaou, x1000)

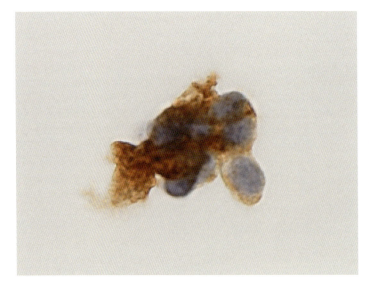

Figure 5. The cytoplasm of carcinoma cells is positive for CD10. (Immunostaining, LBC, x1000)

List of Differential Diagnoses:
1. Benign: Hyperplastic nodule
2. Indeterminate: Follicular neoplasm
3. Malignant: Poorly differentiated carcinoma
4. Malignant: Papillary carcinoma
5. Malignant: Metastatic carcinoma

Pathological Findings

The carcinoma was multinodular, occupying the entire right lobe, but it did not invade into the surrounding connective tissue (Figure 6). The lesions were solid, whitish, and associated with focal hemorrhagic and cystic areas. The carcinoma cells showed alveolar and trabecular growth patterns and the stroma was highly vascular (Figure 7). The cytoplasm was clear (Figure 7). The nuclei exhibited prominent irregularity. Immunohistochemical examination revealed CD10 positivity (Figure 8). Ki-67 (MIB-1) labeling index was more than 80%. Victoria-blue HE stain demonstrated multiple vascular invasions. There were no carcinoma cells at the resected margin of the isthmian side. Central and right lateral lymph nodes exhibited metastatic RCC.

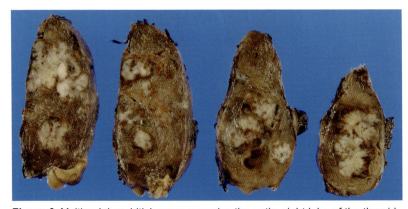

Figure 6. Multinodular whitish mass occupies the entire right lobe of the thyroid.

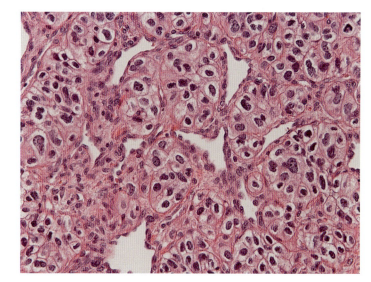

Figure 7. The carcinoma cells show clear cytoplasm and nuclear irregularity. (HE, x200)

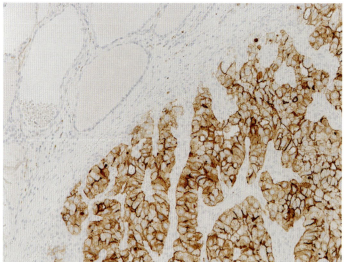

Figure 8. The cell membrane of carcinoma cells is positive for CD10. (Immunostaining, x100)

Differential Diagnoses

Metastatic thyroid carcinoma in patients with extensive metastatic foci is not rare (1, 2), and the lesions are usually multifocal and variable in size. By contrast, clinically significant metastatic thyroid carcinoma is rare. The lesions may be solitary and, necessitating differentiation from primary thyroid tumors (1). Carcinomas originating in surrounding organs tend to involve a single lobe and appear as a large mass. The majority of the patients with metastatic lesions in the thyroid are asymptomatic. Rarely, they may masquerade as primary thyroid tumors or be associated with symptoms of hyperthyroidism or subacute thyroiditis (1, 3).

Among surgical cases, the most common carcinoma metastasizing to the thyroid is those of the kidney (25~33%), followed by the lung (16~25%), breast (12~16%), esophagus (4~9%), uterus (3~7%), stomach (4%), and skin (4%) (1,4,5). The average period from diagnosis of the primary carcinoma to metastasis to the thyroid gland is relatively long, e.g., 106 months for those from the kidney, 131 months from the breast, and 132 months from the uterus (5). As a case with a 22-year-interval has been reported, it is crucial to assess the clinical history before an aspiration (4). However, the metastatic thyroid carcinoma may be found as the initial presentation of an occult primary tumor (6, 7).

RCC is clinically the most common malignant tumor metastasizing to the thyroid (1). According to a report by Kobayashi *et al.* who described 10 RCC cases metastasizing to the thyroid, eight cases presented with previous medical histories of nephrectomy for RCC (7). In the remaining two cases, the primary sites were identified after the thyroidectomy. Interestingly, in 80% of the cases, the primary sites were located in the right kidney, and metastatic sites were present in the right lobe of the thyroid. The metastatic lesions are usually multiple. RCC occasionally metastasizes into primary thyroid tumors, such as follicular variant of papillary thyroid carcinoma, follicular adenoma or adenomatous goiter (8). In such cases, the lesions are solitary (9). When the metastatic lesions are confined within the thyroid, a surgical approach for the diseases promises a favorable prognosis (9).

Cytological smears of metastatic RCC are generally bloody and less cellular because of their high vascularity. Carcinoma cells exhibit trabecular, follicular, sheet-like, or solid clusters. The N/C ratio, cytoplasmic staining, and cell border are diverse, depending on the cell types or smearing techniques. The cytoplasm tends to be abundant and clear or faintly staining. Even in clear cell type of RCC, the cytoplasm may be densely stained. Nuclei are centrally or eccentrically located, and their characteristics vary according to the grade (10). Nucleoli are prominent (10), but their sizes vary. Pale cytoplasm and disrupted cell border result in bare nuclei that are small and uniform (1). Intranuclear cytoplasmic inclusions may be observed (11).

Solitary RCC metastasizing to the thyroid is cytologically difficult to distinguish from follicular neoplasm. The differential diagnostic features between metastatic RCC and follicular neoplasm are shown in Table 1. Both tumors exhibit bloody background, trabecular pattern, and weakly stained cytoplasm. The presence of colloid material within the clusters strongly indicates follicular neoplasm. RCC having intranuclear cytoplasmic inclusions needs to be distinguished from papillary thyroid carcinoma. The cytoplasm of RCC is usually more pale than that of PTC, but may be densely stained even in typical clear cell type.

Immunocytochemical staining is useful to distinguish metastatic RCC from follicular neoplasm. RCC is positive for CD10, RCC, and EMA (epithelial membrane antigen), and negative for TTF-1 (thyroid transcription factor 1) and thyroglobulin. Follicular neoplasm shows the opposite pattern. Amongst them, TTF-1 is the most reliable, because the immunostaining exhibits the least false positivity and false negativity (4). As thyroglobulin immunostaining tends to show diffusion artifact from surrounding tissues, the interpretation is frequently difficult (12).

Table 1. Differential diagnoses of metastatic renal cell carcinoma and follicular neoplasm

	Renal cell carcinoma	Follicular neoplasm
Background	Bloody	Bloody, hyaline colloid
Arrangement	Alveolar, trabecular, sheet-like, solid	Small follicular, trabecular, follicle with colloid material
Cell border	Indistinct or distinct	Indistinct
Cytoplasm	Clear to dense	Weakly stained
Nuclei	Round, irregular	Round
Chromatin pattern	Fine to granular	Fine to granular
Intracytoplasmic inclusion	May present	Not present
Nucleoli	Prominent	Variable
Immunostaining		
Thyroglobulin	Negative	Positive
TTF-1	Negative	Positive
CD10	Positive	Negative
RCC	Positive	Negative
EMA	Positive	Negative

TTF-1: thyroid transcription factor 1; EMA: epithelial membrane antigen

References

1. Kini SR. Thyroid Cytopathology; An Atlas and Text. Philadelphia: Lippincott Williams & Wilkins; 2008, p358-63.
2. Pusztaszeri M, Wang H, Cibas ES, et al. Fine-needle aspiration biopsy of secondary neoplasms of the thyroid gland: a multi-institutional study of 62 cases. Cancer Cytopathol 2015; 123:19-29.
3. Rikabi AC, Young AE, Wilson C. Metastatic renal clear cell carcinoma in the thyroid gland diagnosed by fine needle aspiration cytology. Cytopathol 1991; 2:47-9.
4. Nikiforov YE, Biddinger PW, Thompson LD. Diagnostic Pathology and Molecular Genetics of the Thyroid; A comprehensive guide for practicing thyroid pathology. Philadelphia: Lippincott Williams & Wilkins; 2009, p348-56.
5. Nakhjavani MK, Gharib H, Goellner JR, et al. Metastasis to the thyroid gland. A report of 43 cases. Cancer 1997; 79:574-8.
6. Dal FS, Monari G, Barbazza R. A thyroid metastasis revealing an occult renal clear-cell carcinoma. Tumori 1987; 73:187-90.
7. Kobayashi K, Hirokawa M, Yabuta T, et al. Metastatic carcinoma to the thyroid gland from renal cell carcinoma: role of ultrasonography in preoperative diagnosis. Thyroid Res 2015; 8 (open access).
8. Medas F, Calo PG, Lai ML, et al. Renal cell carcinoma metastasis to thyroid tumor: a case report and review of the literature. J Med Report 2013; 7:265.
9. Dionigi G, Uccella S, Gandolfo M, et al. Solitary intrathyroidal metastasis of renal clear cell carcinoma in a toxic substernal mutinodulargoiter. Thyroid Res 2008; 1.
10. Lew M, Foo WC, Roh MH. Diagnosis of metastatic renal cell carcinoma on fine-needle aspiration cytology. Arch Pathol Lab Med 2014; 138:1278-85.
11. Gritsman AY, Popok SM, Ro JY, et al. Renal-cell carcinoma with intranuclear inclusions metastatic to thyroid: a diagnostic problem in aspiration cytology. Diagn Cytopathol 1988; 4:125-9.
12. Kanjanahattakij N, Chayangsu P, Kanoksil W, et al. Pitfall in immunohistochemical staining for thyroglobulin in case of thyroid metastasis from lung carcinoma. Cytol J 2015; 12:27.

Chapter 23

Biochemical Tests of Fine-needle Aspirate as an Adjunct to Cytologic Diagnosis for Patients with Thyroid Cancer or Primary Hyperparathyroidism

Shinya Satoh, Hiroyuki Yamashita and Kennichi Kakudo

Introduction

Fine-needle aspiration cytology (FNAC) represents the main tool in the evaluation of thyroid tumors. However, it is not possible to reach an accurate diagnosis when there are only few cell clusters in the aspirated specimen. The measurement of organ-specific products in the aspirate is a helpful adjunctive method for cyto-morphological diagnosis, similar to that of serum tumor markers. In our practice, thyroglobulin (TG) and/or calcitonin (CT) in the needle aspirate from the neck lymph nodes are often measured when FNAC is performed. Parathyroid hormone (PTH) in the needle aspirate is also measured when localization studies fail to confirm an abnormal parathyroid gland in patients with primary hyperparathyroidism (PHPT).

Sampling Method (please refer to Chapter 30)

Ultrasound (US) is performed with a high frequency (10-12 MHz) probe. Ideally, all FNACs should be performed under US guidance, using a needle of 22-25 gauge needle attached to a 5- to 10-ml syringe. The aspirated specimen obtained from an individual tumor is immediately fixed and submitted for cytological examination. The needle with syringe is washed with 0.5 ml of saline solution, and the washout solution is submitted for biochemical tests.

TG Measurement in the Needle Washout (FNAC-TG)

TG is a 660 kDa dimeric glycoprotein produced and secreted only by the follicular cells of thyroid gland, and stored in the follicular lumen as colloid substance. Therefore, presence of TG in the needle aspirate from a tumor suggests that the tumor is originated from the thyroid gland. It is impossible to diagnose whether a tumor is malignant in thyroid gland based only on the presence of TG in the needle aspirate. However, this method is useful to establish the diagnosis of well-differentiated thyroid carcinoma when using biopsy samples obtained from possible distant metastatic lesions (e.g., enlarged lymph node, lung tumor, or bone tumor). Miyauchi *et al.* reported in 1983 that demonstration of very high content of TG in the aspirate from the neck cystic lymph node supported the diagnosis of metastatic papillary thyroid carcinoma (PTC) (1). In 1992, Pacini *et al.* proposed the measurement of TG in the washout from FNAC for early detection of neck lymph node metastasis in patients with well-differentiated thyroid carcinoma (2), and now this method is used widely among endocrinologists internationally (3, 4).

Case 1:

The patient was a 47-year-old female who had undergone a mastectomy for breast cancer. Postoperative US incidentally revealed a thyroid nodule and enlarged lymph nodes in her right lateral neck (Figure 1). The serum level of TG and anti-TG antibody was 142.7 ng/ml (<35.0) and 15.6 IU/ml (<28), respectively. The cytological diagnosis of the thyroid nodule was PTC. FNAC of the enlarged lymph node demonstrated many epithelial cell clusters on the smear, suggestive of PTC (Figures 2). The TG concentration of the needle washout from the lymph node was more than 500 ng/ml. Histological examination demonstrated metastatic PTC in the lymph node.

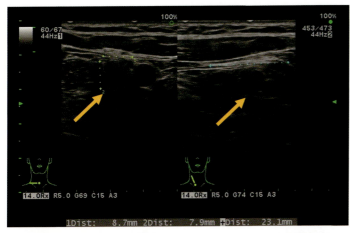

Figure 1. (Case 1) Ultrasound examination of the neck reveals an enlarged lymph node (yellow arrows) in the right lateral neck.

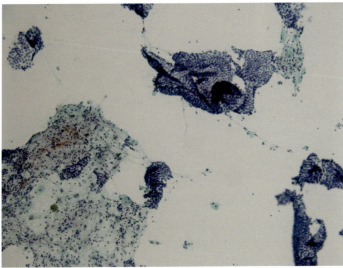

Figure 2. Papillary and monolayered type tissue fragments are observed. (Papanicolaou stain, x100).

Case 2:

A 46-year-old female presented with a six-month history of enlarged neck nodule. US showed a 2.0 cm thyroid nodule and a 3.6 cm enlarged cystic lymph node in her right lateral neck (Figure 3). The serum level of TG and anti-Tg antibody was 246.5 ng/ml (<35.0) and 16.4 IU/ml (<28), respectively. FNAC of the thyroid nodule was unsatisfactory due to the sparse cellularity. FNAC of the cystic lymph node demonstrated only one cell cluster suggestive of PTC in cystic background (Figure 4). The TG concentration of the needle washout was more than 500 ng/ml. The subsequent histological diagnosis revealed PTC with lymph node metastasis.

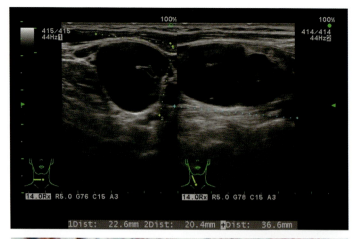

Figure 3. (Case 2) Ultrasound examination of the neck shows a 3.6 cm cystic nodule in the right lateral neck.

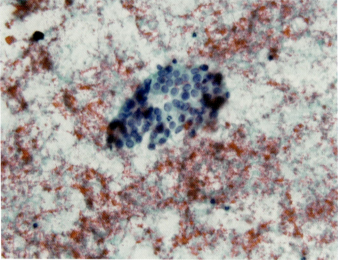

Figure 4. The sole cell cluster suggestive of papillary thyroid carcinoma is seen. Intranuclear grooves and nuclear inclusions are noted. (Papanicolaou stain, x400)

Calcitonin (CT) Measurement in the Needle Washout (FNAC-CT)

CT is a 32-amino acid linear polypeptide hormone produced primarily by the parafollicular (C) cells of thyroid. CT reduces blood calcium concentration, opposing the effects of PTH. Because CT is also an organ-specific product, it has been used as a tumor marker for the diagnosis of medullary (C cell) thyroid cancer (MTC), which produces excess amount of CT compared with normal C-cells, and elevated CT levels after surgery may indicate residual tumor mass and incomplete resection of the tumor. C cells account for about 0.1% of the thyroid epithelial cells and are found mainly around the junction of the upper third and the lower two-thirds of the thyroid lobes. The CT concentration in the needle aspirate is very low even that it is obtained from the C cell rich part. Upon the above physiology, FNAC-CT enables a diagnosis of MTC from not only lymph nodes but also thyroid nodules. In 2007, Boi *et al*. and Kudo *et al.* reported that the measurement of CT in the needle washout solution of FNAC could identify MTC with high sensitivity and specificity (5, 6). Other authors also reported that FNAC-CT could increase the diagnostic accuracy of cytology in the diagnosis of MTC when combining FNAC and FNAC-CT (7, 8).

Case 3:

A 75-year-old female had underwent a total thyroidectomy with neck dissection at the age of 63 because of MTC. Follow-up US detected an enlarged lymph node in the right side of her neck (Figure 5). The serum CT level was 1,847 pg/ml (0.5-4.0 pg/ml). Although FNAC from the lymph node was acellular and inadequate, the CT level of the needle washout solution was extremely high (467,335 pg/ml). The lymph node was removed and histological examination confirmed metastatic MTC.

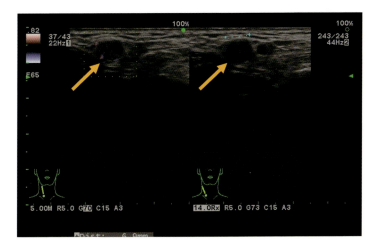

Figure 5. (Case 3) Ultrasound examination of the neck reveals a 7 mm round lymph node (yellow arrows) in the right lateral-posterior neck.

Case 4:

The patient was a 68-year-old female. Magnetic resonance imaging incidentally detected a thyroid nodule and enlarged lymph nodes in her neck (Figures 6 and 7). Because of the suspicion of PTC by US, the TG concentration in the aspirate from the lymph node was measured, but extremely low (4.16 ng/ml). The lymph node was suspected to be metastasis of MTC by cytological examination (Figures 8 and 9). (Please refer to Chapters 15 and 16). Her serum CT level was measured to be 15,400 pg/ml before thyroidectomy. Although we did not have an opportunity to measure CT level of the needle washout in this case, the low level of TG in the lymph node FNA washout was inconsistent with the previous clinical diagnosis of lymph node metastasis from PTC, which helped us to reach a correct cytological diagnosis. Total thyroidectomy with lateral neck dissection was performed, and the final histological diagnosis was MTC (papillary type) (Figure 10) with lymph node metastasis.

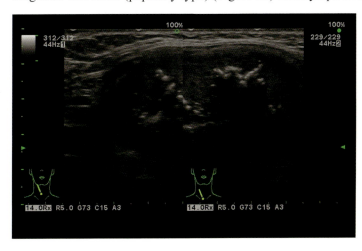

Figure 6. (Case 4) A 40 mm isoechoic nodule with coarse calcification is demonstrated in the right lobe of the thyroid.

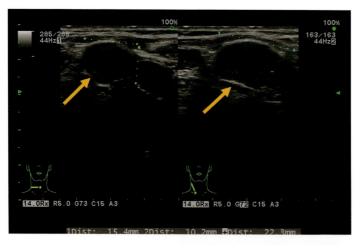

Figure 7. (Case 4) Ultrasound examination of the neck shows a 2.3 cm hypoechoic solid nodule (yellow arrows) in the right lateral neck. This nodule is suspected to be a metastatic lesion in the lymph node from the thyroid nodule.

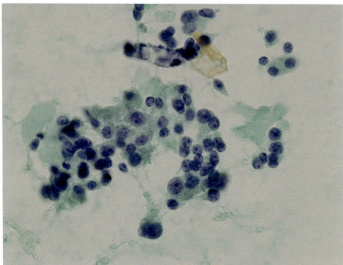

Figure 8. FNA of the enlarged lymph node. The aspirated cells exhibit marked pleomorphism in cell size and shape. A salt-and-pepper chromatin pattern of the nuclei suggesting C cell (medullary) carcinoma is partly seen. (Papanicolaou stain, x400)

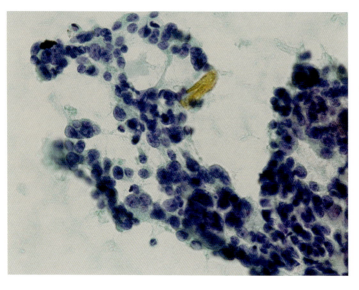

Figure 9. Some of these cells in this aspirate are compactly arranged in a tissue fragment. This cellular pattern may be erroneously interpreted to denote a follicular pattern lesion. (Papanicolaou stain, x400)

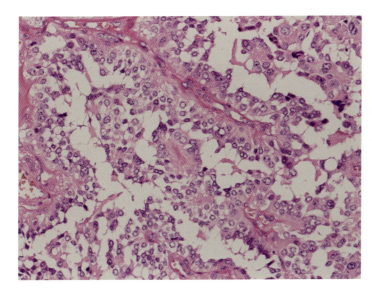

Figure 10. Histological section of the thyroid nodule reveals medullary (C cell) carcinoma, papillary type. The nuclei are oval to round, and the cytoplasm varies from scant to abundant. Note the nuclei of these tumor cells do not show PTC type nuclear features. (HE stain, x200)

PTH Measurement in the Needle Washout (FNAC-PTH)

PTH is secreted by the chief cells of parathyroid glands as a polypeptide containing 84 amino acids. PTH essentially acts to increase blood calcium concentration. PHPT is caused by autonomous and abnormal hypersecretion of PTH from the enlarged parathyroid gland that is histologically diagnosed as adenoma, hyperplasia, or carcinoma. Although surgery of parathyroidectomy offers definitive treatment, resulting in cure in more than 95% of the disease when performed by an experienced surgeon, preoperative localization studies such as US, computed tomography, and technetium-99m sestamibi (MIBI) scintigraphy should be performed to ensure a successful surgery. These localization studies can generally successfully identify one or more abnormal parathyroid gland(s) in almost all patients with PHPT, but there are some cases that abnormal parathyroid(s) fail to be detected with these studies, and often due to the coexistence of thyroid diseases. In such cases, it is possible to obtain confirmation of the parathyroid nature of a suspicious nodule by measuring PTH in the needle washout solution of the nodule. In 1983, Doppman *et al*. reported that the measurement of high concentration of PTH in the aspirate from a neck or mediastinal mass under computed tomography guidance of needle position has provided absolute localization of parathyroid masses (9). Although preoperative localization studies in patients with PHPT change over the time, the usefulness of FNAC-PTH for preoperative localization has been reported (10-12) (please refer to Chapter 18).

Case 5:

The patient was a 59-year-old female with a history of nephrolithiasis. She was incidentally found to have hypercalcemia by a blood test. Her serum calcium level was 11.1 mg/dl (8.8-10.2), and her intact PTH level was 236.6 pg/ml (10-65). In the left thyroid lobe, a 1.5 cm cystic nodule was detected with US (Figure 11). MIBI scintigraphy showed an increased uptake in the left lower pole of the thyroid (Figure 12). Since US findings of the nodule were not typical as an intrathyroid parathyroid adenoma, an FNAC was performed and the smear was submitted for cytological examination (Figure 13). The needle washout solution was also submitted for PTH measurement and the PTH level was more than 5000 pg/ml. Partial lobectomy was performed based on the preoperative diagnosis of intrathyroid parathyroid ademoma. After lobectomy, her serum calcium and intact PTH levels returned to the normal range. An intrathyroid parathyroid adenoma, separated from the thyroid tissue by a fibrous capsule, was confirmed by histological examination (Figures 14 and 15)

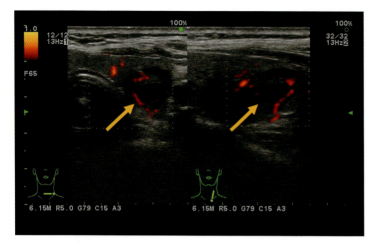

Figure 11. Ultrasound examination of the neck reveals a 1.5 cm cystic nodule in the left lower pole of thyroid.

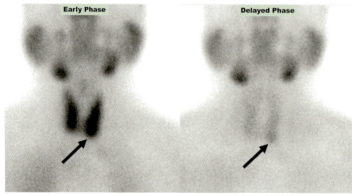

Figure 12. Technetium-99m sestamibi scintigram shows an increased uptake in the left lower pole of thyroid.

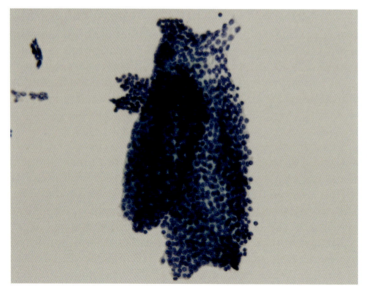

Figure 13. FNA of the cystic nodule in thyroid. The syncytial tissue fragment consists of small cells with extreme crowding and overlapping of the round nuclei. (Papanicolaou stain, x100)

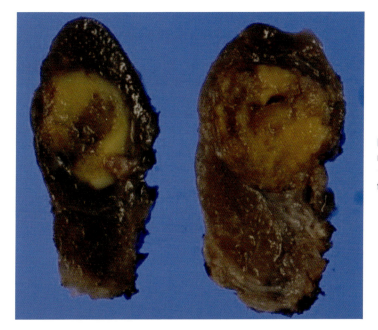

Figure 14. Cut surface of the resected thyroid. A solid nodule, 12 mm x 10 mm, is found within the resected thyroid tissue.

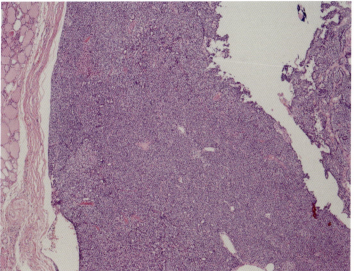

Figure 15. A parathyroid adenoma composed of chief cells with solid growth, and surrounded by fibrous capsule and thyroid parenchyma. (HE stain, x20)

Take Home Message

The measurement of TG and CT concentrations in aspiration needle washout solution is a simple and useful method for the diagnosis of PTC and MTC. As the measurement of PTH in aspiration needle washout solution is useful to confirm the parathyroid tumor, this method should be considered, especially when re-operation is scheduled for patients with recurrent or persistent PHPT.

References

1. Miyauchi A, Takai S, Morimoto S, et al. Fine needle aspiration of neck tumor. Application of cytological, bacteriological and hormonal examinations. Nihon Geka Gakkai Zasshi 1983; 84:667-73.
2. Pacini F, Fugazzola L, Lippi F, et al. Detection of thyroglobulin in fine needle aspirates of nonthyroidal neck masses: a clue to the diagnosis of metastatic differentiated thyroid cancer. J Clin Endocrinol Metab 1992; 74:1401-4.
3. Cunha N, Rodrigues F, Curado F, et al. Thyroglobulin detection in fine-needle aspirates of cervical lymph nodes: a technique for the diagnosis of metastatic differentiated thyroid cancer. Eur J Endocrinol 2007; 157:101-7.
4. Boi F, Baghino G, Atzeni F, et al. The diagnostic value for differentiated thyroid carcinoma metastases of thyroglobulin (Tg) measurement in washout fluid from fine-needle aspiration biopsy of neck lymph nodes is maintained in the presence of circulating anti-Tg antibodies. J Clin Endocrinol Metab 2006; 91:1364-9.
5. Boi F, Maurelli I, Pinna G, et al. Calcitonin measurement in wash-out fluid from fine needle aspiration of neck masses in patients with primary and metastatic medullary thyroid carcinoma. J Clin Endocrinol Metab 2007; 92:2115-8.
6. Kudo T, Miyauchi A, Ito Y, et al. Diagnosis of medullary thyroid carcinoma by calcitonin measurement in fine-needle aspiration biopsy specimens. Thyroid 2007; 17:635-8.
7. Trimboli P, Cremonini N, Ceriani L, et al. Calcitonin measurement in aspiration needle washout fluids has higher sensitivity than cytology in detecting medullary thyroid cancer: a retrospective multicenter study. Clin Endocrinol (Oxf) 2014; 80:135-40.
8. de Crea C, Raffaelli M, Maccora D, et al. Calcitonin measurement in fine-needle aspirate washouts vs. cytologic examination for diagnosis of primary or metastatic medullary thyroid carcinoma. Acta Otorhinolaryngol Ital 2014; 34:399-405.
9. Doppman JL, Krudy AG, Marx SJ, et al. Aspiration of enlarged parathyroid glands for parathyroid hormone assay. Radiology 1983; 148:31-5.
10. MacFarlane MP, Fraker DL, Shawker TH, et al. Use of preoperative fine-needle aspiration in patients undergoing reoperation for primary hyperparathyroidism. Surgery 1994; 116:959-64.
11. Marcocci C, Mazzeo S, Bruno-Bossio G, et al. Preoperative localization of suspicious parathyroid adenomas by assay of parathyroid hormone in needle aspirates. Eur J Endocrinol 1998; 139:72-7.
12. Yabuta T, Tsushima Y, Masuoka H, et al. Ultrasonographic features of intrathyroidal parathyroid adenoma causing primary hyperiparathyroidsm. Endocr J 2011; 58:989-94.

Chapter 24

Infectious Thyroiditis

Claire W. Michael and Xin Jing

Brief Clinical History

A 39-year-old man who presented to the emergency room with tachycardia, headache associated with retrobulbar pain, nausea, vomiting, and fatigue. His blood pressure was 160/90 mm Hg. The patient had a medical history significant for type 1 diabetes mellitus for 27 years complicated by end stage renal disease. He received a renal transplant eight years prior to presentation and subsequently a pancreatic transplant. During his work-up, it was found that he had a painless enlarged thyroid (1).

Laboratory Tests

He had normal blood cell count of 8100 cells per microliter with lymphopenia and relative monocytosis (neutrophils 67.8%, lymphocytes 11.2% and monocytes 19.9%). Thyroid function test indicated hyperthyroidism (FT_4, 3.8 ng/dl and TSH <0.01 mU/L). Testing for anti-thyroglobulin antibodies and anti-thyroid peroxidase was negative. Because of his persistent headache, a lumbar puncture was performed.

Radiological Tests

Thyroid uptake of radioactive iodine performed on the third day of admission was 0.7% (normal range, 7-30). Whole body scan after administration of 185 MBq of gallium-citrate exhibited intense uptake in the thyroid gland at 24 hours.

Ultrasound Findings

Ultrasonography (US) performed on day 5 revealed a diffusely heterogeneous asymmetrically enlarged thyroid, three times the normal, with the right lobe larger than the left. Fine needle aspiration (FNA) of the right lobe was performed.

Cytological Findings:

A rapid onsite assessment was performed during US-guided FNA of the right thyroid. Air-dried Diff-Quick-stained conventional smears performed on site revealed highly cellular smears containing clusters of follicular cells with relatively more cytoplasm than expected in a background of scatted lymphocytes and multinucleated giant cells, and few fragments of colloid (Figure 1). Examining the smears at high magnification, the pathologist also noticed that occasional follicular cells both loose in the background and within the clusters were unusually vacuolated containing pink rounded to oval structures surrounded by a halo, consistent with fungal spores (Figure 2). Also noted were scattered multinucleated giant cells occasionally ingesting colloid and focal granulomas (Figures 3-5). Ethanol-fixed smears stained with Papanicolaou stain exhibited similar findings (Figure 6). Grocott's methenamine silver nitrate fungal stain (GMS) demonstrated fungal spores morphologically, consistent with Cryptococcus neoformans (Figure 7).

Simultaneous cytological examination of the cerebrospinal fluid (CSF) revealed similar spores confirmed by CSF cryptococcal antigen titer of 1:1024 and a serum antigen titer of 1:512 as well as positive blood cultures.

Clinical Management:
The patient was consequently treated with amphotericin B and flucytosine. His thyroid function transitioned to hypothyroid and eventually euthyroid.

List of Differential Diagnoses:
1. Infectious thyroiditis
2. Autoimmune lymphocytic thyroiditis/Hashimoto's thyroiditis
3. Subacute granulomatous thyroiditis (De Quervain)

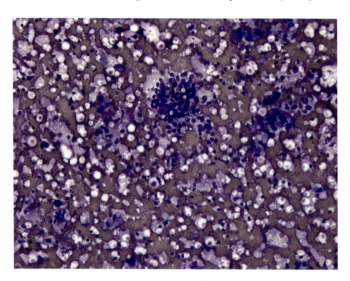

Figure 1. Cellular smear containing aggregates of follicular cells in a highly vacuolated background containing scattered histiocytes and lymphocytes. Even at this magnification the vacuoles contain small rounded to oval pink structures. (Conventional smear, Diff-Quik stain, x200)

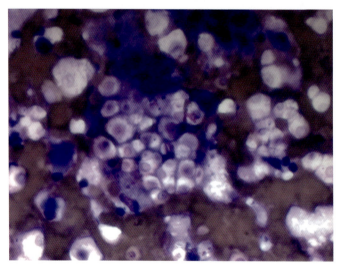

Figure 2. Higher magnification showing that the follicular cells and background histiocytes are highly vacuolated. The vacuoles contain small well-defined round to oval structures surrounded by a halo, consistent with cryptococcal fungal spores. (Conventional smear, Diff-Quik stain, x600)

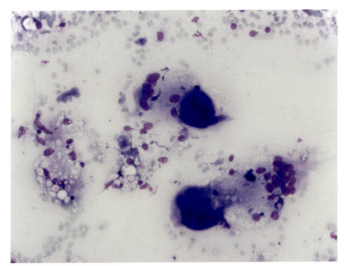

Figure 3. Scattered multinucleated histiocytes occasionally ingesting colloid and with intracytoplasmic spores. Also note the few scattered epithelioid spindled histiocytes and scattered lymphocytes. (Conventional smear, Diff-Quik stain, x400)

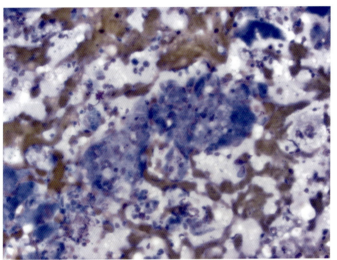

Figure 4. Aggregated multinucleated histiocytes with intracytoplasmic spores in the background of inflammatory cells, histiocytes and small fragments of colloid. (Conventional smear, Diff-Quik stain, x600)

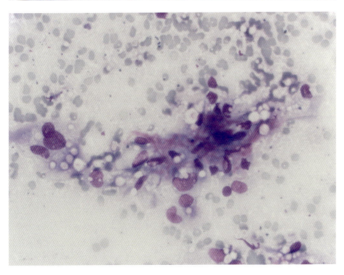

Figure 5. A loose granuloma consisting of aggregated epithelioid histiocytes containing and surrounded by fungal spores. (Conventional smear, Diff-Quik stain, x600)

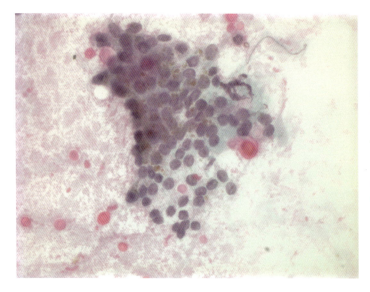

Figure 6. A follicular cluster with intracytoplasmic rounded pink structures surrounded by a halo, consistent with cryptococcal spores with surrounding capsules. Similar spores are also seen in the background. (Conventional smear, Papanicolaou stain, x600)

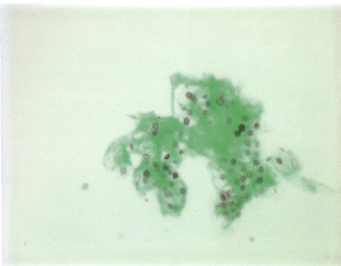

Figure 7. Spores stained as black rounded structures. (ThinPrep, Grocott's methenamine Silver stain, x400)

Discussion:

The thyroid gland is generally resistant to infection because of its fibrous capsule separating it from other structures of the neck, its rich blood supply and lymphatic drainage, and its content of hydrogen peroxide and iodine, which serve as bactericidal agents.

Infectious thyroiditis is the least common cause of thyroiditis. The most common cause is suppurative thyroiditis primarily due to bacterial infections with less than 600 cases reported in the literature. The most common causative organisms are Staphylococcus aureus, Streptococcus pyogenes, Staphylococcus epidermis and Streptococcus pneumonia in descending order. However, many infections are polymicrobial and the offending bacteria are widely variable depending on the immune status of the patient. Infections are most commonly due to either direct extension in the neck or iatrogenic inoculation due to trauma or needle such as post FNA (please refer to Chapter 26). Predisposing factors include congenital anomalies such as persistent thyroglossal duct cyst or piriform sinus fistula (please refer to Chapter 32, mini-test case 8), immunosuppression, and old age. Patients are usually euthyroid throughout the course of their disease. Ultrasound examination demonstrates a homogeneous echo-texture of the thyroid with superimposed anechoic or hypo-echoic nodule. The presence of abscess would present as peripheral hyper-vascularity with no significant interval vascular flow (2, 3). Other rare causes of suppurative thyroiditis including Salmonella typhimurium and Nocardia have been reported (4, 5). Diagnosis can be established by FNA, which will reveal purulent exudate and confirmed by cultures. Rare examples of viral related subacute thyroiditis presenting as hyperthyroidism and heterogeneously enlarged thyroid have also been reported (6, 7).

Fungal related thyroiditis has been reported in less than 70 cases. The patients generally suffered comorbidities contributing to an immunosuppressed status. At least 40 cases were related to Aspergillus, of which 25 cases were diagnosed postmortem in patients with disseminated infection and history of hematological or lympho-reticular malignancies. Fifteen cases were diagnosed antemortem by FNA (8). A wide range of other fungal induced thyroiditis has also been reported in the remaining cases, predominantly diagnosed by FNA (9). Cryptococcal thyroiditis has been reported in a total of four cases including the above described case. All but this case died during the course of their disease (1).

In general, most patients presented with diffusely enlarged heterogeneous thyroid gland and hyperthyroidism although few presented with hypothyroidism or euthyroidism. The hyperthyroidism is presumed to be related to the destruction of thyroid follicles and release of colloid. The clinical picture is usually indistinguishable from subacute thyroiditis such as local tenderness, fever, dysphagia, and dysphonia. Few cases presented with no tenderness. US- guided FNA is currently accepted as the best diagnostic modality. Smears usually reveal a granulomatous process with scattered lymphocytes and epithelioid histiocytes. The extent of necrosis and number of follicular cells could vary among cases. Fungal spores or hyphae can be easily detected or may require diligent search of the necrotic debris particularly in the case of necrotizing lesions (please refer to Chapter 26).

Differential diagnosis should include autoimmune lymphocytic thyroiditis (LT) and subacute thyroiditis, i.e. De Quervain (DQT) (please refer to Chapter 11). Smears in active LT may be highly cellular and contain either a diffuse lymphocytic infiltrate, Hürthle cell hyperplasia or a combination of both (please refer to Chapter 13). The follicular/Hürthle cell aggregates may be infiltrated by lymphocytes. Few multinucleated giant cells sometimes with ingested colloid may be detected in the background. Colloid may be seen but usually not a conspicuous feature (Figure 8) (10). In contrast, smears from DQT tend to be low in cellularity and present with few disrupted follicles infiltrated by lymphocytes or neutrophils (please refer to Chapter 11). Epithelioid histiocytes rather than well-formed granulomas are characteristic. Few droplets of hard colloid may be detected (11). Neither overt necrosis nor micro-organisms are features seen in either disease.

Take Home Message

Fungal thyroiditis is a very rare disease. However, it should be considered in the differential diagnosis of a thyroid FNA from an immunosuppressed patient presenting with a diffusely enlarged heterogeneous thyroid, thyrotoxicosis and smears containing lymphocytes, epithelioid histiocytes, or necrosis.

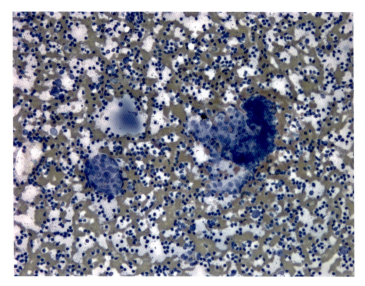

Figure 8. Lymphocytic thyroiditis exhibiting tightly cohesive follicular and Hürthle cell clusters in a background of numerous lymphocytes and a rare fragment of colloid. (Conventional smear, Diff-Quik stain, x200)

References:
1. Avram AM, Sturm CA, Michael CW, et al. Cryptococcal thyroiditis and hyperthyroidism. Thyroid 2004; 14(6):471-4.
2. Bravo E, Grayev A. Thyroid abscess as a complication of bacterial throat infection. J Radiol Case Rep 2011; 5(3):1-7.
3. Sheng Q, Lv Z, Xiao X, et al. Diagnosis and management of pyriform sinus fistula: experience in 48 cases. J Pediatr Surg 2014; 49(3):455-9.
4. Carriere C, Marchandin H, Andrieu JM, et al. Nocardia thyroiditis: unusual location of infection. J Clin Microbiol 1999; 37(7):2323-5.
5. Su DH, Huang TS. Acute suppurative thyroiditis caused by Salmonella typhimurium: a case report and review of the literature. Thyroid 2002; 12(11):1023-7.
6. Assir MZ, Jawa A, Ahmed HI. Expanded dengue syndrome: subacute thyroiditis and intracerebral hemorrhage. BMC Infect Dis 2012; 12:240.
7. Kawano C, Muroi K, Akioka T, et al. Cytomegalovirus pneumonitis, activated prothrombin time prolongation and subacute thyroiditis after unrelated allogeneic bone marrow transplantation. Bone Marrow Transplant 2000; 26(12):1347-9.
8. Nguyen J, Manera R, Minutti C. Aspergillus thyroiditis: a review of the literature to highlight clinical challenges. Eur J Clin Microbiol Infect Dis 2012; 31(12):3259-64.
9. Goldani LZ, Zavascki AP, Maia AL. Fungal thyroiditis: an overview. Mycopathologia 2006; 161(3):129-39.
10. Rathi M, Ahmad F, Budania SK, et al. Cytomorphological Aspects of Hashimoto's Thyroiditis: Our Experience at a Tertiary Center. Clin Med Insights Pathol 2014; 7:1-5.
11. Shabb NS, Salti I. Subacute thyroiditis: fine-needle aspiration cytology of 14 cases presenting with thyroid nodules. Diagn Cytopathol 2006; 34(1):18-23.

Chapter 25

Necrotic Background in Thyroid FNA Cytology: Anaplastic Transformation or Infarction in Papillary Carcinoma

Kennichi Kakudo, Shinya Satoh, Yusuke Mori, and Hiroyuki Yamashita

Brief Clinical Summary

A 23-year-old female presented with a sudden onset of neck pain (radiating to the right ear) and swelling persisting for two days. She had a thyroid nodule in the right side of her neck with tenderness to palpation. The interpretation of the fine needle aspiration (FNA) cytology of this thyroid nodule at another hospital more than two years ago was benign and a surgical treatment was not rendered. Her thyroid function tests were in normal range at presentation, showing TSH, 1.14 mIU/ml; fT3, 2.81 pg/dl; and fT4, 1.20 ng/dl. The white blood cell count was elevated to 12720/mL.

Ultrasound Findings

Ultrasound showed a well-circumscribed solid nodule, 13 mm x 10 mm, in the right lobe of thyroid. The nodule was hypovascular and heterogeneous in echoic texture (Figure 1). Neither calcification nor cystic change was found. Ultrasound-guided FNA cytology was applied to the nodule.

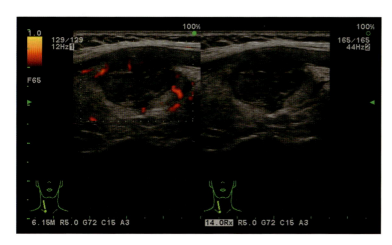

Figure 1. A well-circumscribed nodule, 13 x 10 mm in size, is demonstrated in the right lobe of thyroid. The nodule is hypoechoic with heterogeneous texture, suggesting necrosis.

Cytological Findings

Cytology revealed inflammatory cells with isolated, loosely cohesive atypical epithelial cells in the necrotic background. This case was characterized by numerous granulocytes, histiocytes, lymphocytes, and degenerated cell debris (Figure 2). The epithelial cells were loosely cohesive or individually dispersed with poorly defined cytoplasm matted in the inflammatory cells (Figure 3). These epithelial cells had a larger nucleus than degenerated granulocytes and lymphocytes, with a small to inconspicuous nucleolus (Figure 4). Nuclear features of papillary thyroid carcinoma (PTC) were not appreciated in these isolated cells. Some of them had a dense cyanophilic wide cytoplasm, simulating squamous cell differentiation or spindle-shaped malignant cells (red arrows in Figures 3 and 4), but being different from well differentiated thyroid carcinoma cells of follicular thyroid carcinoma (FTC) or PTC type. Loosely cohesive atypical cells were often observed (Figures 3, 4 and 5). At the same time, there were tightly cohesive follicular cell clusters in syncytial sheet clusters (Figures 5 and 6), overlapping sheet-like clusters (cellular swirls) or large trabecular clusters with nuclear crowding. Nuclear irregularity and nuclear groove (yellow arrow) as shown in Figure 6 gave an impression of suspicious PTC type malignancy. Nuclear cytoplasmic inclusion was rare and not convincing. Foreign body type multinuclear giant cells were often observed (Figure 6). Neither psammoma bodies type calcification nor amyloid deposits were found.

List of Differential Diagnoses
1. Malignant: PTC with necrosis
2. Malignant: Cystic PTC
3. Malignant: PTC with anaplastic transformation
4. Malignant: PTC with subacute thyroiditis
5. Malignant: Poorly differentiated carcinoma
6. Malignant: Undifferentiated carcinoma
7. Malignant: Metastatic (secondary) carcinoma to the thyroid
8. Benign: Acute infectious thyroiditis

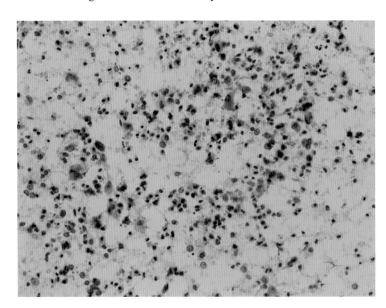

Figure 2. Tumor necrosis with degenerated cell debris, granulocytes, histiocytes, and lymphocytes in the smear background. (Papanicolaou stain, x100)

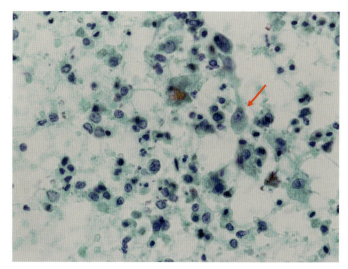

Figure 3. There are many degenerated tumor cells with wide cytoplasm (red arrow) and ill-defined cytoplasm. They appear as isolated and dispersed cells. (Papanicolaou stain, x400)

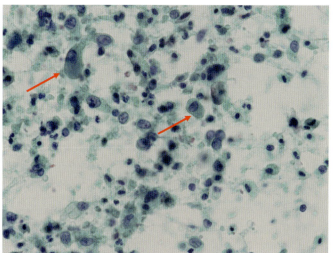

Figure 4. There are many degenerated tumor cells with wide cytoplasm (red arrow) and ill-defined cytoplasm. These epithelial cells have a larger nucleus than that of degenerated epithelial cells, granulocytes and lymphocytes. These tumor cells present a vesicular nucleus with a small nucleolus. (Papanicolaou stain, x400)

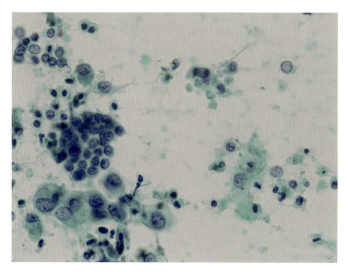

Figure 5. Both tightly arranged syncytial type clusters and loosely cohesive large cells with dense cytoplasm are shown. (Papanicolaou stain, x400)

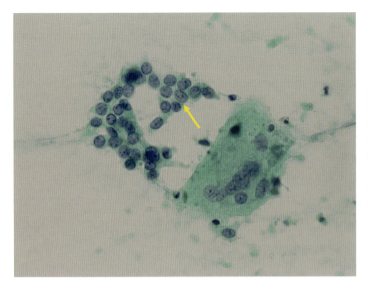

Figure 6. The cells of syncytial type clusters have ovoid nuclei that show powdery chromatin, inconspicuous nucleoli and nuclear grooves (yellow arrow). A foreign body type multinucleated cell is seen nearby. (Papanicolaou stain, x400)

Differential Diagnosis:

From the Figures 5 and 6, many readers of this book might reach easily to a diagnosis of PTC type malignancy. Because of the necrotic background in this case, you might suspect a much more aggressive malignancy such as undifferentiated carcinoma (UC) or poorly differentiated carcinoma (PDC) in which tumor necrosis is often found (1) (please refer to Chapter 21). Atypical cells with dense cyanophilic cytoplasm and spindle-shaped malignant cells as shown in Figures 3, 4, and 5 might be a worrisome cytological features for UC, primary squamous cell carcinoma of the thyroid or metastatic carcinoma to the thyroid. However, UC usually occurs in elderly patients and UC in a 23-year-old patient is extremely rare (1). Please refer to Figure 6 (UC) of Chapter 16 for your comparison, where monstrous giant cells with bizarre nuclei and multiple prominent nucleoli are shown. Nuclear atypia of UC is incomparably higher than that of this case. For more details of PDC, please refer to Chapter 21. Squamous metaplasia may occur in PTC and should be differentiated from primary squamous cell carcinoma with high-grade nuclear features (please refer to Chapters 4, 5, and 7 for squamous metaplasia in PTC, and Chapter 22 for high grade metastatic (secondary) carcinoma to thyroid gland).

Necrosis can be found in certain types of inflammation, and caseous necrosis of tuberculosis type is extremely rare in thyroid gland. Hashimoto thyroiditis (please refer to Chapter 13), subacute granulomatous thyroiditis (please refer to Chapter 11) and acute infectious thyroiditis (please refer to Chapter 24) were denied at histological examination.

Infarction in a thyroid nodule after FNA has been reported as a rare complication and is explained in the following explanatory notes. Although this patient had a past medical history of FNA biopsy more than 2 years ago, this should not be a direct cause of necrosis in this patient, because of very fresh changes in the nodule. Both viable PTC type malignant cells and pyknotic epithelial cells underwent degeneration (a fresh ischemic change of acute infarction) are shown in Figure 7. Table 1 lists several complications attributable to thyroid FNA biopsy (please refer to Chapter 26).

Table 1. Complications and adverse events in thyroid FNA cytology

1. Thyroid gland swelling
2. Infarction and involution of nodule
3. Acute hemorrhage
4. Upper airway obstruction due to hematoma
5. Infection
6. Needle tract seeding (implantation)
7. Histologic changes after FNA simulating capsular invasion (pseudoinvasion) in benign follicular adenoma

Histologic Diagnosis: PTC with massive necrosis, probably due to spontaneous infarction.

The cut surface of the right lobe is shown in the Figure 8, where an ill-defined nodule, 13 x 10 mm in size, was noted. Yellowish white necrotic areas were found within the nodule. The tumor capsule and surrounding thyroid parenchyma were fibrotic and the thyroid gland was adhesive to the surrounding muscle tissue (Figure 8).

Acute coagulative necrosis was found in more than 90% of the tumor area (Figure 9) and histologically viable tumor nests with papillary growth were identified in the periphery of the necrotic tumor (Figure 10). Fibrosis in the nodule was minimal and it was judged that this tumor necrosis was in a subacute phase and was not attributable to FNA carried out more than 2 years ago. It was estimated that this ischemic necrosis probably started from 2 to 4 weeks prior to surgery, probably at the onset of neck pain (18 days prior to lobectomy), due to unknown etiology rather than iatrogenic cause, such as FNA cytology.

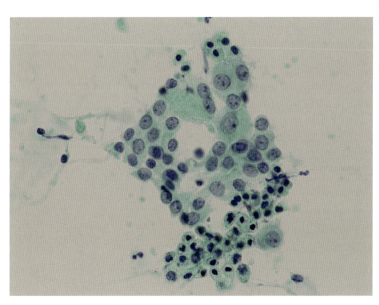

Figure 7. Two types of epithelial cells in a cluster: viable tumor cells with large oval nuclei (upper field) and degenerated small cells with condensed chromatin (lower field). (Papanicolaou stain, x400)

Explanatory Notes

Spontaneous infarction of thyroid neoplasms occurs infrequently as a complication of FNA biopsy (Table 1) (2-6). Jones *et al*. examined a series of 200 thyroid FNAs and reported that necrosis around the needle tract was histologically evident. In one of these cases, necrosis with involution of the nodule was observed. They have concluded that FNA can induce necrosis and apparent clinical regression of thyroid neoplasms (2, 3). Incidence of infarction

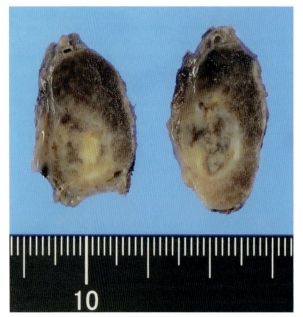

Figure 8. The cut surface of the right lobe of the thyroid gland after formalin fixation. An ill-defined nodule, 13 x 10 mm in size, is noted in the right lobe, with patchy yellowish white areas (necrosis) within the nodule, and fibrosis involving its capsule and surrounding thyroid parenchyma.

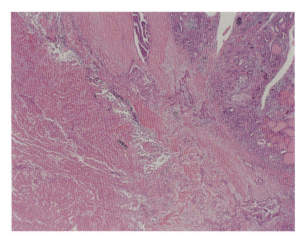

Figure 9. An invasive papillary carcinoma with massive necrosis is shown. Note papillary growth of viable cancer nests at the center of upper field and coagulative necrosis without nuclei (shadow cells) in more than half of this field (lower left). Non-neoplastic thyroid parenchyma in the upper right field shows inflammatory infiltration and mild fibrotic change. (HE stain, x40)

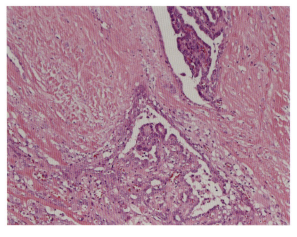

Figure 10. A high magnification of Fig. 9 demonstrates residual foci of conventional papillary carcinoma. (HE stain, x200)

after FNA was reported to be 12/620 (1.9%) and the mean time interval between the last FNA and surgery was 52 days (range 13-133 days) in a series of surgically treated patients with PTC (4). Layfield and Lones pointed out that FNA-related tumor infarction might cause diagnostic problems including: 1) infarction may obscure the nature of neoplasms, making histological confirmation difficult; and 2) FNA of an infarcted nodule may have difficulties in obtaining diagnostic material, potentially resulting in a false negative diagnosis (5).

In the presenting case, the patient's pain started one day prior to the last FNA examination and neither prior trauma nor other events were reported in her past history, therefore, the last FNA procedure could not be the causative factor and other infarction-inducing factor(s) unrelated with FNA might contribute to the massive tumor necrosis in this patient. Hypovascularity on ultrasound examination supported this hypothesis, however histological examination failed to demonstrate any occlusive vascular changes, such as thrombus or emboli.

Pain in the thyroid gland is a rare symptom. Subacute thyroiditis is the most common cause of painful thyroiditis and rarely associated with Hashimoto thyroiditis (7-9) (please refer to cytological features of subacute thyroiditis of Chapter 11 and Hashimoto thyroiditis of Chapter 13).

Pain has been reported very rarely as a complication of FNA biopsy. Chen *et al.* reported a case of painful PTC with secondary infection after FNA (10). Neither suppurative inflammation nor specific granulomatous inflammation was found in the presenting case at histological examination.

References

1. DeLellis RA, Lloyd RV, Heitz PU, et al. World Health Organization Classification of Tumours: Pathology and genetics. Tumours of Endocrine Organs, IARC Oress, Lyon, France, 2004.
2. Jones JD, Pittman DL, Sanders LR. Necrosis of thyroid nodules after fine needle aspiration. Acta Cytol 1985; 29:29-32.
3. Das DK, Janardan C, Pathan SK, et al. Infarction in a thyroid nodule after fine needle aspiration: report of 2 cases with discussion of the cause of pitfalls in the histopathologic diagnosis of papillary thyroid carcinoma. Acta Cytolo 2009; 53:571-5.
4. Liu YF, Ahmed S, Bhuta S, et al. Infarction of papillary thyroid carcinoma after fine-needle aspiration: case series and review of literature. JAMA Otolaryngol Head Neck Surg 2014; 140:52-7.
5. Layfield LJ, Lones MA. Necrosis in thyroid nodules after fine needle aspiration biopsy. Report of two cases. Acta Cytol 1991; 35:427-30.
6. Pinto RG, Couto F, Mandreker S. Infarction after fine needle aspiration. A report of four cases. Acta Cytolo 1996; 40:739-41.
7. Nishihara E, Ohye H, Amino N, et al. Clinical characteristics of 852 patients with subacute thyroiditis before treatment. Intern Med 2008; 47:725-939.
8. Frdem N, Erdogan M, Ozbek M, et al. Demographic and clinical features of patients with subacute thyroiditis: results of 169 patients from a single university center in Turkey. J Endocrinol Invest 2007; 30:546-50.
9. Onoda N, Kato Y, Seki T, et al. Increased thyroid blood flow in the hypoechoic lesions in patients with recurrent, painful Hashimoto's thyroiditis at the time of acute exacerbation. Endocri J 2008; 56:65-72.
10. Chen HW, Tseng FY, Su DH, et al. Secondary infection and ischemic necrosis after fine needle aspiration for a painful papillary thyroid carcinoma: a case report. Acta Cytol 2006; 50:217-20.

Chapter 26

Complications of Fine Needle Aspiration Biopsy

Yasuhiro Ito and Mitsuyoshi Hirokawa

Fine needle aspiration (FNA) biopsy is the most useful technique available to diagnose thyroid nodules. Recent progress in ultrasound-guided FNA has enabled us to detect even very small thyroid nodules. Although FNA is generally a safe technique, several complications have been reported. In this chapter, the prominent complications of FNA are described (please refer to Table 1. Complications and adverse events in thyroid FNA cytology in Chapter 25).

Disturbance on Histological Diagnosis

Histological alterations from FNA biopsy (FNAB) often affect the pathological diagnosis. This phenomenon is also designated as "worrisome histologic alterations following fine needle aspiration of the thyroid" (WHAFFT), and is considered a serious clinical problem. For example, nuclear atypia, vascular changes, capsular pseudoinvasion, infarction and metaplasia often induce misdiagnosis of FNA (1-4) (please refer to Chapter 25). Figure 1 demonstrates inflammation due to FNA resembling the anaplastic transformation in papillary carcinoma. Pandit *et al*. showed that WHAFFT lesions were present in 38% of pathological specimens (1). Rosemary *et al*. demonstrated that these changes were found in 68 of 96 thyroidectomy specimens and peaked within 20 to 40 days after FNA. These changes can also be pitfalls in diagnosing repeat FNA specimens (3). The disappearance of tumor cells after FNA has also been reported (5).

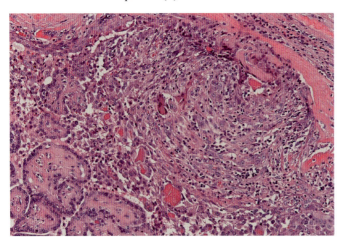

Figure 1. A well-differentiated thyroid carcinoma, which could easily be misdiagnosed as undifferentiated change because of the inflammation caused by FNA. (HE stain, x200)

Dissemination due to FNAB for Parathyroid Adenoma/Hyperplasia

In contrast to the thyroid, FNAB is contraindicated for neck nodules suspected of parathyroid adenoma or hyperplasia. Parathyroid cells are much more easily disseminated than thyroid follicular cells, and can cause serious problems. If nodules are suspected of association with a pathologic parathyroid by ultrasound, measurement of parathyroid hormone, ionized calcium and other biochemical examinations, including urinary examinations, then imaging studies such as sestamibi scintigraphy and computed tomography (CT) should be performed in advance (please refer to Chapter 23). As an exception, FNA for parathyroid with PTH measurement of needle lavage is performed when parathyroid adenoma/hyperplasia is difficult to be identified because of, for example, coexisting multinodular goiter, but this should be done only if surgery is planned for the near future (please refer to Chapter 23).

Needle Tract Implantation of Tumor Cells

Needle tract implantation of neoplastic cells in the subcutaneous or intra-strap muscle layer has been reported as one of the important complications of FNA. In papillary carcinoma, it appears in 0.14% of patients 2 to 131 months after FNA (6). This phenomenon is more likely to occur in papillary carcinoma with poorly differentiated lesions or in cases where the lesion extends beyond the thyroid. Also, the interval between FNA and appearance of implantation is shorter in cases with clinical node metastasis (N-positive) or a high Ki-67 labeling index. These findings indicate that needle tract implantation in papillary carcinoma is likely to occur in cases with aggressive features (please refer to Chapter 8). However, all such cases have been controlled by re-operation.

More recently, it was reported that 45% of papillary carcinoma patients showing subcutaneous or intra-strap muscular recurrence had a distant recurrence simultaneously with or after the appearance of subcutaneous or intra-strap muscular recurrence. It is therefore important that, although local control of needle tract implantation is not difficult, physicians should be on the lookout for distant recurrence at the time of or after the detection of needle tract implantation by constantly checking thyroglobulin levels and conducting imaging studies (7).

Although the incidence is much lower, needle tract implantation was also reported in follicular neoplasm (8). Normally, follicular neoplasm is treated by hemithyroidectomy. In the reported case, the pathological diagnosis was follicular adenoma. However, in such a case, total thyroidectomy with subcutaneous tumor resection should be performed, as such lesions should be regarded as clinically malignant.

Acute Thyroid Hemorrhage and Hematoma

Acute hemorrhage and hematoma are among the most important complications, and can even become fatal when airway obstruction occurs. Hor *et al.* reported a case of bilateral thyroid hematomas causing acute airway obstruction in a hypertensive patient with end-stage renal disease taking aspirin (9). Kakiuchi *et al.* demonstrated a fatal case that underwent not only FNA but also core needle biopsy (CNB) (10). According to a review by Polyzos *et al.*, the incidence of blood extravasation-related complications during or after FNA ranged from 1.9 to 6.4%, but such high incidences are possibly due to varying definitions or recording bias (11). Needless to say, CNB carries a higher risk of acute hemorrhage than FNA. In routine care at our hospital, acute hemorrhage and hematoma are extremely rare events. We ask patients to press the insertion site of needles at least 15 min - even longer, 20 min, for patients taking thrombolytic agents. In the latter case, after 20 min, co-medicals always check whether bleeding or swelling is present and only then are patients allowed to leave the hospital. Such careful attention can minimize the incidence of blood extravasation-related complications after FNA.

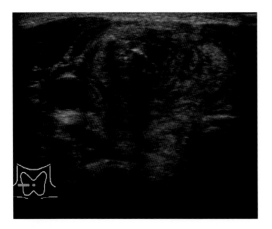 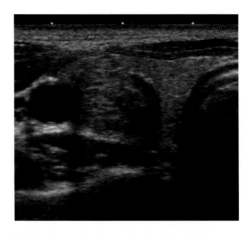

Figure 2. A typical example of acute edema induced by FNA in the side of nodule. A: After FNA and B: before FNA.

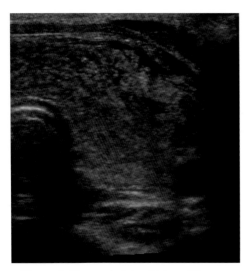 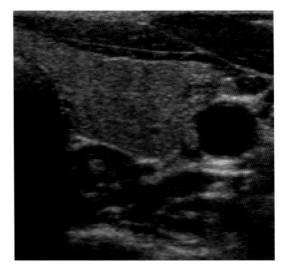

Figure 3. The contralateral lobe of the same case as shown in Figure 2. A: After FNA and B: before FNA.

Acute Edema of the Thyroid

Acute edema of the thyroid can be observed after FNA (Figure 2). The reason why this occurs remains unclear, but it may be related to an allergic reaction of the thyroid to needles. The thyroid is diffusely and often bilaterally swollen immediately after FNA (Figure 3), and patients complain of a swelling sense and/or spontaneous pain. The incidence of such reaction is not high, at about 0.1% or even less. Generally, it is cured by neck cooling, but steroid administration might be occasionally necessary.

Transient Vocal Cord Paralysis

Tomoda *et al.* reported a transient vocal cord paralysis in 0.036% of FNA cases. In this report, all were recovered within 6 months (12). The mechanism of vocal cord paralysis after FNA remains unclear, but it may occur because of stretching or pressing of the recurrent nerve due to hemorrhage or fluid leakage. Alternatively, the needle may partially injure the recurrent laryngeal nerve. When patients complain of hoarseness and/or aspiration after FNA, consultation with an otolaryngologist is desirable.

Acute Suppurative Infection

Although very rare, some case reports have been published regarding acute suppurative infection after FNA (13) (please refer to Chapter 24). The representative complaints are high fever reaching 39.0 °C, painful cervical swelling with or without redness of the skin; in laboratory data, leukocytosis and elevation of C-reactive protein are shown.

Pneumothorax

Pneumothorax was reported in 6.3% of FNA of tumors in the upper mediastinum (14). Although it is much rare for FNA of neck tumors, it can occur in FNA of the lateral lymph node near the venous angle when pleura are located cranially. Thoracic drainage might be necessary for the therapy.

Cutaneous Sinus Formation

This is an extremely rare event. One report of a patient who underwent FNA for recurrent multinodular goiter after thyroidectomy 17 years ago showed sinus formation superior to the thyroidectomy incision. Reoperation of the sinus tract was performed for a cure (15).

Although there are many kinds of complications of FNA, their incidences are very low. Since FNA remains the most useful technique for diagnosis, the risk of these complications should not deter us from performing FNA in patients with thyroid nodules. We have to note that, although FNA can show various complications, it is fundamentally a safe technique to diagnose thyroid nodules and decide the indications and the range for surgery.

References

1. Pandit AA, Phulpager MD. Worrisome histologic alterations following fine needle aspiration of the thyroid. Acta Cytol 2001; 45: 173-8.
2. Bolat F, Kayaselcuk F, Nursal TZ, et al. Histopathological changes in thyroid tissue after fine needle aspiration biopsy. Pathol Res Pract 2007; 203:641-5.
3. Racavarren RA, Houser PM, Yang J. Potential pitfalls of needle tract effect on repeat thyroid fine-needle aspiration. Cancer Cytopathol 2013; 121:155-64.
4. Liu TF, Ahmed S, Bhuta S, et al. Infarction of papillary thyroid carcinoma after fine-needle aspiration. JAMA otolaryngol Head Neck Surg 2014; 140:52-7.
5. Eze OP, Cai G, Baloch ZW, et al. Vanishing thyroid tumors: a diagnostic dilemma after ultrasonography-guided fine-needle aspiration. Thyroid 2013; 23:194-200.
6. Ito Y, Tomoda C, Uruno T, et al. Needle tract implantation of papillary thyroid carcinoma after fine-needle aspiration. World J Surg 2005; 29:1544-9.
7. Ito Y, Hirokawa M, Higashiyama T, et al. Clinical significance and prognostic impact of subcutaneous or intrastrap muscular recurrence of papillary thyroid carcinoma. J Thyroid Res 2012; 2012:819797.
8. Ito Y, Asahi S, Matsuzuka F, et al. Needle tract implantation of follicular neoplasm after fine-needle aspiration biopsy: report of a case. Thyroid 2006; 16:1059-62.
9. Hor T, Lahiri SW. Bilateral thyroid hematomas after fine-needle aspiration causing acute airway obstruction. Thyroid 2008; 18:567-9.
10. Kakiuchi Y, Idota N, Nakamura M, et al. A fatal case of cervical hemorrhage after fine needle aspiration and core needle biopsy of the thyroid gland. Am J Forensic Med Pathol 2015; 36:207-9.

11. Polyzos SA, Anastasilakis AD. Systematic review of cases reporting blood extravasation-related complications after thyroid fine-needle biopsy. J Otolaryngol Head Neck Surg 2010; 39:532-41.
12. Tomoda C, Takamura Y, Ito Y, et al. Transient vocal cord paralysis after fine-needle aspiration biopsy of thyroid tumor. Thyroid 2006; 16: 697-9.
13. Yldar M, Demirpolat G, Aydin M. Acute suppurative thyroiditis accompanied by thyrotoxicosis after fine-needle aspiration: Treatment with catheter drainage. J Clin Diagn Res 2014; 8:ND12-ND14.
14. Linder J, Olsen G, Johnston W. Fine-needle aspiration biopsy of the mediastinum. Am J Med 1988; 81:1005-8.
15. Akbaba G, Omar M, Polat M, et al. Cutaneous sinus formation is a rare complication of thyroid fine needle aspiration biopsy. Case Rep Endocrinol 2014; 2014:923438.

Chapter 27

Cytological Features of Papillary Carcinoma on LBC Preparation, Comparison with Conventional Preparation

Ayana Suzuki

Case Report

The patient was a 66-year-old female complaining of dysphagia for one year. She visited another hospital and a calcified mass was pointed out in the left lobe of the thyroid by ultrasonographic examination (UE). She was referred to our hospital for further examination of the mass. The UE performed in the Kuma Hospital revealed a mass measuring 26 x 16 mm in the left lobe of thyroid. The mass was mainly hypoechoic and contained band-like or dot-like high-echoic areas, indicating calcification. The margin of the mass was ill-defined and irregular, indicating the infiltrative nature (Figure 1). Color Doppler ultrasound showed both intranodular and perinodular hypervascularity. Aspiration cytology for the mass was performed, and both conventional and Liquid-Based Cytology (LBC) preparations were prepared. The needle washout fluid with CytoRich™ RED collection fluid (BD, Burlington, NC) was used for LBC materials. LBC preparation was prepared with the SurePath hand method (BD, Burlington, NC). Cytological report was malignancy, papillary thyroid carcinoma (PTC). She underwent total thyroidectomy with paratracheal neck dissection.

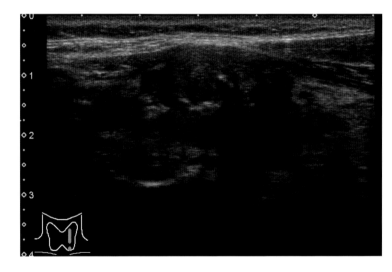

Figure 1. A hypoechoic mass with high-echoic areas indicating calcification. (Ultrasound B-mode image)

Cytological Findings

The conventional preparation was cellular. The background was clean and ropy colloid was scattered. Rounded atypical cells appeared as papillary clusters or a monolayered sheet-like pattern (Figure 2). The cytoplasm was rounded and weakly stained in lightgreen. The nuclei were compactly arranged and showed a few of grooves. A small number of intranuclear cytoplasmic inclusions (NCI) were observed (Figure 3). Nuclear chromatin was powdery to fine granular. Nucleoli were indistinct and darkly stained (Figure 3) (please refer to Tables 1 and 2 of Chapter 3).

The LBC preparation was also cellular. The background was clean and a few bizarre-shaped multinucleated giant cells were observed. The atypical cells showed papillary or monolayered sheet-like pattern. Some clusters adhered to ropy colloid (Figure 4). Compared with conventional preparations, the N/C ratio was higher; the sizes of nuclei and cytoplasm were decreased; the cytoplasmic staining was denser; and the cell border was more distinct; but the nuclei were not crowded. Intercellular window-like spaces were present in monolayered sheet-like clusters (Figure 5). The nuclear grooves and convoluted nuclei were easily observed (Figure 6). A few of NCIs were observed. The chromatin was not powdery but fine granular. The nucleoli were apparent, red in color, and occasionally associated with perinucleolar halo (Figure 7).

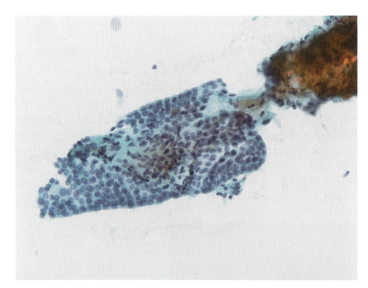

Figure 2. The stromal component exists within a papillary cluster that is composed of atypical cells. (Papanicolaou, conventional preparation, x200)

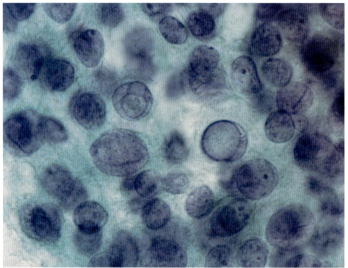

Figure 3. Intranuclear cytoplasmic inclusions and nuclear grooves are seen. Nuclear chromatin is powdery to finely granular. Nucleoli are darkly stained. (Papanicolaou, conventional preparation, x1000)

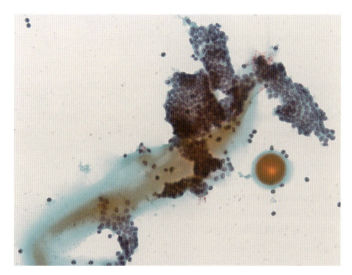

Figure 4. The papillary clusters are intimately mixed with ropy colloid. (Papanicolaou, LBC, x200)

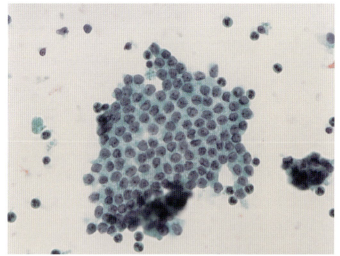

Figure 5. Intercellular window-like spaces are present in the monolayered sheet-like cluster. (Papanicolaou, LBC, x400)

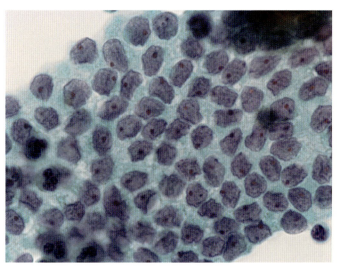

Figure 6. The irregular-shaped and convoluted nuclei are apparent. The chromatin is not powdery but fine granular. The nucleoli are stained red in color and occasionally accompanied by perinucleolar halo (arrows). (Papanicolaou, LBC, x1000)

Pathological Findings

The tumor was located in the upper portion of the left thyroid, and measured 20 x 15 mm. On the cut surface, it was solid, white in color, and associated with calcification. The margin was irregular and the tumor invaded into the surrounding fibroadipose tissue (Figure 7). Microscopically, the atypical cells showed papillary and follicular growth patterns. There was inspissated colloid within the follicles. The atypical cells showed nuclear findings characteristic of papillary carcinoma, including grooves, overlapping, ground glass appearance, and intranuclear cytoplasmic inclusions (Figure 8) (please refer to Chapters 3-7). The stroma was fibrotic and calcification was scattered. Ki-67 labeling index was less than 1%. There was no evidence of nodal metastasis.

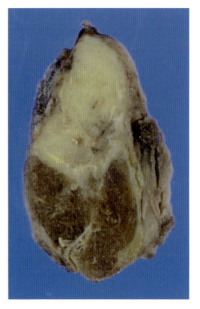

Figure 7. A solid tumor invading into the surrounding tissue is present at the upper portion of the thyroid.

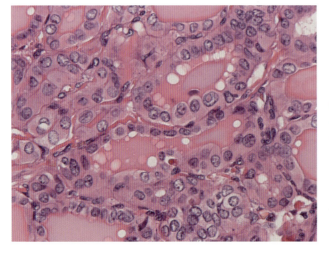

Figure 8. The carcinoma cells show nuclear grooves and intranuclear cytoplasmic inclusions. (HE, x400)

Differential Diagnoses

Liquid-based cytology (LBC) is a new technique to collect the cytological samples and smear them thinly. This technique has been developed in the gynecological field. It is generally known that LBC is useful for reducing unsatisfactory preparations and improving the diagnostic accuracy (1, 2) (please refer to Chapter 30). Recently, LBC is becoming increasingly popular for the non-gynecological cytology including thyroid aspirates (3, 4). Currently, there are mainly two systems for LBC: 1) filtrate and collect vacuum-packed cells on a membrane and then transfer to the glass slide, and 2) centrifuge and sedimentate through a density gradient. Cells are distributed thinly with the former, whereas thickly with the latter (7, 8).

LBC for thyroid aspiration cytology has been becoming popular increasingly, and both filtration and centrifugation methods have been used (1-17). Rossi *et al.* reported that LBC decreases inadequate cases and improves diagnostic sensitivity (5). The method exhibits accuracy equal to that of conventional methods because of its excellent cell preservation and the decrease in blood components that mask follicular cells (4, 6).

There are a number of morphological changes inherent to the LBC preparations. The cytological findings vary depending on the methods (7-9). In addition, they may be changed according to the fixatives (8-9). Therefore, when we observe and understand the cytology of LBC, we should pay attention to the method and fixative. Unless otherwise noted, hereinafter, we describe the cytological findings of PTC prepared with SurePath method using CytoRich^{TM} RED (Table 1).

LBC methods produce slides having a cleaner background and higher cellularity than the conventional slide methods (10). The amounts of colloid and red blood cells are diminished because of proteolytic and hemolytic abilities of fixatives (6, 10, 11). A collagenous stroma that is composed of collagenous connective tissue not associated with PTC cells is easily observed with LBC preparations of PTC cases (Figure 10). The phenomenon may be also caused by a proteolytic behavior of CytoRich^{TM} RED (6). Similarly, naked capillaries tend to be visible on LBC preparations (Figure 11) (6).

LBC methods produce a more three-dimensional configuration for both single cells and clusters than conventional preparations (Figure 4) (7). Isolated cells tend to be decreased. The frequencies of trabecular and hobnail-like patterns are higher. In contrast, papillary pattern and tissue fragments are lower (6). The presence of the intercellular window-like spaces appears to be limited to LBC preparations (Figure 5). It is thought that they are caused by shrinkage of the cytoplasm (6). The findings are seen in two-third of PTC with LBC preparations, but are rarely seen with conventional preparations (6).

The cell shape is well preserved and highlighted with LBC preparations (6). Therefore, tall cell variant, whose height is more than three times as tall as their width, is more easily recognized (12) (please refer to Figure 6 in the Chapter 8). The N/C ratio is higher, the sizes of the nuclei and cytoplasm are more decreased, the cytoplasm is more densely stained, and the cell border is distincter, but the nuclei are not crowded (11, 13, 14). The nuclear features characteristic of PTC, including an irregular nuclear shape, nuclear grooves (Figure 6), and NCIs are easily recognized (15-17). In our study, the incidence of ground glass nuclei in PTC was 0.6%, and most of the nuclei presented granular chromatin pattern (6). We should pay attention to the fact that ground glass nuclei are not a diagnostic clue of PTC in the LBC preparations prepared with SurePath method using CytoRich^{TM} RED.

Nuclear irregularity or angulated nuclear membrane has been described with LBC preparations (7, 10, 15). We call them "convoluted nuclei" (Figure 6) in which zigzag irregularity occupies more than half of nuclear membrane (6). In our study, the convoluted nuclei were observed in 41.0% of PTC cases with LBC preparations (6). The finding was present in 2.5% of PTC with the conventional preparations, and in 3.6% of adenomatous goiters and 0% of follicular neoplasms with LBC preparations. The convoluted nuclei might be a new clue of PTC using LBC preparations (Figure 6).

Papillary carcinoma cells frequently present prominent red nucleoli (11). With conventional preparations, the nucleoli are more darkly stained. Eosinophilic nucleoli are not only observed in PTC, but also in adenomatous goiter or follicular neoplasms in LBC preparations (6). The red nucleoli seen in PTCs are occasionally associated with perinucleolar halo (Figure 6). As the halo is not observed in adenomatous or hyperplastic nodules and in follicular neoplasms, its presence may be useful in differential diagnosis.

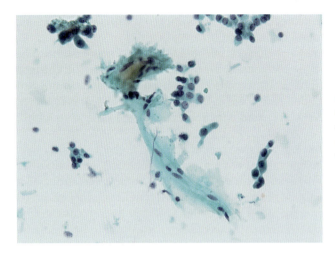

Figure 9. Collagenous stroma without carcinoma cells found in papillary carcinoma. Note spindle-shaped nuclei indicating fibroblasts within the connective tissue. (Papanicolaou, LBC, x200)

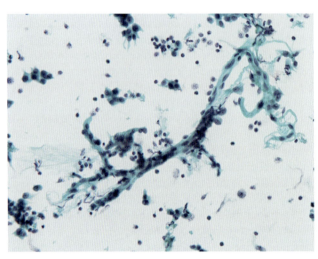

Figure 10. Naked capillaries seen in papillary carcinoma. They are not associated with connective tissue or carcinoma cells. (Papanicolaou, LBC, x200)

Table 1. Cytological features of papillary carcinomas on LBC (SurePath), compared with conventional preparations

Background	Decrease in red blood cells and colloid
	Collagenous stroma
Arrangement	More 3-dimensional
	More preserved histological structure
	Decrease in isolated cells
Intercellular spaces	Present
Overlapping nuclei	Diminished
Cytoplasm	Decreased in size, more densely stained
Nuclei	Decreased in size
Nuclear groove	Present
Nuclear cytoplasmic inclusion	Present
Chromatin pattern	Granular
	Indistinct ground-glass appearance
Convoluted nuclei	Present
Nucleoli	Eosinophilic, perinucleolar halo

References

1. Nandini NM, Nandish SM, Pallavi P, et al. Manual liquid based cytology in primary screening for cervical cancer - a cost effective preposition for scarce resource settings. Asian Pac J Cancer Prev 2012; 13:3645-51.
2. Akamatsu S, Kodama S, Himeji Y, et al. A comparison of liquid-based cytology with conventional cytology in cervical cancer screening. Acta Cytol 2012; 56:370-4.
3. Argon A, Uyaroglu MA, Nart D, et al. The effectiveness of the liquid-based preparation method in cerebrospinal fluid cytology. Acta Cytol 2013; 57:266-70.
4. Rossi ED, Morassi F, Santeusanio G, et al. Thyroid fine needle aspiration cytology processed by ThinPrep: An additional slide decreased the number of inadequate results. Cytopathol 2010; 21:97-102.
5. Rossi ED, Raffaelli M, Zannoni GF, et al. Diagnostic efficacy of conventional as compared to liquid-based cytology in thyroid lesions: evaluation of 10,360 fine needle aspiration cytology cases. Acta Cytol 2009; 53:659-666.
6. Suzuki A, Hirokawa M, Higuchi M, et al. Cytological Characteristics of Papillary Thyroid Carcinoma on LBC Specimens, Compared with Conventional Specimens. Diagn Cytopathol 2014; 43:108-13.
7. Jung CK, Lee A, Jung ES, et al. Split sample comparison of a liquid-based method and conventional smears in thyroid fine needle aspiration. Acta Cytol 2008; 52:313-9.
8. Zhao FH, Hu SY, Bian JJ, et al. Comparison of ThinPrep and SurePath liquid-based cytology and subsequent human papillomavirus DNA testing in China. Cancer Cytopathol 2011; 119:387-94.
9. Fadda G, Rossi ED. Liquid-based cytology in fine-needle aspiration biopsies of the thyroid gland. Acta Cytol 2011; 55:389-400.
10. Kim DH, Kim MK, Chae SW, et al. The usefulness of SurePath™ liquid-based smear in sonoguided thyroid fine needle aspiration; a comparison of a conventional smear and SurePath™ liquid-based cytology. Korean J Cytopathol 2007; 18:143-52.
11. Mygdakos N, Nikolaidou S, Tzilivaki A, et al. Liquid based preparation (LBP) cytology versus conventional cytology (CS) in FNA samples from breast, thyroid, salivary glands and soft tissues. Our experience in Crete (Greece). Roman J Morphol Embryol 2009; 50:245-50.
12. Lee SH, Jung CK, Bae JS, et al. Liquid-based cytology improves preparative diagnostic accuracy of the tall cell variant of papillary thyroid carcinoma. Diagn Cytopathol 2013; 42:11-7.
13. Ali SZ, Cibas ES. The Bethesda System for reporting thyroid cytopathology: definitions, criteria and explanatory notes. New York: Springer; 2010, p178.
14. Afify AM, Al-Khafaji BM. Cytologic artifacts and pitfalls of thyroid fine-needle aspiration using ThinPrep: A comparative retrospective review. Cancer 2001; 93:179-86.
15. Geers C, Bourgain C. Liquid-based FNAC of the thyroid a 4-year survey with SurePath. Cancer Cytopathol 2011; 119:58-67.
16. Malle D, Valeri RM, Pazaitou K, et al. Use of a thin-layer technique in thyroid fine needle aspiration. Acta Cytol 2006; 50:23-7.
17. Fischer AH, Clayton AC, Bentz JS, et al. Performance differences between conventional smears and liquid-based preparations of thyroid fine-needle aspiration samples. Arch Pathol Lab Med 2013; 137:26-31.

Chapter 28

Pitfalls in Immunocytochemical Study Using Fine Needle Aspiration Samples

Junko Maruta

Introduction

Immunostaining of histopathological specimen is carried out using formalin-fixed paraffin-embedded tissues with or without antigen retrieval. Meanwhile, immunostaining of fine needle aspiration (FNA) smears is usually carried out using 95% alcohol-fixed specimens. The immunostaining results obtained with histopathological specimens and those with cytological specimens may be discrepant or even contradictory due to the differences in fixatives, fixation methods, and/or antigen activation treatment. An automated immunostaining instrument in our hospital is used for the special care in fixation of cytological smears. For FNA smears, alcohol fixation is used, which is followed by further fixation with phosphate buffered formalin solution, and an antigen activation treatment. Useful immunostaining markers in thyroid cytology are shown in Table 1.

Table 1. Useful immunostaining markers for the diagnosis of thyroid tumors

	Positive	Negative
Normal follicular epithelial cells	Thyroglobulin (cytoplasm), thyroid transcription-1 (nuclear), PAX8 (nuclear)	
Papillary carcinoma	CK 19 (cytoplasm),	
Cribriform variant papillary carcinoma	β-Catenin (nuclear, cytoplasm), estrogen receptor (nuclear), progesteron receptor (nuclear)	
Hyalinizing trabecular adenoma	MIB-1 (Ki-67, cell membrane)	CK 19 (cytoplasm)
Medullary (C cell) carcinoma	Calcitonin (cytoplasm), chromogranin A (cytoplasm), CEA (cell membrane and cytoplasm)	Thyroglobulin (cytoplasm)
Anaplastic carcinoma	*p53* protein (nuclear)	
Proliferation potency	MIB-1 (nuclear)	
ITET/CASTLE*	CD5 (cell membrane), *p63* protein (cytoplasm), c-kit (CD117) (cytoplasm)	Thyroglobulin (cytoplasm), calcitonin (cytoplasm)
Metastatic carcinoma	CD10 for renal cell carcinoma	Thyroglobulin (cytoplasm), thyroid transcription-1 (nuclear)

*ITET/CASTLE: Intrathyroid epithelial thymoma/Carcinoma showing thymus-like differentiation

Methods

1. Protocol for immunohistochemistry using formalin-fixed paraffin-embedded specimens

Immunohistochemical study is performed with 4-μm serial sections prepared from formalin-fixed, paraffin-embedded tissue blocks. Immunostaining is carried out with an automated immunostainer, the Ventana Benchmark XT device (Ventana, Tucson, AZ), using a streptavidin-biotin-peroxidase kit with 3,3'-diamino-benzidine (LSAB, Ventana).

1) Deparaffinization
2) Wash with buffer solution
3) Antigen retrieval with activation solution specialized for the equipment at 95 °C for 30 minutes
4) Wash with buffer solution
5) Delayed inhibitor
6) Wash with buffer solution
7) Primary antibody incubation at 37 °C for 30 minutes
8) Wash with buffer solution
9) Streptavidin-biotin-peroxidase kit with 3,3'-diamino-benzidine at 37 °C for 8 minutes
10) Wash with buffer solution
11) Hematoxylin nuclear counterstaining at 37 °C for 8 minutes
12) Wash with buffer solution
13) Post-counterstain (lithium carbonate) at 37 °C for 4 minutes
14) Wash with buffer solution
15) Wash with water
16) Dehydration with 100% alcohol and clearing with xylene
17) Mount with Marinol

2. Protocol for immunocytochemistry using cytological specimens

Immunocytochemical study is carried out using 95% alcohol-fixed smears from FNA. Alcohol fixation is used, followed by additional fixation with 20% phosphate buffered formalin solution for 30 minutes, and antigen retrieval with activation solution specialized for the equipment at 95 °C for 30 minutes. This procedure is followed by the steps from 2) to 17) in the protocol for tissue section immunohistochemistry. This protocol can also be used for staining decolorized Papanicolaou-stained smears and those from cell transfer technique (1-3).

3. An example of fixation effects on immunohistochemical results

As an example, MIB-1 (Ki-67) immunostaining of papillary thyroid carcinoma is presented to explain how the fixation causes differences in the results.

In the histopathological specimen of a papillary carcinoma, only few cells were positively stained (nuclear antigen), showing a MIB-1 labeling index of 1.3% (Figure 1). However, in the alcohol-fixed cytological specimen from the same case, MIB-1 was negatively stained, showing a MIB-1 index of 0% (Figure 2). When the alcohol fixation was followed by an additional step of formalin fixation (double fixation), MIB-1 was also negatively stained, showing a MIB-1 index of 0% (Figure 3). On the other hand, when the specimen with alcohol fixation was followed by formalin fixation and antigen activation treatment, some tumor cells became positively stained with MIB-1 (Figure 4), showing a MIB-1 index of 1.3%, which was identical to that of the histological specimen (Figure 1). However, when the specimen with alcohol fixation alone went through the activation treatment, MIB-1 was positively stained, but at the same time the cellular details were demolished (Figure 5). For other antigens of immunostaining, such as cell membrane and cytoplasm antigens, formalin fixation and antigen activation treatment often produce more favorable results. An example stained with CK19 is shown in Figure 6.

Conclusion

For the purpose to obtain reliable and optimal results in immunostaining with cytological specimens, it is essential to formulate the standard staining conditions and to implement a regular protocol. Please refer to Table 2 for the immunohistochemical illustrations in other Chapters in this Book.

Table 2: Please refer to the following chapters for immunohistochemistry as examples.

Markers	Chapters and illustration numbers	Positive antigen localization
β-Catenin	Chapter 9 (Figures 11 and 14)	Nucleus and cytoplasm
Calcitonin	Chapter 15 (Figure 2A), Chapter 16 (Figures 7 and 10), S-Chapter 5 (Figure 18)	Cytoplasm
Carcinoembryonic antigen (CEA)	Chapter 16 (Figure 11)	Cell membrane and cytoplasm
Chromogranin A	Chapter 18 (Figure 15)	Cytoplasm
CD5	Chapter 17 (Figures 7-9)	Cell membrane
CD10	Chapter 22 (Figures 4 and 7)	Cell membrane and cytoplasm
CD23	Chapter 14 (Figure 8)	Cytoplasm
CD68	Chapter 11 (Figure 3G)	Cytoplasm
Cytokeratin AE1/AE3	Chapter 14 (Figure 9)	Cytoplasm
Cytokeratin 19	Chapter 28 (Figure 6)	Cytoplasm
Estrogen receptor	Chapter 9 (Figures 13 and 15)	Nucleus
GATA-3	Chapter 18 (Figure 18)	Nucleus
Ki-67 (MIB-1)	Chapter 12 (Figures 8 and 11), Chapter 16 (Figure 12), and Chapter 28 (Figures 1, 4 and 5)	Cell membrane of HTT but in nucleus of others
Parathyroid hormone	Chapter 18 (Figure 14)	Cytoplasm
PAX8	Chapter 18 (Figure 17)	Nucleus
p53	Chapter 21 (Figure 9)	Nucleus
Thyroglobulin	Chapter 9 (Figure 12), Chapter 11 (Figure 3H)	Cytoplasm
Thyroid transcription-1 (TTF1)	Chapter 18 (Figure 16)	Nucleus

References

1. Maruta J, Hashimoto H, Yamashita H, et al. Value of thyroid specific peroxidase and Ki-67 stains in preoperative cytology for thyroid follicular tumors. Diagn Cytopathol 2015; 43(3):202-9.
2. Brown GC, Tao LC. Restoration of broken cytology slides and creation of multiple slides from a single smear preparation. Acta Cytol 1992; 36(2):259-63.
3. Sherman ME, Jimena-Joseph D, Grang MD, et al. Immunostaining of small cytologic specimens. Facilitation with cell transfer. Acta Cytol 1994; 38(1):18-22.

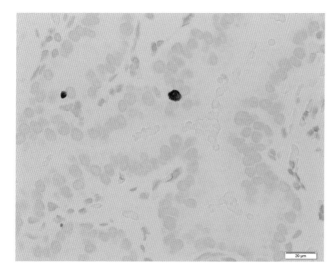

Figure 1. MIB-1 staining of a histological specimen with formalin fixation and antigen activation treatment (x400).

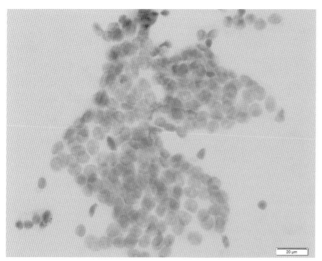

Figure 2. MIB-1 staining of a cytological specimen with alcohol fixation alone (x400).

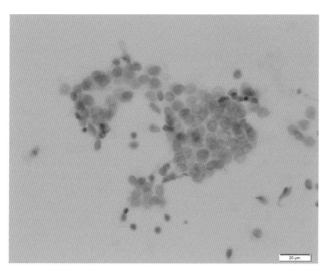

Figure 3. MIB-1 staining of a cytological specimen with alcohol and formalin double fixation (x400).

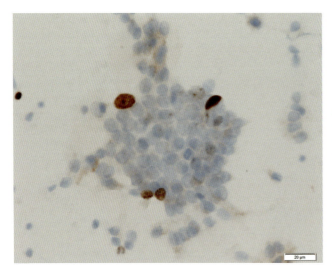

Figure 4. MIB-1 staining of a cytological specimen with alcohol and formalin double fixation as well as antigen activation treatment (x400).

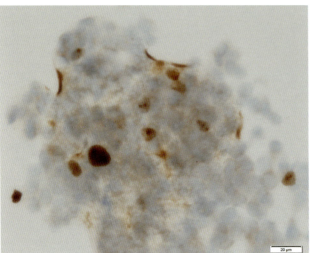

Figure 5. MIB-1 staining of a cytological specimen with alcohol fixation and antigen activation treatment. Note poor morphological details and higher non-specific staining. (x400)

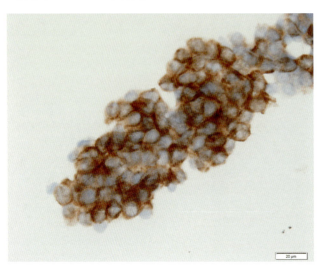

Figure 6. CK19 staining of a cytological specimen with alcohol and formalin double fixation as well as antigen activation treatment (x400).

Chapter 29

Pitfalls in Molecular-based Diagnosis Using Thyroid Aspirates

Toru Takano

The ATA Guidelines and Molecular Tests in Thyroid Cytology
　　　The 2015 ATA management guidelines for adult patients with thyroid nodules and differentiated thyroid cancer have recommended for cases with AUS/FLUS cytology that after consideration of worrisome clinical and sonographic features, investigations such as repeat FNA or molecular testing may be used to supplement malignancy risk assessment in lieu of proceeding directly with a strategy of either surveillance or diagnostic surgery (recommendation 15 as a weak recommendation with a moderate-quality evidence) (1). For cases with FN/SFN cytology, after consideration of clinical and sonographic features, molecular testing may be used to supplement malignancy risk assessment data in lieu of proceeding directly with surgery (recommendation 16 as a weak recommendation with a moderate-quality evidence) (1). Although the diagnostic surgery is the long-established standard for patients with FN/SFN nodules in most Western countries, the ATA guidelines sifted to more conservative clinical managements.

　　　As more than 70% of thyroid cancers harbor at least one known genetic alteration, molecular tests for a panel of somatic mutations are a powerful adjunct to morphological diagnosis. Several studies on *BRAFV600E* mutation, *RET/PTC* rearrangements, or *RAS* mutations in thyroid FNA samples have suggested that detection of these gene abnormalities could provide a conclusive diagnosis. When indeterminate aspirates were analyzed for the presence of *BRAF* and *RAS* mutations and for *RET/PTC* and *PAX8-PPARγ* (peroxisome proliferator-activated receptor gamma) gene rearrangements, mutations have been found in 16% of cases (2-5). These genetic markers have a high specificity and a high predictive value, therefore helping identify which indeterminate nodules are malignant (6).
However, Trimboli *et al.* concluded differently that the role of the BRAF mutation to detect or exclude cancers in the indeterminate nodule was marginal, because the BRAF mutation rate in the indeterminate nodules was low to 4.6% (43/1361 cases) in their meta-analysis of 8 studies (7). The ATA guideline has also stated that there is currently no single optimal molecular test that can definitively rule in or rule out malignancy in all cases of indeterminate cytology (1).

Commercially Available Tests
　　　　Another approach is the use of gene expression signatures, which achieves a high sensitivity and a high negative predictive value (8). This sensitive preoperative test allows accurate identification of benign nodules and the prevention of purely diagnostic surgery. There are two commercially available methods, the Afirma gene expression classifier (AGEC) and the ThyroSeq next-generation sequencing assay (9, 10).
　　　　AGEC is a proprietary diagnostic assay developed by Veracyte Inc (San Francisco, CA). It relies on the "benign gene expression fingerprint" to identify those indeterminate FNAs with a high negative predictive value. The assay analyzes the mRNA expression of a panel of 167 genes and is essentially a "rule-out" test for thyroid cancer. Of these 167 genes, 142 are involved in the main classifier (benign *vs.* malignant) and the remaining 25 genes filter out rare neoplasms.
　　　　The multi-gene ThyroSeq next-generation sequencing assay examines point mutations

in 14 genes and 42 types of gene fusions occurring in thyroid cancer, in addition to 8 genes to evaluate the cell composition. A sensitivity of 90.9%, specificity of 92.1%, positive predictive value of 76.9% and negative predictive value of 97.2% were demonstrated by Nikiforov et al. following analysis of 465 AUS/FLUS nodules (10).

However, these diagnostic kits using thyroid aspirates are very expensive, about three to ten thousand dollars, since they analyze a large number of targets, and are not covered by the health insurance in Japan. In addition, it is not suitable to use them for cancer screening since they show a low sensitivity for detecting thyroid carcinoma. At present, these kits are only used in a limited number of countries, thus, it is quite difficult for the author to recommend them in this textbook. Considering that the current cytological examination provides a reliable diagnosis for the majority of thyroid tumors and cost only about 20 dollars, such expensive diagnostic kits are not likely to be introduced as routine clinical tests in other countries. Rather, a molecular-based diagnosis targeting a small number of genes, such as the *TFF3*(trefoil factor 3)-based testing (please see below), might be initially introduced as an adjunct to cytology in the near future.

Changing Concept of Thyroid Carcinogenesis

Cancer has long been hypothesized that it develops through a mechanism of multi-step carcinogenesis or an adenoma-carcinoma sequence. However, the recent clinical evidence on thyroid carcinoma, such as from the Korean thyroid cancer epidemic, observation trials of papillary thyroid microcarcinoma (PTMC), and the Fukushima Health Management Survey, is clearly inconsistent with this hypothesis (11-13). First, thyroid carcinomas arise not from thyroid follicular cells in adults, but from some unknown origins that only present in infants. In other words, small thyroid carcinomas are already established during the infantile period. Second, the majority of thyroid tumors never progress into tumors with higher malignant features. In other words, the characteristics of each thyroid tumor strictly depend on its cellular origin, and the accumulating genetic changes are not always responsible for the malignant characteristics of cancer cells. These ideas are now summarized as the fetal thyroid cell carcinogenesis (14, 15). These marked changes in the basic concept of thyroid carcinogenesis mean that the targets of molecular-based diagnosis of thyroid carcinoma should be re-evaluated.

Differentiation of Follicular Thyroid Carcinoma from Adenoma

The most important molecular-based diagnosis in thyroid cytology is how to identify follicular carcinoma (FTC), because other types of carcinoma can be easily distinguished from benign tumors by conventional cytological examinations. There have been many studies reporting optimistic molecular targets for diagnosing FTC but, to date, none of them has been established as a diagnostic tool for clinical use.

Because most thyroid researchers have believed in multi-step carcinogenesis, and almost all of these targets were carcinoma-specific because, in multi-step carcinogenesis, FTC are derived from follicular adenomas by accumulating genetic alternations or through the overexpression of oncogene-related products.

However, recent data using microarrays have proved that FTC could be classified into at least two different groups by gene expression, leading to questions about some previous studies with favorable results using carcinoma-specific genes (16). On the other hand, follicular adenoma consists of a single group, suggesting that adenoma-specific genes are promising targets for differential diagnosis. Among these genes, trefoil factor 3 (*TFF3*) mRNA is regarded as the most promising, because its expression level is high in thyroid tumors and the expression difference between malignant and benign is more marked than that for other candidate genes (17). Clinical trials of *TFF3*-based diagnosis are ongoing in some countries, including Japan and Germany (18, 19).

The next pitfall to be considered is the fifteen percent issue in the pathological diagnosis of FTC (20). Recent studies have proved that the pathological diagnosis using the current WHO criteria has a high interobserver variation (21). Thus, at least 15% of the cases show a discrepancy between the pathological diagnosis and the biological characteristics of the tumor. This phenomenon is called "the fifteen percent issue" in FTC, which results in a marked discrepancy between pathological and molecular-based diagnosis. In fact, *TFF3*-based diagnosis using tumor tissues also showed a discrepancy to the pathological diagnosis at a rate of around 20% for minimally invasive FTC without metastasis, but it showed almost perfect agreement for widely invasive FTC and minimally invasive FTC with metastasis (17-19). Thus, molecular tests on FA/FTC lineage tumors remain in research level, and ideal molecular targets should be established not only based on diagnostic accuracy but also the sensitivity in diagnosing clinically evident malignant cases.

Mature and Immature Cancer

It should be taken into consideration that the majority of thyroid carcinomas are not lethal, even though they have invasive or metastatic potential. Thus, we have to determine not only whether a tumor is malignant but also whether it is lethal.

In an observation trial of PTMC, no patient died from cancer (12). This finding revealed that lethal thyroid cancer is different from PTMC. In other words, PTMC does not progress to lethal carcinoma. The prognosis of thyroid cancer for patients under the age of 40 is extremely favorable, whereas lethal cancer appears suddenly to be relatively large or exhibits evident metastasis in patients over 40 years of age due to its rapid growth. Such tumors eventually lead to a poor prognosis. Tumors associated with a favorable prognosis represented by PTMC are called mature cancer, whereas those associated with a poor prognosis that appear suddenly in the elderly is called immature cancer in the fetal carcinogenesis theory by Takano (14). However, the morphological differences under microscopy of these two types of cancer have not been established. Thus, the prognosis of differentiated thyroid cancer in patients over 40 years old is quite difficult to be assessed.

Molecular-based distinction between the two types of cancer also remains in research level. Some studies reported that the point mutation in the *BRAF* gene is a good indicator of poor prognosis associated with papillary carcinoma (22). However, some other studies raised questions about such a conclusion (23). Furthermore, the prevalence of the *BRAF* mutation markedly differs even in studies on same areas and on the populations with same ethnic background, which raises serious concerns about the technical reliability of *BRAF* mutation analysis (24). Another possible candidate prognostic indicator is the mutation of *TERT* gene. Some studies showed that the thyroid tumors with *TERT* gene mutation were associated with a poorer prognosis than in those without mutation (25). However, since the prevalence of *TERT* gene mutation shows a strong positive correlation with the patients' age, also an important indicator of poor prognosis in thyroid cancer patients, thus the significance of *TERT* gene mutation is not well established.

When considering the fetal cell carcinogenesis hypothesis, the prognosis associated with thyroid cancer cannot be determined by analyzing genetic alternations. The fate of thyroid cancer is strictly determined by its cellular origin (15). A patient with a tumor derived from a differentiated fetal cell or mature cancer shows a good prognosis, whereas a patient with a tumor derived from an undifferentiated fetal cell such as a stem cell or immature cancer shows a poor prognosis. In fetal cell carcinogenesis, a tumor mass is formed by the proliferation of an undifferentiated cell and these proliferating tumor cells differentiate into well-developed mature cells. Thus, a tumor derived from undifferentiated stem cells can be viewed morphologically as a differentiated tumor when containing only a small number of cancer stem cells, since it is not possible to distinguish it from a tumor consisting of only differentiated tumor cells.

A tumor containing cancer stem cells is definitely associated with a poor prognosis. However, it is not possible to identify such a tumor due to the difficulty in detecting a small portion of immature cells in a tissue using the conventional pathological or molecular-based methods. Identification of a minor proportion of tumor cells in FNA smear samples has a certain limitation because they contain only small numbers of tumor cells.

Preparation of Aspirated Samples

Thyroid aspirates usually contain considerable numbers of normal cells other than thyroid tumor cells. Especially, contamination of peripheral blood cells can interfere with the results of molecular-based diagnosis. Pretreatment of the aspirated sample to purify thyroid tumor cells is inevitable in molecular-based diagnosis. We have developed a simple method to collect tumor cells efficiently (18). Since thyroid tumor cells tend to form clusters, they can be purified by passing through a mesh filter after the sample has been treated with an anti-coagulant (Figure 1). Blood cells pass through the filter, while large clusters of tumor cells remain on the filter. For the extraction of nucleic acids in tumor cells, the filter is washed with a degenerating reagent to lyse cells.

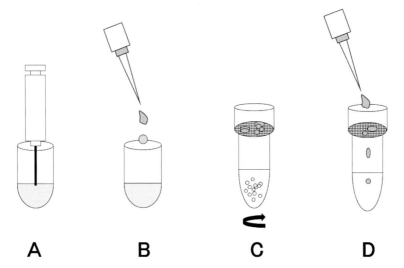

Figure 1. Preparation of the thyroid aspirate by mesh filtration. The aspirate is dispersed into medium containing an anti-coagulant (A), and then the nucleic acid stabilizer is added (B). Following mesh filtration (C), cells remaining on the filter are lysed by adding a degenerating solution (D).

Take Home Message

Some molecular-based diagnostic kits using thyroid aspirates are now available commercially. Because they are extremely expensive and show limited sensitivity in diagnosing thyroid carcinoma, they are not likely to replace cytological examination. Clinical trials of new diagnostic methods based on the new concept of thyroid carcinogenesis, fetal cell carcinogenesis, are now ongoing. Since these methods, such as the *TFF3*-based diagnosis, are cheap and show high sensitivity for diagnosing thyroid carcinoma, it is expected they will be firstly introduced into clinical practice as an adjunct to cytology in the near future.

References

1. Haugen BR, Alexander EK, Bible KC, et al. American Thyroid Association management guidelines for adult patients with thyroid nodules and differentiated thyroid cancer. Thyroid 2015; 26:1-134.
2. Sapio MR, Posca D, Raggioli A, et al. Detection of RET/PTC, TRK and BRAF mutations in preoperative diagnosis of thyroid nodules with indeterminate cytological findings. Clin Endocrinol 2007; 66: 678-83.
3. Jo YS, Huang S, Kim YJ, et al. Diagnostic value of pyrosequencing for the BRAF V600E mutation in ultrasound-guided fine-needle aspiration biopsy samples of thyroid incidentalomas. Clin Endocrinol 2009; 70:139-44.
4. Hyeon J, Ahn S, Shin JH, et al. The prediction of malignant risk in the category 'atypia of undetermined significance/follicular lesion of undetermined significance' of the Bethesda System for Reporting Thyroid Cytopathology using subcategorization and BRAF mutation results. Cancer Cytopathol 2014; 122: 368-76.
5. Cantana S, Capezzone M, Marchisotta S, et al. Impact of proto-oncogene mutation detection in cytological specimens from thyroid nodules improves the diagnostic accuracy of cytology. J Clin Endocrinol Metab 2010; 95:1365-9.
6. Nikiforov YE, Ohori NP, Hodak SP, et al. Impact of mutational testing on the diagnosis and management of patients with cytologically indeterminate thyroid nodules: a prospective analysis of 1056 FNA samples. J Clin Endocrinol Metab 2011; 96: 3390-7.
7. Trimboli P, Treglia G, Condorelli E, et al. BRAF-mutated carcinomas among thyroid nodules with prior indeterminate FNA report: a systematic review and meta-analysis. Clin Endoclinol (Oxf) 2016; 84:315-20.
8. Eszlinger M, Paschke R. Molecular fine-needle aspiration biopsy diagnosis of thyroid nodules by tumor specific mutations and gene expression patterns. Mol Cell Endocrinol 2010; 322:29-37.
9. Alexander EK, Kennedy GC, Baloch ZW, et al. Preoperative diagnosis of benign thyroid nodules with indeterminate cytology. N Engl J Med 2012; 367:705-15.
10. Nikiforov YE, Carty SE, Chiosea SI, et al. Impact of the multi-gene ThyroSeq next-generation sequencing assay on cancer diagnosis in thyroid nodules with atypia of undetermined significance/follicular lesion of undetermined significance cytology. Thyroid 2015; 25:1217-23.
11. Ahn HS, Kim HJ, Welch HG. Korea's thyroid-cancer "epidemic" - screening and overdiagnosis. New Engl J Med 2014; 371:1765-7.
12. Ito Y, Miyauchi A, Kihara M, et al. Patient age is significantly related to the progression of papillary microcarcinoma of the thyroid under observation. Thyroid 2014; 24: 27-34.
13. Suzuki S. Childhood and adolescent thyroid cancer in Fukushima after the Fukushima Daiichi nuclear power plant accident: 5 years on. Clin Oncol 2016; 28: 263-71.
14. Takano T. Fetal cell carcinogenesis of the thyroid: a hypothesis for better understanding of gene expression profile and genomic alternation in thyroid carcinoma. Endocr J 2014; 51: 509-15.
15. Takano T. Molecular classification of thyroid tumor: A proposal based on the fetal cell carcinogenesis hypothesis. J Basic Clin Med 2015; 4:81-6.
16. Wojtas B, Pfeifer A, Jarzab M, et al. Unsupervised analysis of follicular thyroid tumours transcriptome by oligonucleotide microarray gene expression profiling. Endokrynol Pol 2013; 64: 28-34.
17. Takano T, Miyauchi A, Yoshida H, et al. High-throughput differential screening of mRNAs by serial analysis of gene expression: decreased expression of trefoil factor 3 mRNA in thyroid follicular carcinomas. Br J Cancer 2004; 90:1600-5.
18. Yamada H, Takano T, Kihara M, et al. Measurement of TFF3 mRNA in aspirates from thyroid nodules using mesh filtration: the first clinical trial in 130 cases. Endocr J 2012; 59: 621-30.
19. Karger S, Krause K, Gutknecht M, et al. ADM3, TFF3 and LGALS3 are discriminative molecular markers in fine-needle aspiration biopsies of benign and malignant thyroid tumours. Br J Cancer 2012; 106: 562-8.

20. Takano T. The fifteen percent issue in molecular-based diagnosis of follicular thyroid carcinoma. Pathol Int 2011; 61:165-6.
21. Cipriani NA, Nagar S, Kaplan SP, et al. Follicular thyroid carcinoma: How have histologic diagnosis changed in the last half-century and what are the prognostic implications? Thyroid 2015; 25:1209-16.
22. Xing M. Prognostic utility of BRAF mutation in papillary thyroid cancer. Mol Cell Endocrinol 2010; 321:86-93.
23. Ito Y, Yoshida H, Maruo R, et al. BRAF mutation in papillary thyroid carcinoma in a Japanese population: its lack of correlation with high-risk clinicopathological features and disease-free survival of patients. Endocr J 2009; 56:89-97.
24. Guerra A, Sapio MR, Marotta V, et al. The primary occurrence of BRAFV600E is a rare clonal event in papillary thyroid carcinoma. J Clin Endocrinol Metab 2012; 97:517-24.
25. Xing M, Liu R, Liu X, et al. BRAF V600E and TERT promoter mutations cooperatively identify the most aggressive papillary thyroid cancer with highest recurrence. J Clin Oncol 2014; 32: 2718-26.

Chapter 30

Techniques of Thyroid Fine-Needle Aspiration

Hongxun Wu

Thyroid nodules are common, approximately 2% to 22% of biopsied and resected thyroid nodules are malignant, and only a small percentage of them exhibit aggressive behavior. Fine-needle aspiration (FNA) is a standard test to determine proper management. High quality FNA samples obtained by technically-skilled operators should be representative of the lesion for further interpretation. This chapter emphasizes on thyroid FNA techniques, and pre-/post- management in detail, as well as the issues related to specimen adequacy.

Routine FNA Procedure

At our institute, the patients taking antithrombotic therapy are requested to suspend the medication for an appropriate period of time before FNA. For the patients taking aspirin, FNA is performed as usual and the increased risk of bleeding complications is informed. We recommend pressing on the biopsy site for a longer period than usual. The detailed procedure and the possible complications are explained to patients. (please refer to Chapter 26) The patient is questioned about the possible allergies, and told not to talk, cough, and swallow during biopsy. The informed consent is signed.

Conventional and color Doppler ultrasound scans are performed to understand the location, size, and sonographic features of the nodule(s) for determining which nodule is to be biopsied. Color Doppler imaging is used to observe and locate any large vessels in and around the nodule to avoid vascular injury.

The patient is placed supine with his or her neck extended (Figure 1). The patient's head turns away from the side to be biopsied to allow easy access for the operator to perform biopsy. The patient's neck is prepared with povidone iodine (alcohol) swabs. Local anesthetic is not used. Rapid on-site cytological assessment is not available (please refer to Chapter 31). A 23-gauge needle (23G is standard in China and Japan, while 25G is popular in Europe and USA) is used with an attached 5-mL disposable syringe in our practice in China (Figure 2). The operator, using a freehand biopsy technique, places the needle immediately above the transducer, inserts the needle adjacent to the side of the midpoint of the transducer, and angles the needle back toward the transducer. The angle varies depending on the depth of the nodule biopsied. With this perpendicular approach (Figure 3), the needle is advanced toward the nodule under ultrasound guidance. When employing the capillary technique, once the needle is within the target region of the nodule, the operator moves the needle back and forth at about 2 to 3 oscillations per second while rotating the needle on its axis to create an evenly distributed vacuum force. Aspiration is applied when it is necessary.

The operator obtains four smears by extracting two samples from each nodule. The FNA specimens are directly smeared on slides and fixed in 95% ethyl alcohol. Subsequently, the needle and syringe are washed with 1 ml of normal saline solution, and the rinsed sample is used for tumor marker measurement of washout fluids, such as calcitonin (please refer to Chapter 23). The excess FNA samples can also be processed as a specimen to aid in the molecular testing.

Points

The smear slides should be labeled clearly with patient's name and specimen source. Place an order in the electronic record system. The order should indicate which nodule was biopsied, as well as its location and size, brief sonographic features (echogenicity, composition, shape, margin, and presence and type of calcification), and the background structure described on the current ultrasound scan. The perfect FNA results can be predicated upon continuity of the contribution by a team of experienced physicians skilled at good communication for their findings.

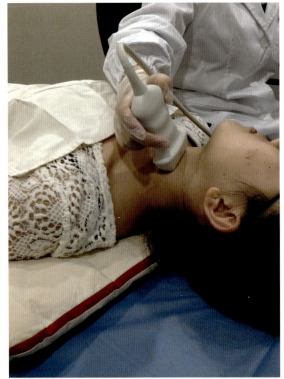

Figure 1. Patient positioning. The patient lies on his/her back with a pillow under shoulders and neck extended. The operator locates at the shoulder of patient.

Figure 2. 2A: Tools for fine-needle aspiration; and 2B: Spring-action core needle biopsy gun.

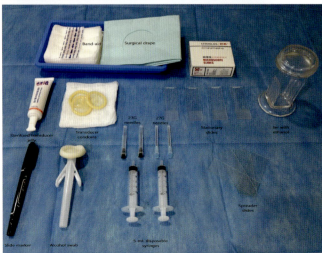

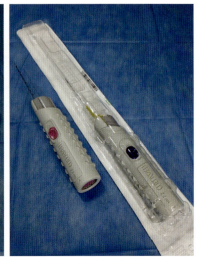

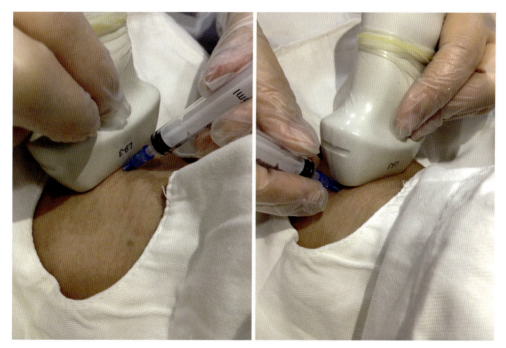

Figure 3. 3A: Perpendicular approach; and 3B: Parallel approach.

Factors influencing Diagnostic Accuracy of FNA

The diagnostic accuracy of FNA has been known to vary depending on the experience of the operator, intrinsic sonographic features of the nodule, FNA techniques, and cytology interpretation.

Intrinsic Sonographic Features

Several more locations should be selected for sampling to ensure obtaining representative samples of a heterogeneous large nodule. The needle tip localization is greatly depended on the judgment of the operator.

In the past two decades, some studies have focused on the association between the sonographic features and the nondiagnostic results in cytology. A cystic portion greater than 50%, a nodule with less than 5 mm in diameter, and hypoechogenicity are the independent factors affecting nondiagnostic results (1). In a study by Degirmenci *et al.*, the nondiagnostic results have been shown to be more frequent in hypoechoic nodules than non-hypoechoic nodules, although the difference is not statistically significant (2); the findings are consistent with the study by Wu *et al.*, which has suggested that the nondiagnostic results are observed more frequently in hypoechoic sites of a nodule with avascularity in color Doppler ultrasound and hard pattern in ultrasound elastography (3). One possible explanation is that a combination of aforementioned features may be necessary to predict fibrosis of the target region. Thus, it is difficult to obtain sufficient samples in nodules with severe fibrosis or dense calcification. In clinical practice, regions with these features should be excluded when choosing sample locations for FNA. Theoretically, regions with suspicious calcification should be sampled. In some studies, whether calcification is present and its type have been indicated not independent factors for predicting nondiagnostic results. While the present data suggest that it is dilemma to obtain sufficient specimens in the nodule with rim calcification.

Points

The cellularity of a nodule influences mostly its intrinsic sonographic features. When selecting a region for sampling, the operator should fully take into account the intrinsic features that are helpful to improve the adequacy of thyroid FNA. These features are also helpful to determine which sampling technique, FNA or fine needle capillary (FNC), is applied.

Needle Size and Utilization of Core Biopsy

Many studies have focused on what size of needles could provide better specimens for adequate cytopathology. The lumen diameter of the needle is an independent factor for nondiagnostic results. A well-accepted viewpoint is that a larger needle (22-23G) can provide samples with more cells, although the correlation between the gauge of the needle and the quality of specimen has been debated. In a study by Ucler *et al.*, the effect of increasing the needle diameter used for FNA was investigated and the investigators have demonstrated that the larger needle was superior to the smaller needle (25-27G) for specimen adequacy and diagnostic accuracy (4). Increasing the gauge of needle for nodules with prior nondiagnostic results is recommended.

Many studies have reported a significantly lower nondiagnostic rate with core needle biopsy (CNB) than repeat FNA, showing that the performance of CNB in conjunction with FNA is helpful in improving adequacy rate (5-7). The advantage of CNB is providing more adequate specimen for evaluation, which is not readily available by FNA (7). Unsuccessful penetration into the peripheral calcification as well as restricted intra-nodular movement of the needle yields an inadequate specimen. However, the powerful spring action of CNB might make it easier to penetrate the calcification and ensure collecting sufficient specimens for subsequent analysis.

In some studies, inconclusive rate for CNB (17.6%) has been reported to be significantly lower than that for repeat FNA (37.3%) for AUS/FLUS nodules. The higher diagnostic rate of CNB is mainly attributed to more tissues obtained, providing histopathologic information of the lesion (including the fibrous capsule) as well as the surrounding thyroid parenchyma (8). In addition, CNB could provide tissue samples that enable immunohistochemical staining for differential diagnosis. For diagnosis of follicular carcinoma, as we know, evaluation of the entire nodular capsule is required to detect the presence of capsular/vascular invasion. Sampling tissues showing malignant invasion is not easy. Although the sensitivity of CNB may be superior in the diagnosis of non-follicular thyroid lesions, e.g. papillary thyroid carcinoma, CNB is not enough for a definitive diagnosis or to exclude follicular carcinomas. A specific recommendation has not yet been established on using CNB as a follow-up tool for nodules with nondiagnostic results. As a cost-effective and simple technique, FNA remains the best method for initial evaluation, and CNB has been suggested to use as a potential complementary diagnostic tool.

Points

Once a core needle is inserted into a hypervascular nodule, it often fills with blood immediately, which makes it difficult to obtain adequate specimen. In some circumstances, even though the procedure is performed by a skilled operator and an adequate number of cells may be present in a bloody sample, interpretation of the contaminated specimen is still problematic. Because of the potential complications including bleeding or post-biopsy hematomas, CNB is not recommended for use. A large fine needle (23G) in conjunction with liquid-based preparation obviates the concern. When biopsy materials are directly deposited into preservative liquid, the redundant red blood cells are removed by lysis, which enhances the FNA diagnostic rate (please refer to Chapter 27).

Comparison between Sampling Techniques

The sample may be obtained with application of either aspiration action technique (FNA) or capillary action technique (fine needle capillary, FNC). In the procedure of FNA, once the needle is placed into the target region, the operator moves the needle back and forth as well as applies suction. The plunger of the syringe is then slowly released and the needle is withdrawn. For FNC, only a fine needle is used without negative suction as done in FNA. The hub of needle is held between the thumb and forefinger, and the needle is inserted into the lesion and then moved back and forth while being rotated on its axis. As soon as aspirate appears in the hub through capillary action, the needle is withdrawn and attached to the air-filled syringe. The contents are then expelled onto the slides. With this method, the materials ascend spontaneously to the needle by capillary action.

The number of nondiagnostic or unsatisfactory specimens greatly depends on the sampling techniques. For a reliable cytological diagnosis, the adequacy of specimen is essential, which is determined by the amount of cellular material, preservation of cellular architecture, degree of cellular degeneration, degree of cellular trauma, and presence or absence of blood contamination (9-11). The advantages of both FNA and FNC methods have been reported in the literature. In general, we think FNC is better because of less blood contamination in the background, maintenance of cellular architecture, and less cellular degeneration and trauma to cells. Regarding the amount of cellular yield, it is found to be better by FNA as compared to by FNC. However, the problem of blood-contaminated samples is that it is difficult for cytopathologists to interpret. It has been demonstrated that negative suction used in FNA could disrupt the nodule structure. Thus, performance of FNC following FNA results in an increased frequency of inadequate specimens. It is interesting that a few studies have come to the conclusion that the diagnostic yields of FNA and FNC are almost identical, and there is no significant benefit for FNA (12-13).

Points

Both techniques have their own advantages and disadvantages, and neither is absolutely superior to the other. Although it depends upon the operator to select the technique, we propose FNC should be performed first for sampling. FNA is only suggested when the amount of cellular material is inadequate.

Rotation of the needle around the long axis adds a shearing component to the cutting action of the trailing edge of needle, and this approach might improve cellular yield. The dwell time within the nodule must be reduced as much as possible. Rapid sampling action may diminish bloody obscuration.

FNC for small nodules will increase the chance of inadequate specimens. Extensive fibrosis is more frequently detected in small nodules. It is hard for the fine needle to penetrate to a firm nodule and sample the nodule using the capillary technique. Even under the ultrasound guidance, targeting and needle excursion are problematic for this technique. Thus, FNC is not recommended for this situation.

Direct Smear (DS) vs. Liquid-based Cytology (LBC) Preparation

In a DS, the materials are extruded onto slides directly and then fixed with 95% ethyl alcohol for Papanicolaou stain. DS is a regular preparation method for thyroid cytology, however, its quality is highly dependent on the operator who performed the smear. For operators who are not trained in the smear techniques, LBC procedure is easy and reasonable. The aspirate is deposited directly into the preservative liquid, thus obtaining a thin layer of representative cells on a single slide. The procedure can be repeated safely when the smear shows low cellularity with on-site assessment.

Most studies have reported that LBC produces more clear nuclear details and background, but there is no significant difference in the adequacy rate and diagnostic accuracy between LBC and DS. A better cell morphology is attributed to fewer nuclei overlap presented by LBC. It is also found that hemorrhage and necrosis are reduced in LBC as compared with DS. Decrease of obscuring background elements makes it easy for cytological interpretation (14). In general, LBC preserves adequate cellularity with sufficient cellular details for diagnostic purposes. However, some authors have stated that LBC alone for thyroid FNA diagnosis is inferior to DS due to its lower sensitivity (15) (please refer to Chapter 27).

Another advantage of LBC over DS in the diagnosis of follicular lesions is the possibility to apply ancillary techniques such as immunocytochemistry, flow cytometry, and molecular analysis, which are helpful in refining the diagnosis of a follicular lesion. It is possible to differentiate benign from malignant by evaluating the markers regardless of the presence of capsular or vascular invasion. In addition, the residual sample in the fixative solution after cytological diagnosis can be safely stored at room temperature for up to six months (16).

One of the most important changes occurring in LBC compared to DS is the lack of watery colloid, which has been considered a major problem for interpretation. Sparsely cellular DS specimens are frequently identified as adequate on the basis of abundant colloid, and thus, the removal of colloid in LBC processing has the potential to obscure the diagnosis of benign nodules (17).

It is true that papillary thyroid carcinoma is more easily recognized with DS than with LBC, because the pristine nuclear morphology is more clearly displayed with DS. Conversely, benign goiter appears to be more easily recognized with LBC (18). In addition, a combination of DS and LBC will lead to increase in definitive diagnosis of papillary thyroid carcinoma. The morphological differences between the two methods, such as smaller fragments in LBC and cell dyshesion, are challenges for pathologists to review (19) (please refer to the Table 1 of Chapter 27).

Points

Split sample can be used for processing thyroid FNA with the LBC technique: a part of the aspirated materials is smeared onto slides for DS, and the residual is deposited in a solution for LBC. In an attempt to avoid uneven distribution of materials, direct to vial, two separate samplings, are recommended; the first smears onto slides for DS and the second rinses in the solution for LBC. The rate of unsatisfactory LBP might also been attributed to the split sample technique used in acquiring needle rinse materials, which likely accounts for insufficient cellularity. With the direct-to-vial method, all of the materials are submitted for cytological analysis. The average cellularity with the direct-to-vial method is generally higher than that with the split-sample method, and the rates of inadequacy and false positivity are decreased significantly.

In conclusion, despite the advantages, including low cost, simple procedure, high overall accuracy, decreased background noise, presentation of uniform cells, prominent nucleoli and preserved fine nuclear details, are noted in LBC, the procedure is usually considered as an adjunct to DS, and it is not recommended to use alone.

Smear Preparation

The aspirated material is expressed onto a stationary slide by using an air-filled syringe to extrude material. Alternatively, operator can gently express a drop of aspirate onto a stationary slide. The method selection mainly depends on the nature of the material. A drop may be easily expressed without force if the aspirated material is abundant and fluid. If the material is scant, or viscous, the material should be forcefully expelled. The latter method can result in splattering of the material off the slide, which is not easy for control of the smear process (20).

The operator holds a stationary slide in one hand, a spreader slide in the other hand to make the smear. The spreader slide is gently lowered over the droplet, which will spread out slightly by capillary action. The spreader slide is then gently pulled straight back in one smooth motion, down the length of the stationary slide (20). Repeat the above procedure with additional drops of material to create 2-4 slides. We prefer to immediately fix the slides with 95% ethanol for Papanicolaou staining in our practice.

Points

When smearing the slide, do not apply pressure to the aspirated material. Do not lift either end of the spreader slide until smear preparation is complete.

Fixation

Wet fixation is a routine process by placing the freshly prepared smears immediately in fixative solutions for a defined period of time. Fixation can keep cells and tissue away from putrefaction and degeneration caused by bacteria and autolytic enzymes present in the cells, and preserve the cell morphology as close as possible to the living state. As a dehydrating agent, 95% ethanol is the ideal fixative recommended for cytological specimen.

Wet-fixed smears are superior to air-dried smears in quality with regard to nuclear and cytoplasmic preservation, preventing the drying artefacts presented in the latter, the drying artefacts lead to difficulty in interpretation (please refer to Chapter 31). When the smears are fixed in 95% ethanol immediately, the cells are killed rapidly and uniformly. With an increased air-dried duration, the staining quality of the smears becomes more unsatisfactory. There is no doubt that rehydration of the air-dried smears, by immersing the air-dried smears in normal saline for 30 seconds followed by fixation in 95% ethanol, can lyse the red blood cells and obtain a clear background. However, there is no significant difference between the two methods in cytology diagnosis.

Points

All alcohol fixatives should be discarded after each use. A minimum of 30 minutes fixation is essential. Prolonged fixation for several days or even few weeks will not affect the morphology of cells.

When delayed fixation occurs due to improper training of the staff, and the air drying is less than 30 minutes, it seems a plausible choice with subsequent rehydration of the air-dried smears, which yields results comparable to those of wet-fixed smears.

An educational video for optimal FNA techniques is available online at the Papanicolaou Society of Cytopathology home page (www.papsociety.org) and educational sessions at:
(http://www.thyroidmanager.org/chapter/fine-needle-aspiration-biopsy-of-the-thyroid-gland/).

References

1. Moon HJ, Kwak JY, Kim EK, et al. Ultrasonographic characteristics predictive of nondiagnostic results for fine-needle aspiration biopsies of thyroid nodules. Ultrasound Med Biol 2011; 37:549-55.
2. Degirmenci B, Haktanir A, Albayrak R, et al. Sonographically guided fine-needle biopsy of thyroid nodules: the effects of nodule characteristics, sampling technique, and needle size on the adequacy of cytological material. Clin Radiol 2007; 62:798-803.

3. Wu H, Zhang B, Zang Y, et al. Ultrasound-guided fine-needle aspiration for solid thyroid nodules larger than 10 mm: correlation between sonographic characteristics at the needle tip and nondiagnostic results. Endocrine 2014; 46:272-8.
4. Ucler R, Kaya C, Çuhacı N, et al. Thyroid nodules with 2 prior inadequate fine-needle aspiration results: effect of increasing the diameter of the needle. Endocr Pract 2015; 21:595-603.
5. Samir AE, Vij A, Seale MK, et al. Ultrasound-guided percutaneous thyroid nodule core biopsy: clinical utility in patients with prior nondiagnostic fine-needle aspirate. Thyroid 2012; 22:461-7.
6. Choi SH, Baek JH, Lee JH, et al: Thyroid nodules with initially non-diagnostic, fine-needle aspiration results: comparison of core-needle biopsy and repeated fine-needle aspiration. Eur Radiol 2014; 24:2819-26.
7. Yeon JS, Baek JH, Lim HK et al. Thyroid nodules with initially nondiagnostic cytologic results: the role of core-needle biopsy. Radiology 2013; 268:274-80.
8. Choi YJ, Baek JH, Ha EJ, et al. Differences in risk of malignancy and management recommendations in subcategories of thyroid nodules with atypia of undetermined significance or follicular lesion of undetermined significance: the role of ultrasound-guided core-needle biopsy. Thyroid 2014; 24:494-501.
9. Romitelli F, Di Stasio E, Santoro C, et al. A comparative study of fine needle aspiration and fine needle non-aspiration biopsy on suspected thyroid nodules. Endocr Pathol 2009; 20:108-13.
10. Mair S, Dunbar F, Becker PJ, et al. Fine needle cytology - is aspiration suction necessary? A study of 100 masses in various sites. Acta Cytol 1989; 33:809-13.
11. Kamal MM, Arjune DG, Kulkarni HR. Comparative study of fine needle aspiration and fine needle capillary sampling of thyroid lesions. Acta Cytol 2002; 46:30-4.
12. Maurya AK, Mehta A, Mani NS, et al. Comparison of aspiration vs. non-aspiration techniques in fine-needle cytology of thyroid lesions. J Cytol 2010; 27:51-4.
13. Mahajan P, Sharma PR. Fine-needle aspiration versus nonaspiration technique of cytodiagnosis in thyroid lesions. JK Sci 2010; 3:120-2.
14. Pawar PS, Gadkari RU, Swami SY, et al. Comparative study of manual liquid-based cytology (MLBC) technique and direct smear technique (conventional) on fine-needle cytology/fine-needle aspiration cytology samples. J Cytol 2014; 31:83.
15. Hyeyoon C, Eunjung L, Hyunjoo L, et al. Comparison of diagnostic values of thyroid aspiration samples using liquid-based preparation and conventional smear: one-year experience in a single institution. APMIS 2013; 121:139-45.
16. Yassa L, Cibas ES, Benson CB, et al. Long-term assessment of a multidisciplinary approach to thyroid nodule diagnostic evaluation. Cancer 2007; 111:508-16.
17. Nagarajan N, Schneider EB, Ali SZ, et al. How do liquid-based preparations of thyroid fine-needle aspiration compare with conventional smears? an analysis of 5475 specimens. Thyroid 2015; 25: 308-13.
18. Fischer AH, Clayton AC, Bentz JS, et al. Performance differences between conventional smears and liquid-based preparations of thyroid fine-needle aspiration samples: analysis of 47076 responses in the College of American Pathologists Interlaboratory Comparison Program in Non-Gynecologic Cytology. Arch Pathol Lab Med 2013; 137:26.
19. Mygdakos N, Sylvia N, Anna T, et al. Liquid based preparation (LBP) cytology versus conventional cytology (CS) in FNA samples from breast, thyroid, salivary glands and soft tissues. Our experience in Crete (Greece). RGME 2009; 50:245-50.
20. Fine needle aspiration preparation of direct smears. http://www.pathlabsofark.com/fnadirectsmears.html, 2007-10.

Chapter 31

Standard and Rapid Stains in Fine-Needle Aspiration Cytology and Rapid On-Site Evaluation

Takashi Koshikawa

Standard Stains in Fine-Needle Aspiration (FNA) Cytology

Two different fixations are used in FNA cytology: wet-fixation by ethanol and air-dried fixation. Wet-fixed smears are mainly stained by Papanicolaou (PAP) staining (1), but some of them also by Hematoxylin-Eosin (HE) staining. On the other hand, air-dried smears are stained with May-Gruenwalds-Giemsa (MGG), Giemsa (2), or Wright staining (3). MGG stain is also called Pappenheim stain in Germany, where Dr. Pappenheim invented and reported this method in 1911 (4). MGG stain is one of the Romanowsky stains, which is characterized by Romanowsky effects, i.e., polychromatic effects caused by the mixture of methylene blue, methylene azur, and eosin in the staining solution (5).

The cytological findings between PAP and MGG stains are quite different. Both stains have their own advantages and disadvantages (6). The characteristic features of both stains are shown in Tables 1 and 2. The air-dried cells on MGG smears are flattened on the glass and appear approximately 1.5 times larger than cells wet-fixed by ethanol. This is one of the most distinctive features of air-dried MGG smears. Dry materials are good for MGG staining, while wet materials are good for PAP staining. Peeling off of smeared cells from the glass sometimes occurs with PAP staining, but seldom with MGG staining. Squamous differentiation or nuclear features such as nuclear grooves and nuclear cytoplasmic inclusions are easily recognized on PAP smears. On MGG smears, on the other hand, cytoplasmic granules or extracellular materials such as basement membrane substance, myxoid ground substance, etc., are easily recognized by Romanowsky effects. Both stains seem to complement each other's disadvantages.

A cytologist's preference on staining methods depends on his/her cytological training background (6). Cytologists with training in gynecological cytology prefer Pap smears, while those with a hematological background prefer air-dried MGG smears. However, it is strongly recommended to use PAP and MGG stains together in FNA cytology, because cytologists can obtain much more useful findings for cytological diagnosis from a FNA specimen in this manner.

Table 1. Comparison of the Pap and MGG stain characteristics

	PAP Stain	MGG Stain
Fixation	Wet-fixed by ethanol	Air-dried by cool wind
Dry material	Drying artifacts seen	Well preserved
Wet material	Well preserved	Swelling artifacts seen
Peeling artifacts	Sometimes occur	Seldom
Cell size	Similar to that of tissue sections	About 1.5 times larger than Pap or H&E
Cytoplasm	Hard to see cytoplasmic granules	Easy to see cytoplasmic granules
Nucleus	Similar to tissue sections	Different from Pap or H&E
Nucleoli	Always clear	Not always clear
Cell clusters	Easy to see each cell	Hard to see each cell
Stromal components	Poorly shown	Often shown by metachromasia

Table 2. Advantages of both Pap and MGG stains

	PAP Stain	MGG Stain
Nucleus and Cytoplasm	Squamous differentiation (squamous cell carcinoma)	Secretory granules
	Nuclear grooves and cytoplasmic inclusions (thyroid papillary carcinoma)	Neuroendocrine granules (endocrine tumors)
		Lipofuscin granules (seminal vesicle, thyroid, etc.)
		Bile pigment
		Marginal vacuoles (hyperthyroidism)
		Cytoplasmic crystals (alveolar soft part sarcoma)
Extracellular materials	Psammoma bodies	Extracellular mucin (mucinous carcinoma)
		Colloid (thyroid)
		Amyloid (thyroid medullary carcinoma, etc.)
		Basement membrane substance (capillary vessels, adenoid cystic carcinoma, etc.)
		Myxoid ground substance (mixed tumor, fibroadenoma, etc.)
		Chondroid ground substance (cartilage, chondroma, etc.)
		Osteoid (bone, osteosarcoma, etc.)
		Lymphogranular bodies (lymphocyte or lymphoma)
		Cholesterol crystals (cystic change)

Rapid Stains in FNA Cytology and Rapid On-site Evaluation (ROSE)

Rapid stains in FNA cytology are used for ROSE. Cytological smears are usually air-dried and stained by rapid Romanowsky stain, such as Diff-Quik stain (7). Other stains, such as rapid PAP or rapid H&E stains, are also available for ROSE (8-9), but Diff-Quik stain is the easiest and most convenient in my experience. Cytologists working with ROSE are recommended to be familiar with Romanowsky smears. Diff-Quik stain is based on the modification of the Wright-Giemsa stain and is commercialized as a rapid staining kit. Diff-Quik staining kit consists of three solutions (fixative, red-colored solution 1 containing eosin G, and blue-colored solution 2 containing thiazine dye). Air-dried smears can be stained very quickly in a few minutes, and they exhibit beautiful Romanowsky effects (Figures 1-2). After staining, the excess water is wiped out from the glass, and the smear is ready for on-site microscopic examination by cytologists. They can make a tentative diagnosis there, but the final diagnosis is usually not made on-site. It should be made after examining the wet-fixed, regularly prepared PAP smears. The primary purpose of ROSE is not to make a diagnosis on-site, but to confirm the specimen adequacy.

Specimen adequacy influences diagnostic results of FNA cytology. ROSE is a method to confirm a specimen adequacy on the spot in FNA examinations. The practice of ROSE improves the specimen adequacy rate, and also the diagnostic accuracy. ROSE is used in various fields, such as endoscopic ultrasound-guided FNA (EUS-FNA) of pancreas (9), FNA of thyroid (11), and endobronchial ultrasound-guided transbronchial FNA (EBUS-TBNA) of lung (12). The introduction of ROSE results in a high specimen adequacy rate of more than 90%. In my experience, the specimen adequacy rate by application of ROSE is 98.9% for the thyroid and 95.0% for the pancreas (EUS-FNA). The diagnostic accuracy also improves to 92.8% for the thyroid and 95.6% for the pancreas. ROSE may also decrease the incidence of repeat FNA examinations (7). ROSE is a really important aid for FNA cytology to improve the diagnostic results. As mentioned above, the main purpose of ROSE is to evaluate the specimen adequacy, not to make a cytological diagnosis on-site, therefore not only cytologists but also cytotechnologists can perform ROSE.

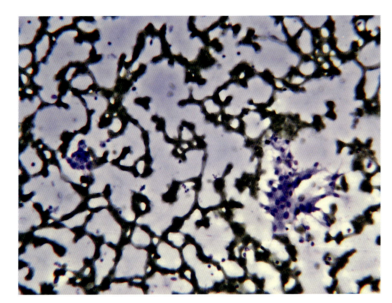

Figure 1. Benign adenomatous nodule of the thyroid. (Diff-Quik, x200)

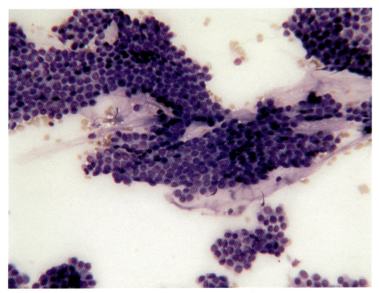

Figure 2. Thyroid papillary carcinoma. (Diff-Quik, x200)

References

1. Papanicolaou GN. A new procedure for staining vaginal smears. Science 1942; 95:438-9.
2. Giemsa G. Eine Vereinfachung und Vervollkommnung meiner Methylenazur-Methylenblau-Eosin-Färbemethode zur Erzielung der Romanowsky-Nochtschen Chromatinfärbung. Centralblatt für Bakteriologie 1904; 37:308-11.
3. Wright JH. A rapid method for the differential staining of blood films and malarial parasites. J Med Res 1902; 7(1):138-44.
4. Pappenheim A. "Panchrom", eine Verbesserung der panoptischen Universalfarbloesung fuer Blutpraeparate jeder Art nebst Ausfuehruengen ueber metachromatische Farbstoffe und die mrtachromatisch Potenz des polychromen Methlenblau (Unna). Folia Haematologica 1911; 11:194-223.
5. Romanowsky D. Zur Frage der Parasitologie und Therapie der Malaria. St. Petersburg Med Wochenschr 1891; 16:297-302, and 307-15.
6. Vielh WP. The Techniques of FNA Cytology. In Orell SR, Sterrett GF, Walters MN-I, Whitaker D, eds. Manual and Atlas of Fine Needle Aspiration Cytology. Churchill Livingstone, London, 1999; p9-27.
7. Silverman JF, Frable WJ. The use of the Diff-Quik stain in the immediate interpretation of fine-needle aspiration biopsies. Diagn Cytopathol 1990; 6:366-9.
8. Yang GC, Alvarez II. Ultrafast Papanicolaou stain. An alternative preparation for fine needle aspiration cytology. Acta Cytol 1995; 39(1):55-60.
9. Jörundsson E, Lumsden JH, Jacobs RM. Rapid staining techniques in cytopathology: a review and comparison of modified protocols for hematoxylin and eosin, Papanicolaou and Romanowsky stains. Vet Clin Pathol 1999; 28:100-8.
10. Collins BT, Murad FM, Wang JF, et al. Rapid on-site evaluation for endoscopic ultrasound-guided fine-needle biopsy of the pancreas decreases the incidence of repeat biopsy procedures. Cancer Cytopathol 2013; 121:518-24.
11. Witt BL, Schmidt RL. Rapid onsite evaluation improves the adequacy of fine-needle aspiration for thyroid lesions: a systematic review and meta-analysis. Thyroid 2013; 23:428-35.
12. Alsharif M, Andrade RS, Groth SS, et al. Endobronchial ultrasound-guided transbronchial fine-needle aspiration. Anat Pathol 2008; 130:434-43.

Chapter 32:

Case Study and Mini-Tests
(Multiple choice questions and differential diagnosis)

Kennichi Kakudo, Masahiko Ura, Keiko Inomata, Ayana Suzuki, Yun Zhu,
Zhiyan Liu, Yubo Ren, Xin Jing and Shinya Satoh

Case 1:
A female patient, 57 years old, was found to have a1.5 x 1.5 cm thyroid nodule in her left lobe. A FNA cytology was performed (Case 1 Figures 1-3).

Please select the most suitable diagnosis from the following choices.
1. Low-risk Indeterminate Category (Follicular lesion of undetermined significance: FLUS)
2. High-risk Indeterminate Category (Hurthle Cell Neoplasm)
3. Suspicious for Poorly Differentiated Carcinoma
4. Suspicious for C cell (medullary) Carcinoma
5. Malignant (Papillary carcinoma, oxyphilic cell type)
6. Malignant (Metastatic Carcinoma)

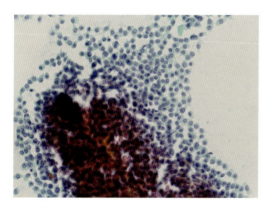

CASE 1 Figure 1

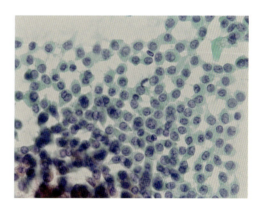

CASE 1 Figure 2

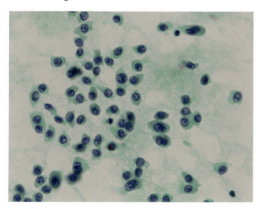

CASE 1 Figure 3

Case 2:
A 78 years old male patient noticed a rapidly growing neck mass. A FNA cytology was performed (Case 2 Figures 1-3).

Please select the most suitable diagnosis from the following choices.
1. Inadequate (Cyst fluid)
2. Benign, Abscess (Acute infectious thyroiditis)
3. Benign, Necrosis and degeneration (Infarct) of hyperplastic nodule
4. Low-risk Indeterminate (AUS, Thy 3a or TIR 3A)
5. Suspicious for Malignant lymphoma
6. Malignant, Cystic papillary carcinoma
7. Malignant, Undifferentiated carcinoma

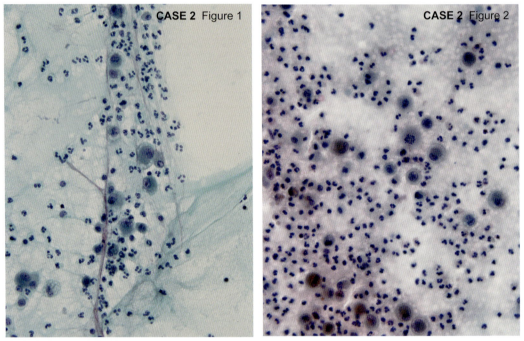

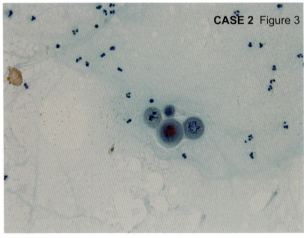

Case 3:
A 41 years old female patient was found to have a 2.5x1.5 cm thyroid nodule in her left lobe of the thyroid. A FNA cytology was performed (Case 3 Figures 1 and 2).

Please select the most suitable diagnosis from the followings.
1. Benign, Adenomatous nodule
2. Low-risk Indeterminate Category (AUS/FLUS, Thy 3a or TIR 3A)
3. High-risk Indeterminate Category (FN, Thy 3f or TIR 3B)
4. Suspicious for Papillary Carcinoma, follicular variant
5. Malignant, Papillary Carcinoma, conventional

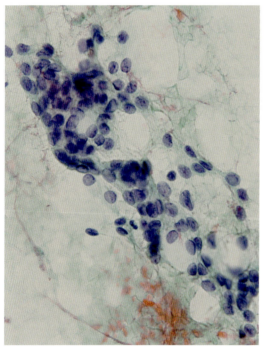   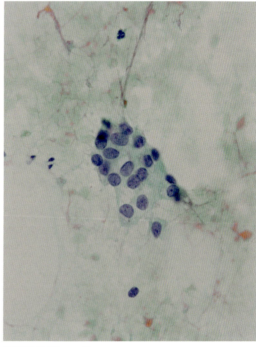

CASE 3 Figure 1   CASE 3 Figure 2

Case 4:
A female patient of 78 years old was found to have a mass lesion in her thyroid. A FNA cytology was performed (Case 4 Figures 1 and 2).

Please select the most suitable diagnosis from the following choices.
1. Low-risk Indeterminate Category (Follicular lesion of undetermined significance)
2. High-risk Indeterminate Category (Follicular Neoplasm)
3. Suspicious for Poorly Differentiated Carcinoma
4. Malignant (Papillary carcinoma)
5. Malignant (Metastatic carcinoma)

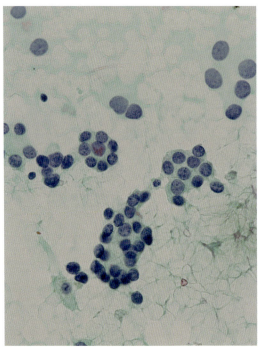

CASE 4 Figure 1

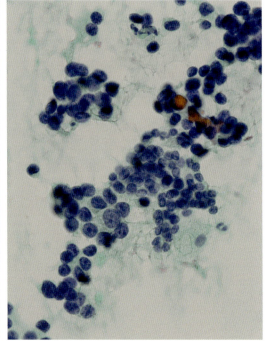

CASE 4 Figure 2

Case 5:

A 31 years old female patient was found to have a cystic mass in her left thyroid lobe (Case 5 Figures 1 and 2)

Please select the most suitable diagnosis from the following choices.
1. Inadequate (Cyst) (Thy 1c or TIR 1C)
2. Benign, Cystic Adenomatous Nodule (Thy 2c or TIR 3C)
3. Low-risk Indeterminate (AUS, Thy 3a or TIR 3A)
4. Suspicious for Cystic Papillary Carcinoma
5. Malignant, Cystic papillary carcinoma

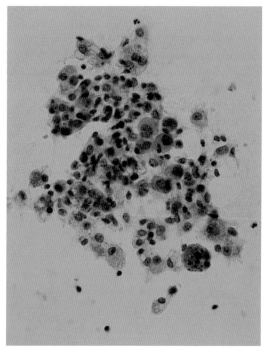

CASE 5 Figure 1

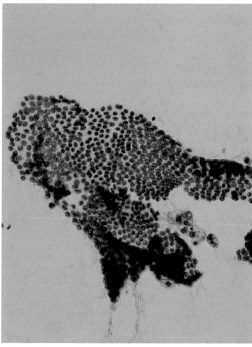

CASE 5 Figure 2

Case 6:
A 20 years old female patient visited at Yamashita Clinic for thyroid enlargement.
Ultrasound examination disclosed a diffuse enlargement of the thyroid with psammomatous calcification (Case 6 Figure 1). FNA cytology was obtained from a hypoechoic nodule from the right lobe (Case 6 Figures 2 and 3).

Please select the most suitable diagnosis from the following choices.
1. Benign: Hashimoto Thyroiditis
2. Indeterminate: Hashimoto Thyroiditis, PTC cannot rule out.
3. High-risk Indeterminate Category (Follicular Neoplasm)
4. Suspicious for Papillary Carcinoma
5. Suspicious for Malignant Lymphoma

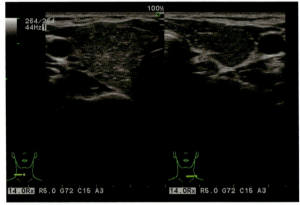

CASE 6 Figure 1

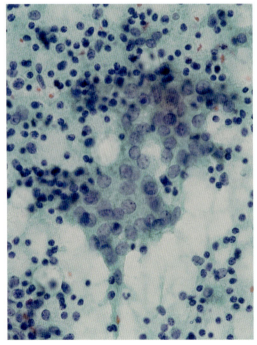

CASE 6 Figure 2

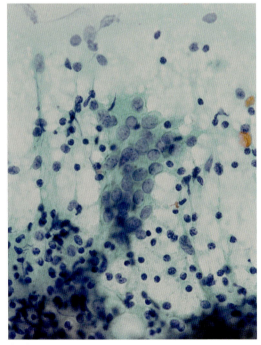

CASE 6 Figure 3

Case 7:
A 55 years old female found to have an 8 mm thyroid nodule at ultrasound examination of carotid arteries. A FNA aspiration biopsy was carried out (Case 7 Figures 1 and 2).

Please select the most suitable diagnosis from the following choices.
1. Benign: Hashimoto Thyroiditis
2. Low-risk Indeterminate Category (AUS, Thy 3a or TIR 3A)
3. High-risk Indeterminate Category (Follicular Neoplasm)
4. Suspicious for Papillary Carcinoma
5. Suspicious for C cell (medullary) Carcinoma

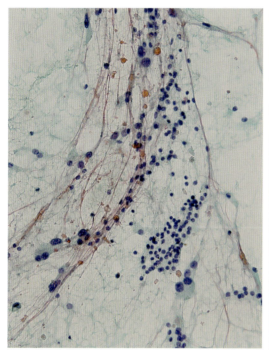
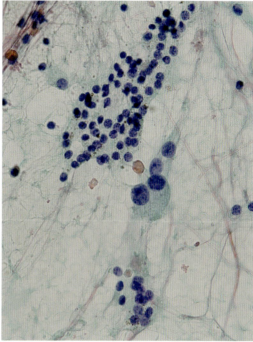

CASE 7 Figure 1   CASE 7 Figure 2

Case 8:
This is a 46-years-old male with a nodule in the left lobe of the thyroid. A FNA cytology was performed (Case 8 Figure 1 and 2).

Please select the most suitable diagnosis from the following choices.
1. Benign, Chronic thyroiditis
2. Benign, Lateral cervical cyst
3. Benign, Esophageal diverticulum
4. Benign, Piriform sinus fistula
5. Malignant, Anaplastic carcinoma

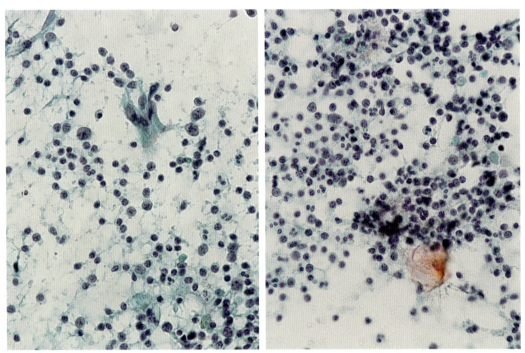

CASE 8 Figure 1   CASE 8 Figure 2

Case 9:
A 66-year-old male patient noticed a neck mass. A FNA cytology was performed. (Case 9 Figures 1-3).

Please select the most suitable diagnosis from the following choices.
1. High-risk Indeterminate Category (Follicular Neoplasm with bizarre nuclei)
2. Suspicious for Malignancy (Undifferentiated Carcinoma)
3. Malignant (C cell Carcinoma)
4. Malignant (Poorly Differentiated Carcinoma)
5. Malignant (Parathyroid Carcinoma).

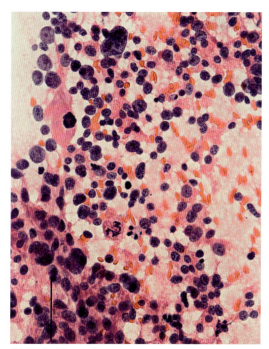

CASE 9 Figure 1

CASE 9 Figure 2

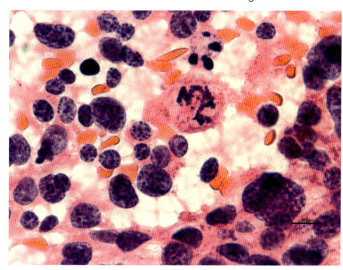

CASE 9 Figure 3

Case 10:

A 61 year-old female was self-referred to the ENT clinic due to neck mass. An ultrasound exam detected multiple thyroid nodules and the dominant one was located at the isthmus, measuring 2.2 x 1.6 x 1.2 cm. No other lab tests performed. An ultrasound-guided fine needle aspiration was performed with rapid on-site evaluation (ROSE) (Case 10 Figures 1 and 2).

What is your diagnosis?
1. Suspicious /positive for papillary thyroid carcinoma
2. Suspicious/positive for Hurthle cell neoplasm
3. Hurthle cell lesion of undetermined significance
4. Lymphocytic (Hashimoto's thyroiditis)
5. Metastatic carcinoma

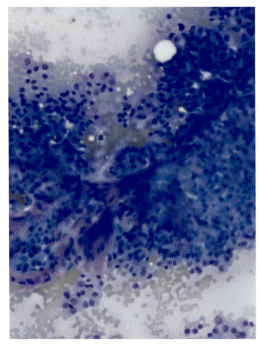

CASE 10 Figure 1

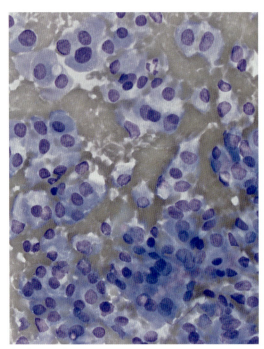

CASE 10 Figure 2

Diagnoses and Explanatory Notes

Case 1 (Case 1A-Figures 1-3):

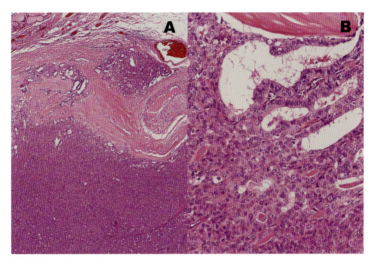

CASE 1A Figure 1

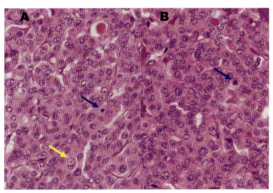

CASE 1A Figure 2

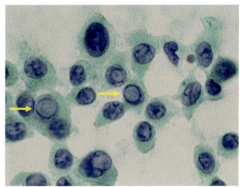

CASE 1A Figure 3

Diagnosis: Both 3 (Suspicious for Poorly Differentiated Carcinoma) and 5 (Malignant, Papillary carcinoma, oxyphilic cell type) are acceptable.

This was a case of invasive encapsulated carcinoma (Case 1A, Figure 1) with predominant solid/trabecular growth (Case 1A, Figures 1 and 2), and a minor papillary growth was found in the periphery of the tumor (Case 1A, Figures 1A and 1B). Increased mitoses (blue arrows) were noted (Case 1A, Figures 2A and 2B). No insular growth or tumor necrosis was found. Papillary thyroid carcinoma type nuclear features (nuclear inclusions and grooves) (yellow arrow) were observed in a few cells (Case 1A, Figure 2A). Answer No.5: Malignant (Papillary carcinoma, oxyphilic cell type) is also acceptable. The nuclear characteristics differed from those of neuroendocrine carcinoma (salt and pepper) type, and typical PTC type nuclear features, including nuclear cytoplasmic inclusions, were noted (Case 1A, Figure 2A: yellow arrow). Please note these are also observed in Case 1A Figure 3 (yellow arrows).

Please refer to Chapter 15 for C-cell (medullary) carcinoma, Chapter 20 for follicular neoplasms, Chapter 21 for poorly differentiated carcinoma, and Chapter 22 for metastatic carcinoma.

Case 2 (Case 2A-Figures 1-3):
Diagnosis: Malignant, Undifferentiated carcinoma

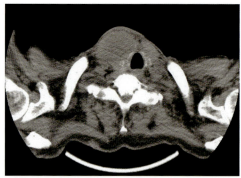
CASE 2A Figure 1

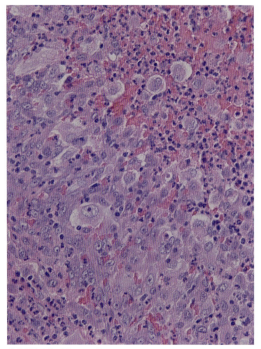
CASE 2A Figure 2

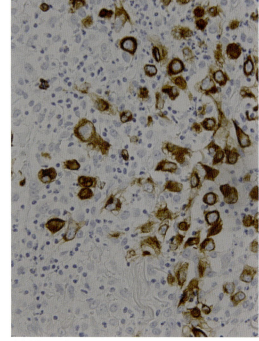
CASE 2A Figure 3

The neck tumor in the thyroid invaded into surrounding anatomic structures (Case 2A Figure 1), including trachea and muscle tissue, and only a wedge biopsy of the tumor was obtained for histopathologic diagnosis (Case 2A Figure 2). The patient died of disease on the 30th hospitalization, and permission for autopsy was not granted. This was a case of an invasive tumor in which granulocytic infiltration and atypical large cells with bizarre nuclei were observed (Case 2A, Figure 2). No epithelial arrangement, such as follicular structure or papillary growth, was found. These atypical cells showed densely stained, broad cytoplasm, resulting in a histiocytic or rhabdoid appearance (Case 2A, Figure 2). Keratin immunohistochemistry revealed the epithelial nature of these atypical cells (Case 2A Figure 3), with high Ki 67 labeling index (30-50%) and p53 positivity.

Please refer to Chapter 7 for cystic papillary carcinoma, Chapter 11 for subacute thyroiditis, Chapters 15 and 16 for C cell carcinoma, Chapter 21 for poorly differentiated carcinoma, Chapter 24 for infectious thyroiditis and Chapter 25 for tumor necrosis.

Case 3 (Case 3A-Figures 1-3):

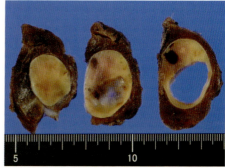
CASE 3A Figure 1

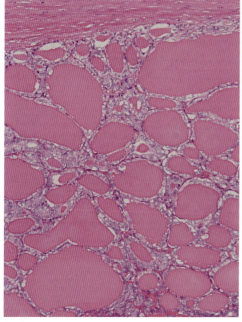
CASE 3A Figure 2

CASE 3A Figure 3

Diagnosis: Non-invasive follicular thyroid neoplasm with papillary-like nuclei (NIFTP) (Synonyms include non-invasive encapsulated follicular variant papillary thyroid carcinoma, well differentiated tumor of uncertain malignant potential and well differential tumor with uncertain behavior) (1-3)

2. Low-risk Indeterminate Category (AUS/FLUS, Thy 3a or TIR 3A) is the most suitable choice.

An encapsulated thyroid nodule was found in the left lobe (Case 3A Figure 1), and was identified as a follicular pattern lesion in both cytology (Case 3 Figures 1 and 2) and histology (Case 3A Figure 2). Neither invasive growth nor papillary growth was found. These enlarged nuclei showed ground glass (pale) chromatin and irregular nuclear contours (Case 3A Figure 3). These worrisome nuclear features of papillary thyroid carcinoma in histology (Case 3A Figure 3) were also observed as irregular nuclei in cytology (Case 3 Figures 1 and 2). No metastatic carcinoma was found in the dissected lymph nodes.

Please refer to Chapters 11 and 13 to evaluate papillary thyroid carcinoma type nuclear features in non-neoplastic lesions, Chapter 6 for precursor lesions, and Chapters 3, 4 and 5 for fully developed papillary carcinoma.

Case 4 (Case 4A-Figures 1 and 2):

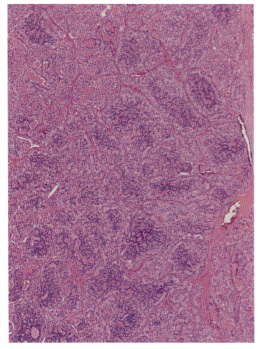 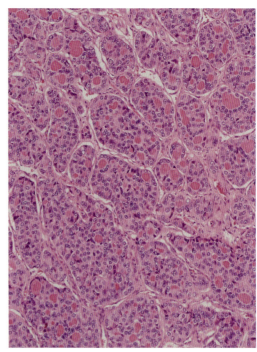

CASE 4A Figure 1   CASE 4A Figure 2

Diagnosis: 2 High-risk Indeterminate Category (Follicular Neoplasm) and 3 Suspicious for Poorly Differentiated Carcinoma are equally acceptable.

Histological Diagnosis: Poorly differentiated carcinoma (widely invasive follicular carcinoma with angio-invasion and insular growth).

A follicular pattern cellular smear is shown in Case 4 Figures 1 and 2. High grade nuclear features were observed, such as large hyperchromatic nuclei and distinct nucleoli (Case 4 Figures 1 and 2). Nuclear enlargement, overlapping, and anisonucleosis were marked in the 3-dimensional follicular clusters (Case 4 Figures 1 and 2). Neither nuclear grooves nor nuclear cytoplasmic inclusions were found, ruling out PTC type malignancy. Metastatic carcinoma and ITET/CASTLE were ruled out due to the presence of microfollicles with colloid production (Case 4 Figures 1 and 2). No mitotic figures were identified in cytology, although they were frequently observed in histology (please refer to Chapter 21). No colloid, necrotic debris, or inflammatory cell infiltration was observed in the smear background.

The tumor occupied the entire left lobe. Histologically prominent insular growth with follicle forming islands were observed (Case 4A Figures 1 and 2). Necrosis and degeneration and marked vascular invasion were noted.

Please refer to Chapters 4, 8, and 10 for aggressive variants of papillary carcinoma, Chapter 16 for giant cell type C-cell carcinoma, Chapter 20 for widely invasive follicular carcinoma, Chapter 21 for poorly differentiated carcinoma, and Chapter 22 for metastatic carcinoma.

Case 5 (Case 5A-Figures 1-3):
Diagnosis: Malignant, Cystic papillary carcinoma
4. Suspicious for Cystic Papillary Carcinoma is also acceptable.

The cystic nodule contained a solid portion (Case 5A, Figure 1) that was identified as a papillary carcinoma with cystic degeneration at histology (Case 5A, Figure 2). Please refer to Chapter 7 and supplement Chapter 3 for cyst and cystic papillary carcinoma. Dispersed atypical cells as shown in Case 5 Figure 1 and a sheet-like cluster in Case 5 Figure 2 were conclusive for papillary thyroid carcinoma type malignancy (please refer to Chapters 4 and 7). These cancer cells are usually identified in cyst fluid from papillary carcinoma, when samples are properly taken from the solid portion of the cyst wall. In some cystic papillary carcinomas, cancer cells with a histiocytoid appearance and broad, vacuolated cytoplasm may be observed, as shown in Case 5A Figure 3, reported by Renshaw (4). This images is from a 36-year-old female patient with cystic papillary carcinoma. Note the nuclear enlargement and irregular nuclear contour with intranuclear cytoplasmic inclusions in addition to the psammoma body type calcifications (Case 5A Figures 3).

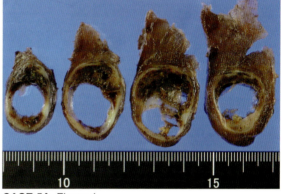

CASE 5A Figure 1

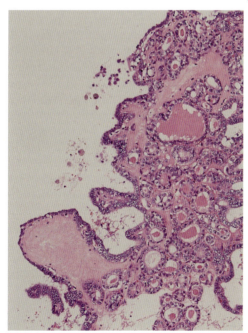

CASE 5A Figure 2

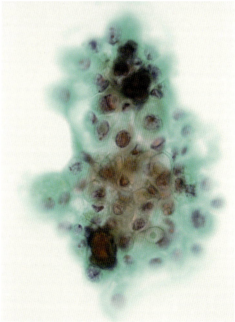

CASE 5A Figure 3

Case 6 (Case 6A-Figures 1 and 2):
Diagnosis: Papillary Carcinoma, diffuse sclerosing variant

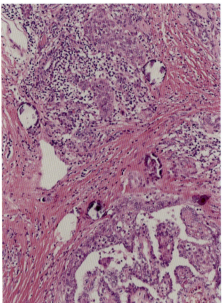

CASE 6A Figure 1

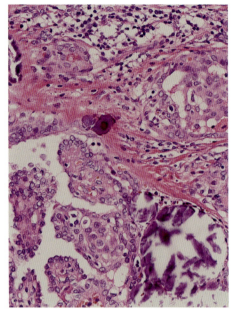

CASE 6A Figure 2

Both 4. Suspicious for Papillary Carcinoma and 2. Indeterminate: Hashimoto Thyroiditis, PTC cannot rule out are acceptable.

A moderate number of follicular cell clusters were observed in the lymphocyte-rich background in Case 6 Figures 1 and 2.
The first differential diagnosis includes papillary thyroid carcinoma and Hashimoto disease, based on the nuclear features of the follicular cells (please refer to Chapters 3, 5, and 13). Mild nuclear enlargement, irregularity of the nuclear membrane, few nuclear grooves, and pale chromatin pattern as shown in Case 6 Figures 2 and 3 suggest suspicious for PTC type malignancy, but are not sufficient for conclusive diagnosis of papillary carcinoma. Suspicious for papillary carcinoma may be the most suitable diagnosis for this case. Together with diffuse psammomatous calcification throughout the entire thyroid (Case 6 Figure 1) and the patient's young age, a sclerosing variant of papillary carcinoma may also be suggested. The second differential diagnosis includes Hashimoto thyroiditis and malignant lymphoma (extranodal marginal zone B cell lymphoma) due to the cytological features of the lymphocytes (please refer to Chapter 14). Presence of a variety of lymphocytes, such as numerous small lymphocytes and few large immature lymphocytes, favors Hashimoto disease more than malignant lymphoma (Case 6 Figures 2 and 3). The third point for differential diagnosis is whether there is presence of neoplastic follicular clusters. Although slightly increased cellularity and overlapping nuclei were observed in Case 6 Figures 2 and 3, the nuclear features did not favor classification into the follicular neoplasm category (please refer to Chapters 19 and 20).
The patient underwent total thyroidectomy and no dominant mass lesion was found in the fibrotic thyroid gland. Invasive papillary carcinoma with psammoma bodies and squamous metaplasia (Case 6A Figures 1 and 2) were found diffusely throughout the thyroid gland, with chronic inflammation and fibrosis.

Case 7 (Case 7A-Figures 1 and 2):
Diagnosis: C cell (medullary) Carcinoma

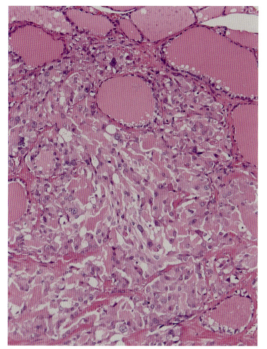
CASE 7A Figure 1

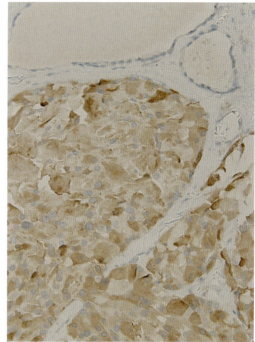
CASE 7A Figure 2

5. Suspicious for C cell (medullary) Carcinoma is the most suitable answer and 2. Low risk Indeterminate Category (AUS, Thy 3a or TIR 3A) is also acceptable.

Two types of cells were observed in the smear (Case 7, Figures 1 and 2): isolated large cells and normal follicular cell clusters with small round nuclei. Due to the small size of the lesion, contamination of surrounding normal follicular cells may have occurred. The isolated large cells had large nuclei and occasionally a giant nucleus eccentrically located in the broad cytoplasm (Case 7 Figure 2). These nuclei displayed a salt and pepper chromatin pattern and distinct nucleoli, which are different from papillary thyroid carcinoma type nuclear features and/or high grade nuclear atypia of undifferentiated carcinoma (please refer to Chapters 15 and 16). No colloid, amyloid substance, necrosis, or cystic change was noted in the smear background.

The cut surface of the thyroid lobe demonstrated an 8 mm solid tumor in the upper pole. The tumor showed solid medullary growth infiltrating into the surrounding thyroid parenchyma, without a capsule. The tumor cells had broad eosinophilic cytoplasm and contained round to oval nuclei with coarse chromatin (Case 7A Figure 1). Immunohistochemistry for calcitonin revealed cytoplasmic positivity, demonstrating the C-cell nature of the case (Case 7A Figure 2). Calcification and amyloid deposits were also noted in the stroma. The patient had no systemic neoplasia syndrome nor family history of neoplastic disease.

Case 8 (Case 8A-Figures 1 and 2):
Diagnosis: 4. Benign, Piriform sinus fistula

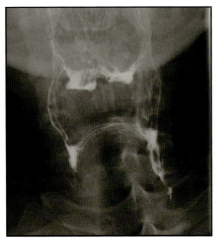

CASE 8A Figure 1

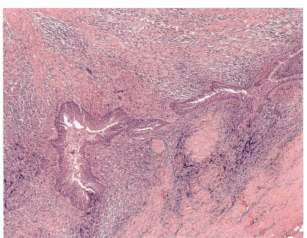

CASE 8A Figure 2

Ultrasound examination showed a hypoechoic, heterogeneous lesion in the dorsal portion of the left lobe of the thyroid. Cytological preparation revealed a large number of lymphocytes and neutrophils. Ciliated columnar cells (Case 8 Figure 1), squamous cells (Case 8 Figure 2), and bacteria were observed.

The presence of squamous cells, bacteria, and neutrophils lead to the differential diagnoses of esophageal diverticulum and piriform sinus fistula. Because lymphocytes and ciliated columnar cells are not seen in the former, the latter is the most acceptable diagnosis in this case. Pleases refer to Supplemental Chapter 4 for thyroglossal duct cyst. The possibility of ciliated cell contamination from the airway was low because of the location of the lesion. Chronic thyroiditis is not associated with neutrophils and can be ruled out (please refer to Chapter 13). The wall of the lateral cervical cyst is composed of squamous cells and lymphocytes, but the latter is not usually obtained by aspiration cytology. Neutrophils, lymphocytes, and squamous cells may appear in anaplastic carcinoma, but neoplastic atypical cells were not seen in this case.

Pyriform sinus fistula (PSF) is a rare congenital internal fistula, arises from the apex of the pyriform sinus of hypopharynx, penetrates the cricothyroid muscle, and terminates in or adjacent to the dorsolateral portion of the left lobe of the thyroid (5). The condition is definitely diagnosed by the detection of the fistula in pharyngoesophageal contrast radiography (Case 8A Figure 1). The condition is frequently accompanied by acute suppurative thyroiditis (please refer to Chapter 24) (5). Therefore, when aspiration cytology from the left upper portion of the thyroid revealed acute inflammatory exudate, the possibility of PSF had to be considered. Microscopically, the internal surface of the fistula was covered by squamous cells (Case 8A Figure 2) or ciliated columnar cells. Lymphocytic infiltration or fibrosis is usually observed around the fistula (Case 8A Figure 2). As a treatment, surgical resection is usually performed, but chemocauterization is currently recommended (6).

Case 9 (Case 9A-Figures 1-3):
Diagnosis: Malignant, Parathyroid Carcinoma

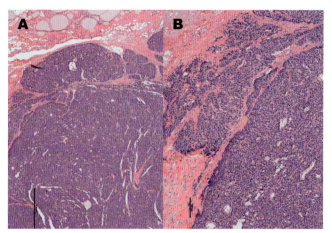

CASE 9A Figure 1

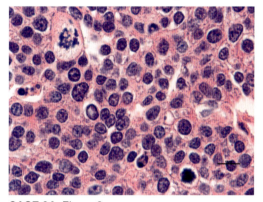

CASE 9A Figure 2

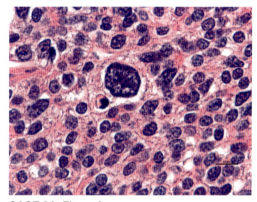

CASE 9A Figure 3

The cells were extremely pleomorphic in size and shape, ranging from medium-size to large or giant size in syncytial tissue fragments or in a dispersed cell pattern (Case 9 Figures 1-3). The nuclei were polygonal with coarsely granular chromatin, containing multiple micro-macronucleoli; mitotic figures were also noted (Case 9 Figures 1 and 3). Due to the mitotic activity and other high grade nuclear features, undifferentiated carcinoma was first suspected. However, the background of the smear was clean without cellular or necrotic debris or inflammatory cells (please refer to Chapter 25). The coarsely granular to salt and pepper-like chromatin (Case 9 Figure 3), dispersed cell pattern, and presence of a few giant cells suggested the possibility of C-cell carcinoma, yet no nuclear inclusions or amyloid in the background were observed, and mitotic activity is often very rare or absent in C-cell carcinoma (please refer to Chapters 15 and 16). Equally important, giant cells and high mitotic activity are also not frequently observed in poorly differentiated carcinoma (please refer to Chapter 21). Parathyroid carcinoma was not initially considered because it is extremely rare. In our practice and limited experience of this type of lesion, parathyroid carcinoma cells might present less distinct cytological features (please refer to Chapter 18). Consequently, ultrasonography and calcitonin and parathyroid hormone serum levels tests were requested. Ultrasound detected a 2.8 x 2.5 x 2.5 cm hypoechoic mass in the right lobe of the thyroid. The patient had osteoporosis associated with hypercalcemia and hyperparathyroidism confirmed by laboratory data. The surgical specimen showed cells containing clear to eosinophilic cytoplasm that were separated by dense bands of fibrosis (Case 9A Figure 1A). Capsular invasion was identified at the periphery of the tumor (Case 9A Figures 1A and 1B). Coarsely granular chromatin, mitotic figures, and giant cells were easily identified (Case 9A Figures 2 and 3), corresponding with the cytological presentations. This case suggested that the accurate diagnosis of parathyroid lesions can be made only in the correct clinical context due to the morphologic overlap between thyroid and parathyroid lesions.

Please refer to Chapters 15 and 16 for C-cell carcinoma, Chapter 18 for parathyroid tumor, Chapter 21 for poorly differentiated carcinoma, and Chapter 25 for necrotic backgrounds in thyroid cytology.

Case 10 (Case 10A-Figures 1-3):
Diagnosis: Nodular hyperplasia with Hurthle cell changes

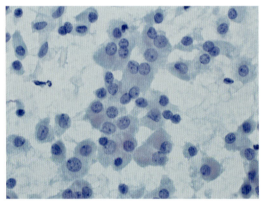

CASE 10A Figure 1

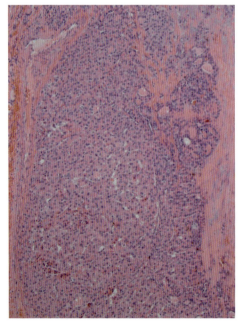

CASE 10A Figure 2

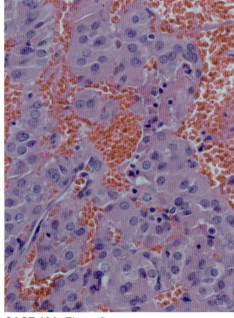

CASE 10A Figure 3

The Diff Quik-stained conventional smears are cellular and consist almost exclusively of Hurthle cells. Many cells arranged as papillary fragments. There are some spindled cells embedded in the fragment, raising the possibility transgressing vessels (Case 10 Figure 1). In addition, single and small clusters of the cells are also appreciated (Case 10 Figure 2). The Pap-stained conventional smears reveal that the cells have abundant granular cytoplasm, round, oval and/or elongated nuclei with relatively smooth nuclear contour, fine to coarse chromatin, prominent nucleoli and occasional intranuclear grooves (Case 10A Figure 1). Although a preliminary diagnosis of suspicious for papillary thyroid was rendered upon the rapid on site evaluation (ROSE) of Diff Quik-stained conventional smears, examination of whole specimen shows no combined features suspicious for papillary thyroid carcinoma, i.e. architectural atypia with syncytial arrangement, marked nuclear enlargement, irregular nuclear outline, powdery chromatin, intranuclear pseudo-inclusion. Occasional intranuclear grooves present and appear thin and incomplete, which can be seen in any benign conditions. It is noteworthy to mention that any of the aforementioned features for papillary thyroid carcinoma alone is not diagnostic for papillary thyroid carcinoma. Overall, Cytologic diagnosis of "Suspicious/positive for Hurthle cell neoplasm" or "Hurthle cell lesion of undetermined significance" is acceptable It was not a complete surprise that the subsequent thyroidectomy revealed nodular hyperplasia with Hurthle cell changes (Case 10A Figures 2 and 3). Importance of sampling involving fine needle aspiration procedure is also reflected in the work up of this case/patient. However, it is beyond the scope of the current discussion. Please refer to Chapter 3 for pitfalls attributed to misdiagnosis of papillary thyroid carcinoma.

References:

1. Nikiforov YE, Seethala RR, Tallini G et al: Nomenclature revision for encapsulated follicular variant of papillary thyroid carcinoma: A paradigm shift to reduce overtreatment of indolent tumors. JAMA Oncol (in press)
2. Liu Z, Zhou G, Nakamura M, Koike E, Li Y et al (2011) Encapsulated follicular thyroid tumor with equivocal nuclear changes, so-called well-differentiated tumor of uncertain malignant potential: a morphological, immunohistochemical, and molecular appraisal. Cancer Sci 102:288-294.
3. Ganly I, Wang L, Tuttle RM et al Invasion rather than nuclear features correlates with outcome in encapsulated follicular tumors: further evidence for reclassification of encapsulated papillary thyroid carcinoma follicular variant. Hum Pathol 46:657-664, 2015.
4. Renshaw AA. "Histiocytoid" cells in fine-needle aspirations of papillary carcinoma of the thyroid. Frequency and significance of an under-recognized cytologic pattern. Cancer Cytopathol. 96: 240-243, 2002.
5. Takai S, Miyauchi A, Matsuzuka F et al: Internal fistula as a route of infection in acute suppurative thyroiditis. Lancet 1(8119):751-752, 1979.
6. Miyauchi A, Inoue H, Tomoda C et al: Evaluation of chemocauterization treatment for obliteration of pyriformis sinus fistula as a route of infection causing acute suppurative thyroiditis. Thyroid 19:789-793, 2009.

Supplemental Chapter 1

The Italian Reporting System for Thyroid Cytology

Guido Fadda

Introduction

The accurate preoperative diagnosis of thyroid nodular lesions represents a real problem for physicians, endocrinologists, and surgeons. The pivotal role of the pathologist is to characterize as best as possible these lesions to enable the patient to receive timely and appropriate treatment. Fine-needle aspiration (FNA) cytology is the only test that can provide a definitive preoperative diagnosis, especially for benign and malignant nodules. Its sensitivity and specificity were reported as 68–98 and 56–100%, respectively, in different studies (1,2).

FNA cytology also represents the most accurate and cost-effective method for distinguishing patients with thyroid nodules who are candidates for surgery from those who

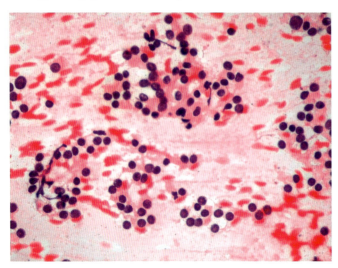

Figure 1. Low-risk indeterminate lesion (TIR 3A). The thyrocytes are monomorphous, and they exhibit scattered microfollicular structures (hematoxylin and eosin stain, ×400).

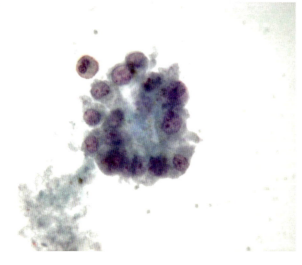

Figure 2. High-risk indeterminate lesion (TIR 3B) displaying a microfollicle lined by follicular cells with mild-to-moderate atypia (ThinPrep, Papanicolaou stain, ×1000).

can be clinically managed. The Italian reporting system for thyroid cytology committee was established in 2011–2014 with the aim of updating the previous Italian Society for Anatomic Pathology and Cytology-Italian Division of the International Academy of Pathology (SIAPEC-IAP) system devised in 2007 (3). The committee that accomplished this task, sponsored by the SIAPEC-IAP in agreement with the endocrinology societies Italian Society of Endocrinology, Association of Medical Endocrinologists, and Italian Association of Thyroid, was composed of 10 experts in thyroid diseases (five pathologists and five endocrinologists). The previous SIAPEC-IAP reporting system was a five-tiered scheme that included the following categories: *TIR 1* - nondiagnostic; *TIR 2* - negative for neoplasia; *TIR 3* - indeterminate/follicular proliferation; *TIR 4* - suspicious for malignant neoplasm; and *TIR 5* - positive for malignancy. The newly devised Italian reporting system (Table 1) (4) introduces the additional subgroup of *TIR 1C* (cystic) in the nondiagnostic group and the subdivision of the indeterminate category (TIR 3 of the previous SIAPEC-IAP system) into *TIR 3A* (low-risk indeterminate lesion, Figure 1) and *TIR 3B* (high-risk indeterminate lesion, Figure 2). The Bethesda Reporting System for Thyroid Cytology (TBRSTC) (5) included six categories. The nondiagnostic, benign, and malignant groups were similar to those in the Italian and British classifications, whereas indeterminate lesions where further subclassified in three diagnostic groups: 1) atypia of undetermined significance/follicular lesion of undetermined significance (AUS/FLUS); 2) follicular neoplasm/suspicious for follicular neoplasm (FN/SFN): and 3) suspicious for malignancy (6).

Table 1. The 2014 Italian reporting system for thyroid cytology (Ref 4)

Code	Diagnostic Category	Risk of malignancy (%)	Suggested actions
TIR 1	Non diagnostic	Non defined	Repeat US-guided FNA after at least 1 month
TIR 1C	Non-diagnostic-cystic	Low (variable on the basis of clinical findings)	Evaluate in the clinical setting and/or repeat FNA
TIR 2	Non malignant/benign	<3	Follow-up
TIR 3A	Low-risk indeterminate lesion (LRIL)	<10*	Repeat FNA/clinical follow-up
TIR 3B	High-risk indeterminate lesion (HRIL)	15-30*	Surgery
TIR 4	Suspicious of malignancy	60-80	Surgery (consider frozen section)
TIR 5	Malignant	>95	Surgery

*The expected rates of malignancy for the TIR 3 subcategories are mainly based on clinical experience and only partially supported by the published data.

The British Thyroid Association together with the Royal College of Pathologists immediately followed TBSRTC in subclassifying FNs into the two subgroups of Thy3a (atypia), corresponding to the Bethesda AUS/FLUS category, and Thy3f (FN), corresponding to the

FN/SFN category of the NCI Conference (7). This reporting scheme was also confirmed in the last update of the British system (8). It is of note that all cases categorized as indeterminate or suspicious and/or malignant in the British system should be referred to the multidisciplinary team to establish the most appropriate clinical management.

The Italian Reporting System 2014

Based on the previous published experiences of the British and American national reporting systems, the Italian committee developed a project with the purposes of i) revising the morphologic criteria of inclusion in each category, and ii) updating the clinical actions with more innovative diagnostic techniques, and iii) validating the new system via a multicenter study. Thus, the 2014 Italian system is different from the previous system, and it features some structural differences in comparison to the aforementioned and Japanese systems (Table 2). The first difference is the different interpretation of nuclear atypia of follicular cells (oncocytic cells are excluded). In fact, architectural atypia remains the basis for distinguishing low-from high-risk lesions (TIR 3A *vs.* TIR 3B), but a significant degree of nuclear atypia warrants the inclusion of a lesion in a suspicious category (TIR 3B or TIR 4), which is immediately submitted for surgical consultation (9-10). Based on this parameter, the Italian committee expects that the frequency of inclusion in the low-risk category (TIR 3A), which does not include cases with severe atypia of thyrocytes, will decrease the risk of malignancy to 5–10%, compared to 5–15% for the homologous categories of the British and American systems. The new Italian reporting system has also included in the suggested actions for the non-diagnostic category (TIR 1) the possibility to use, in cases of repeated non-diagnostic results, the core-

Table 2. Synopsis of the most popular national reporting systems

UK RCPath	Italy	USA BETHESDA	JAPAN THYROID ASSOCIATION
Diagnostic category	Diagnostic category	Terminology	Terminology
Thy1/Thy1c Non-diagnostic for cytological diagnosis Unsatisfactory, consistent with cyst	TIR 1: Non-diagnostic TIR 1C: Cystic	I. Non-diagnostic	Inadequate (non diagnostic)
Thy2/Thy2c Non-neoplastic	TIR 2: Non-malignant/benign	II. Benign	Normal or benign
Thy 3a Neoplasm possible – atypia/non-diagnostic	TIR 3A: Low-risk indeterminate lesion (LRIL)	III. Atypia of undetermined significance (AUS) or follicular lesion u.s. (FLUS)	Indeterminate A. Follicular Neoplasm • A1 favor benign • A2 border-line • A3 favor malignant B. Others (atypia in non-follicular patterned lesions)
Thy3f Neoplasm possible - suggesting follicular neoplasm	TIR 3B: High-risk indeterminate lesion (HRIL)	IV. Follicular neoplasm or suspicious for a follicular neoplasm	
Thy 4 Suspicious of malignancy	TIR 4: Suspicious of malignancy	V. Suspicious of malignancy	Malignancy suspected
Thy 5 Diagnostic of Malignancy	TIR 5: Malignant	VI. Malignant	Malignancy

needle biopsy (CNB) technique. CNB allows the sampling of the lesion with a 20–22-gauge spring-activated needle to obtain a thin biopsy that can be processed as a histologic specimen. This technique has been extensively studied by Korean and Italian groups, and it can be used to obtain material for performing immunohistochemical procedures such as galectin-3, HBME-1, and cytokeratin-19 staining in indeterminate lesions (11-12). Immunocytochemical staining may be also applied to the material processed by liquid-based cytology, which is specifically mentioned in the reporting system even though it is recommended to be used only in institutions with specific experience (13-14).

Indeterminate lesions

Indeterminate lesions remain a controversial subject in the classification of FNA specimens. Numerous studies demonstrated that this category may represent up to 20% of thyroid diagnoses, and it represents the so-called "grey zone" in which both benign and malignant entities are included (15-16). This category may also result in a diagnosis of follicular variant of papillary thyroid carcinoma (PTC) at the histologic examination, as the lack of the distinctive nuclear features of PTC may fall short of a definitive diagnosis of malignancy. This evidence results in a high number of unnecessary surgeries, which may cause additional morbidity and increase healthcare costs. This category reflects the major limit of the morphology and represents the main cause of the reduced diagnostic accuracy of the technique in cases of follicular-patterned neoplasms, for which only capsular or vascular invasion is the cornerstone for the diagnosis of carcinoma.

A recent paper published by an international group (17), based on the studies of groups around the world, particularly Japan (18), introduced the pathologic entity of noninvasive follicular tumor with papillary-like structures (NIFTP). This entity represents the low-malignant potential counterpart of the follicular variant of PTC and is the most important cause of false-negative diagnoses in thyroid cytology. The introduction of NIFTP in histologic practice will likely decrease the risk of malignancy for the diagnostic categories of the thyroid reporting systems (probably excluding the Japan Thyroid Association system (19)) and lead to a revision of the existent Western national reporting systems (20).

If the surgical removal of a nodule diagnosed as an indeterminate lesion is the preferred option, as many as 70% of patients will undergo an unnecessary operation. Based on TBSRTC, the AUS/FLUS category has a 5–15% risk of malignancy, a value that increases to 15–30% in the FN/SFN and Hürthle cell neoplasm groups (21). The 2014 Italian reporting system for thyroid classification (SIAPEC-AIT 2014) introduced the new subclasses of TIR3A and TIR3B, identified on the basis of both architectural and cytologic atypia with the purpose of decreasing the number of unnecessary surgeries.

The TIR 3A subgroup (low-risk indeterminate lesion) is comparable to the AUS/FLUS category of TBSRTC and the Thy3a class of the British Thyroid Association. It is characterized by increased cellularity with numerous microfollicular structures (which represent less than 60% of the overall cellular component) in a background of a poor colloid amount. A mild degree of atypia can sometimes be observed in the nuclei of the follicular cells. The overall proportion of microfollicles, however, is not sufficient for a diagnosis of follicular neoplasm. Degenerative changes may be present, as sometimes observed in nonneoplastic lesions. At times, sparsely cellular samples containing predominantly microfollicular groups, in addition to oncocytic features ("Hürthle cells"), in a background of scant colloid can fulfill the criteria for inclusion in this category.

The TIR 3A category also includes partially compromised specimens (because of preparation artifacts or blood contamination), with cytologic or architectural alterations that can be not confidently classified as either benign or otherwise categorized. This subcategory is expected to have an estimated maximum risk of malignancy of 10%.

The TIR 3B subgroup is similar to the FN/SFN category of TBSRTC and the Thy3f category of the British Thyroid Association. The subgroup includes nodules with an expected risk of malignancy of 15–30%. It is characterized by high cellularity with a predominant microfollicular/trabecular arrangement (>60% of the cell component), with focal cytologic atypia (mostly moderate, rarely severe) suggestive of FN. Samples composed almost exclusively of oncocytes (Hürthle cells - oncocytic neoplasm, Figures 3–4) are included in the TIR 3B subcategory without considering the architectural or cytologic atypia. This subcategory also includes samples characterized by nuclear alterations suggestive of papillary carcinoma that do not permit a reliable exclusion of malignancy but are too mild or focal to be included in the TIR 4 (suspicious for papillary carcinoma) category.

For these reasons, the clinical actions recommended for the TIR 3 subgroups are different. Clinical and sonographic follow-up lesions and repeat FNA within 6 months are the clinical suggestions for TIR 3A, whereas surgery is the most appropriate indication for TIR 3B nodules. However, the surgical or conservative management of these novel subcategories depends upon both the cytologic and clinical data and requires consultation between cytopathologists and clinicians.

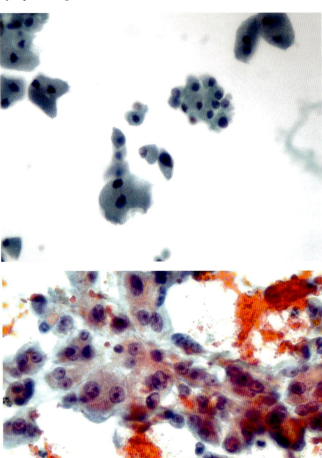

Figure 3. High-risk indeterminate lesion (TIR 3B), oncocytic type (ThinPrep, Papanicolaou stain, ×1000).

Figure 4. High-risk indeterminate lesion (TIR 3B), oncocytic type (Papanicolaou stain, ×500).

Conclusions

The 2014 update of the Italian reporting system was meant as a project for providing Italian cytopathologists a manageable tool for diagnosing thyroid nodules in daily practice. Meanwhile, the assessment of the morphologic criteria for classifying each case in the proper reporting category and the identification of the molecular tests that may help in diagnosing the most difficult (more often indeterminate) cases are reasons for further improvement of the cytologic technique (22-23). The most important point a cytopathologist should remember regarding the cytologic characterization of a thyroid nodule is that the morphologic picture is the most important driver of clinical management (whether surgical or clinical), and it is also the basis for validating all molecular techniques. Finally, in the absence of marked atypical features of follicular cells, the future impact of NIFTP on thyroid cytologic practice should prompt the use of diagnoses of low-risk indeterminate over those of suspicion to avoid an increase in the number of unnecessary surgical procedures.

Acknowledgements:

The author thanks for their invaluable support the members of the Committee for the Update of the Italian Reporting System 2011–2014: Fulvio Basolo, Anna Crescenzi, Andrea Frasoldati, Francesco Nardi, Fabio Orlandi, Lucio Palombini, Enrico Papini, Alfredo Pontecorvi, Paolo Vitti, and Michele Zini.

References

1. Gharib H: Changing trends in thyroid practice: understanding nodular thyroid disease. Endocr Pract. 2004;10:31-39.
2. Yassa L, Cibas ES, Benson CB, Frates MC, Doubilet PM, Gawande AA, Moore FD jr, Kim BW, Nosè V, Marqusee E, Reed Larsen P, Alexander EK: Long-term assessment of a multidisciplinary approach to thyroid nodule diagnostic evaluation Cancer 2007; 111: 508-516.
3. Fadda G, Basolo F, Bondi A, Bussolati G, Crescenzi A, Nappi O, Nardi F, Papotti M, Taddei G, Palombini L Cytologicalclassification of thyroidnodules. Proposal of the SIAPEC-IAP Italian Consensus Working Group. Pathologica 2010; 102(5):405-8.
4. Nardi F, Basolo F, Crescenzi A, Fadda G, Frasoldati A, Orlandi F, Palombini L, Papini E, Zini M, Pontecorvi A, Vitti P. Italian consensus for the classification and reporting of thyroid cytology. J Endocrinol Invest. 2014 Jun;37(6):593-9.
5. Baloch ZW, LiVolsi VA, Asa SL, Rosai J, Merino MJ, Randolph G, Vielh P, DeMay RM, Sidawy MK, Frable WJ. Diagnostic terminology and morphologic criteria for cytologic diagnosis of thyroid lesions: a synopsis of the National Cancer Institute Thyroid Fine-Needle Aspiration State of the Science Conference. Diagn Cytopathol. 2008;36:425-37.
6. Cibas ED, Ali S. The Bethesda The Bethesda system for reporting thyroid cytopathology. Am J Clin Pathol 2009;32:658-665.
7. Lobo C, McQueen A, Beale T, Kocjan G. The UK Royal College of Pathologists Thyroid Fine-Needle Aspiration Diagnostic Classification Is a Robust Tool for the Clinical Management of Abnormal Thyroid Nodules Acta Cytol 2011;55:499–506.
8. Poller DN, Baloch ZW, Fadda G, Johnson SJ, Bongiovanni M, Pontecorvi A, Cochand-Priollet B. Thyroid FNA: New classifications and new interpretations. Cancer Cytopathol. 2016 Jul;124(7):457-66.
9. Vanderlaan PA, Marqusee E, Krane JF Usefulness of Diagnostic Qualifiers for Thyroid. Fine-Needle Aspirations With Atypia of Undetermined Significance Am J Clin Pathol 2011,136:572-577.
10. Castro MR, Espiritu RP, Bahn RS, et al. Predictors of Malignancy in Patients with Cytologically Suspicious Thyroid Nodules. Thyroid. 2011;21:1191-1198.
11. Na DG, Kim JH, Sung JY, Baek JH, Jung KC, Lee H, Yoo H. Core-needle biopsy is more useful than repeat

fine-needle aspiration in thyroid nodules read as nondiagnostic or atypia of undetermined significance by the Bethesda system for reporting thyroid cytopathology. Thyroid 2012;22:468-75.

12. Nasrollah N, Trimboli P, Guidobaldi L CicciarellaModica DD, Ventura C, Ramacciato G, Taccogna S Romanelli F, Valabrega S, Crescenzi A. Thin core biopsy should help to discriminate thyroid nodules cytologically classified as indeterminate. A new sampling technique. Endocrine 2013; 43: 659-665.

13. Fadda, G., Rossi, E.D. Liquid-based cytology in fine-needle aspiration biopsies of the thyroid gland Acta Cytol, 2011; 55 (5): 389-400.

14. Fadda G, Rossi ED, Raffaelli M et al. Follicular thyroid neoplasms can be classified as low and high risk according to HBME-1 and Galectine 3 expression on liquid based fine needle cytology. Eur J Endocrinol 2011; 165; 447-453.

15. Renshaw AA Should "atypical follicular cells" in thyroid fine-needle aspirates be subclassified? Cancer Cytopathol 2010, 118: 186-189.

16. Faquin WC, Baloch ZW. Fine-Needle Aspiration of Follicular Patterned Lesions of the Thyroid: Diagnosis, Management, and Follow-Up According to National Cancer Institute (NCI) Recommendations. Diagnostic Cytopathology. 2010;38:731-739.

17. Nikiforov YE, Seethala RR, Tallini G et al. Nomenclature Revision for Encapsulated Follicular Variant of Papillary Thyroid Carcinoma: A Paradigm Shift to Reduce Overtreatment of Indolent Tumors. JAMA Oncol. 2016 Apr 14 (online).

18. Kakudo K Bai Y, Liu Z, Ozaki T: Encapsulated papillary thyroid carcinoma, follicular variant: a misnomer Pathol Intern 2012; 62: 155-160.

19. Kakudo K, Kameyama K, Miyauchi A, Nakamura H: Introducing the reporting system for thyroid fine-needle aspiration cytology according to the new guidelines of the Japan Thyroid Association Endocr J 2014; 61: 539-552.

20. Baloch ZW, Seethala RR, Faquin WC, Papotti MG, Basolo F, Fadda G, Randolph GW, Hodak SP, Nikiforov YE, Mandel SJ. Noninvasive follicular thyroid neoplasm with papillary-like nuclear features (NIFTP): A changing paradigm in thyroid surgical pathology and implications for thyroid cytopathology. Cancer Cytopathol. 2016 May 20 (online).

21. Straccia P, Rossi ED, Bizzarro T, Brunelli C, Cianfrini F, Damiani D, Fadda G. A meta-analytic review of the Bethesda System for Reporting Thyroid Cytopathology: Has the rate of malignancy in indeterminate lesions been underestimated? Cancer Cytopathol. 2015 Dec;123(12):713-22.

22. Nikiforov YE. Molecular diagnostics of thyroid tumors. Arch Pathol Lab Med 2011; 15: 569-773.

23. Alexander EK, Kennedy GC, Baloch ZW et al. Preoperative diagnosis of thyroid nodules with indeterminate cytology. N Engl J Med 2012, 367: 705 – 15.

Supplemental Chapter 2

How to Follow Fine-needle Aspiration Biopsy-Proven Benign Thyroid Nodules, Active Surveillance *vs.* Diagnostic Lobectomy for Indeterminate Nodules and
Individualized Treatments for Low-risk Thyroid Carcinomas

Kennichi Kakudo

Introduction:

Thyroid nodules are common, and they cause concern due to the possibility of malignancy (1,2). Risk stratification of patients with thyroid nodules is well established in most clinical guidelines (3-6), but how to triage patients for surgery and the optimal surgical protocol for low-risk thyroid carcinoma remain controversial (7-15). Variation in histopathologic diagnoses among pathologists (16-18) and the recent introduction of borderline tumors in thyroid tumor classification systems (19-25) have complicated the interpretation of reported data and conclusions in the literature. This chapter reviews the current literature regarding the prognosis of cytologically benign thyroid nodules, cytologically indeterminate nodules, histologically borderline thyroid tumors, and low-risk thyroid carcinomas. The author of this chapter believes this information will help readers to understand the biological behavior of these lesions and select the most suitable clinical management for patients, which will ultimately reduce overdiagnosis and overtreatment of those tumors (12, 13, 15, 26).

Different approach for patients with thyroid nodules:

Thyroid nodules are common, and they cause concern because of the possibility of malignancy, although relatively few nodules are malignant and thyroid cancers are rarely lethal. Indeed, less than 1% of curatively treated patients with low-risk thyroid cancer will die of thyroid cancer in the next 20 years (13, 27-29). These considerations, as well as unavoidable surgical complications (more than 10% of surgically treated patients experience hypoiparathyroidsm or vocal cord dysfunction, 100% of patients with total thyroidectomy require lifelong thyroid hormone replacement therapy, and patients with radioactive iodine [RAI] treatment often experience salivary gland dysfunction and second primary malignancy) (13, 30,31), justify further risk stratification and conservative clinical management of thyroid nodules in patients (1,2,5,6,13,15,27,32-34). Thyroid fine-needle aspiration (FNA) cytology has an essential role in this process, together with other clinical tests such as molecular tests, ultrasound (US), and measurements of serum thyroglobulin levels and nodule size (3-6,35-39). This risk stratification of the thyroid nodule for surgery is standard practice in Japan, and surgery is usually advised only in patients with indeterminate cytology who have high-risk clinical features (5,10,40,41). This approach reduces the number of operations for clinically benign-looking thyroid nodules and avoids excessive invasive tests (1,2,35,42,43), as encapsulated/well circumscribed thyroid cancer has a better outcome (28,29,42-48). However, the development of The Bethesda System for Reporting Thyroid Cytopathology (TBSRTC) has changed this strategy. The authors of TBSRTC made a different recommendation, namely a definitive diagnostic procedure for all patients with high-risk indeterminate (follicular neoplasm [FN]) nodules, because only histological examination can reveal whether the nodule is a benign follicular adenoma or malignant follicular thyroid carcinoma (FTC) (49,50). Theoretically, diagnostic thyroidectomy (usually lobectomy) is the only method to avoid missing malignancy in patients with indeterminate thyroid nodules and thus prevent legal action by patients. Therefore, diagnostic surgery became the established standard of care for the management of patients with FN nodules in Western practice (3,4,6,49,50). Furthermore, the 2010 AACE/AME/ETA guidelines recommend diagnostic surgery even for cytologically benign nodules when they have been found to grow (4). This was a significant turning point in the treatment of both benign tumors and low-risk thyroid carcinomas. However, further clinical triage of patients with indeterminate nodules for surgery remains the standard practice in Japan (5, 40, 41,43) and other Asian countries (35,42). These different strategies between Western and Eastern countries also make comparisons of the performance of different diagnostic systems for thyroid FNA cytology difficult because resection rates differ between Western and Eastern practices.

Different treatment strategies for patients with low-risk papillary thyroid carcinoma (PTC) (lobectomy or total thyroidectomy plus RAI):

The majority of patients with low-risk PTC are usually treated with lobectomy in Japan (5,10), and some patients with low-risk papillary microcarcinoma (T1, N0, M0, ex0, and <1 cm) are advised to receive active surveillance without surgical intervention (5,32-34). This is a different approach from those of Western practices, in which the majority of patients are treated with total thyroidectomy followed by RAI treatment (3,4,6-15). As a result, the optimal surgical protocol for low-risk PTC remains controversial (5-15).

A new treatment strategy for low risk thyroid carcinomas:

Hay *et al.* and Brito *et al.* from the Mayo Clinic questioned this standard care of low-risk thyroid carcinoma in Western practice (8,13). They commented that patients with these small, localized PTCs have a 99% survival rate after 20 years. They further added that despite their excellent prognosis, these subclinical low-risk cancers are often treated aggressively in Western practice. Although surgery is traditionally viewed as the cornerstone treatment for these tumors, there is less agreement concerning the extent of surgery (lobectomy *vs.* total thyroidectomy) (5-15). Brito *et al.* concluded that nonsurgical, minimally localized, invasive therapies (ethanol ablation and laser ablation) and active surveillance may form part of a more individualized treatment approach for low-risk papillary thyroid tumors (13), although the majority of those patients were treated with total thyroidectomy followed by RAI treatment in Western countries (3-6,11,13,30).

In their commentary on a borderline thyroid tumor, Hodak *et al.* stated that the increasing incidence or "overdiagnosis" of clinically insignificant papillary microcarcinoma, the growing evidence that low-risk cancers do not benefit from RAI therapy, the recent endorsement of thyroid lobectomy as an acceptable surgical option for larger intrathyroidal PTCs, and the emerging data suggesting small intrathyroidal biopsy-proven PTCs may even be safely managed with observation in lieu of surgery suggest that for many patients with thyroid cancer, we may often be violating the important dictum *primum non nocere* (do not harm patients) (15). Total thyroidectomy may be indicated in patients with high-risk features, such as extrathyroid extension, clinical nodal metastasis, and/or distant metastasis, which may necessitate RAI treatment, but total thyroidectomy is associated with greater risks of hypoparathyroidism and recurrent laryngeal nerve injury, as well as a need for lifelong thyroid hormone replacement therapy, than lobectomy (6,9,10,13,15).

Fate of benign thyroid nodules (cytologically proven benign nodules)

To monitor the risk of false-negative cytology and possible progression from a benign nodule to thyroid carcinoma, follow-up with periodic US every 6–18 months is recommended for cytologically benign thyroid nodules with no specified endpoint (3-6).

Kuma *et al.* re-examined 134 patients with thyroid nodules who had benign FNA cytology findings (51). There were 86 single nodules, 14 multiple nodules, and 34 cystic nodules on the first examination. They reported that only one case (0.9% false-negative rate) was found to be malignant, and their most striking finding was that many benign nodules decreased in size or disappeared during the 9–11-year follow-up period. They concluded that no medical or surgical treatment is required if the nodules do not grow, as biopsy-proved benign thyroid nodules remain benign over a prolonged period (51). This observation strongly suggests progression from a benign tumor to thyroid carcinoma rarely occurs. Nakamura *et al.* from the same group recently updated the analyses. They reviewed 542 surgically treated patients with cytologically benign nodules. They confirmed that nodule growth itself is not a risk factor for malignancy in cytologically benign nodules. In their cohort, there were 18 thyroid malignancies (6 PTCs, 11 FTCs, and 1 malignant lymphoma) among 542 benign diagnoses, and their false-negative rate was 3.3% (41).

Lee *et al.* divided 646 patients with FNA benign nodules into two groups, namely 226 patients with short-term follow-up (median, 13 months) and 140 patients with long-term follow-up (median, 57 months), and found two cases of thyroid cancer (4.5% false negative) in 44 patients who underwent surgery (0 of 13 in the short-term follow-up group and 2 of 31 in the long-term follow-up group, p > 0.99). They concluded that after 3 years of follow-up, consideration should be given to ceasing long-term routine follow-up of biopsy-proven benign cytology nodules because no there was improvement in the malignancy detection rate (52).

Ajmal *et al.* examined 263 patients (48 patients underwent immediate thyroidectomy and 215 patients underwent annual US follow-up) with benign FNA cytology and identified two cases of PTC in the immediate thyroidectomy group (4.2% false-negative rate). During follow-up of 215 patients for 3.3 years, 81 (37.6%) patients underwent thyroidectomy, of whom 70 (86.4%) were found to have benign lesions, whereas seven (8.6%), three (4%), and one patient (1.2%) had PTC, FTC, and malignant lymphoma, respectively (53). They concluded that a significant number of benign thyroid nodules grow by more than 5 mm over 3 years, and larger and more rapidly growing nodules were not predictive of malignancy.

Medici *et al.* evaluated 1254 patients with 1819 FNA-proven benign nodules with a median time to first follow-up of 1.4 years (range 0.5–14.1 years). They found the growth of the nodules and the likelihood of repeat FNA were increased with increasing follow-up time. However, malignancy or mortality rates did not differ among the various follow-up intervals. Although the current expert opinion recommends repeat evaluation at 1–2 years, they concluded that this interval can be safely extended to 3 years without increased mortality or patient harm (54).

The findings of these studies indicate that patients with cytologically proven benign nodules have an extremely low risk of developing thyroid cancer (false-negative rates of 1–10%) or progression from benign nodules to malignant tumors. Most importantly, no cancer death due to a false-negative diagnosis was reported in these studies (41,51-55).

Some researchers claimed that prolonged follow-up was appropriate because patients who ultimately underwent thyroidectomy for compressive symptoms or thyroid cancer did so more than 3 years after the initial benign FNA cytology (53), whereas other reports did not favor prolonged follow-up due to the increased healthcare cost and lack of increased detection of malignancy (54). This is likely influenced by different health insurance systems and cultural issues between Western and Eastern societies, as patients with chronic diseases in

Japan usually continue with lifelong health consultations with their attending doctors. Patient may visit their doctors to inform them of their present health conditions (lifelong follow-up) to keep their physicians appraised of their disease condition, and a second visit for follow-up usually only costs the patient $10 of their own money (30% of the total fee) in Japan when no additional clinical tests are necessary.

Watchful follow-up of patients with indeterminate thyroid nodules (active surveillance) or diagnostic surgery:

In Eastern practice, further triage for surgery is usually performed in patients with indeterminate thyroid nodules (35,40,42,43). This is because diagnostic surgery for patients with benign nodules is harmful, and although possible, biologically malignant (lethal) thyroid nodules are rare. In fact, after histological analysis, the majority of FN nodules are revealed to be benign (more than 70% in surgically treated patients from Western countries) (6,49,50, 56,57). Nakamura *et al*. analyzed 409 patients with FN nodules surgically treated between 2011 and 2012 at Kuma Hospital, Japan. They found that FN nodules have a higher risk of malignancy when they grow in size and identified 23 follicular tumors of uncertain malignant potential (FT-UMPs) (28%) and 15 malignancies (18.3%) in 82 patients with growing FN nodules during follow-up, whereas 44 FT-UMPs (13.5%) and 54 malignancies (16.5%) were found in 327 patients with FN nodules who underwent immediate surgery (41).

The clinical management of FN thyroid nodules was modified in the 2015 American Thyroid Association (ATA) guidelines to more conservative management using clinical and sonographic features. Molecular testing may be used to supplement malignancy risk assessment data in lieu of proceeding directly with surgery (6).

Since the introduction of borderline thyroid tumors (FT-UMP, well-differentiated tumor of uncertain malignant potential [WDT-UMP], capsular invasion-only FTC, papillary microcarcinoma, and encapsulated papillary carcinoma) into thyroid tumor classification systems (21-24) and the recent proposal of noninvasive follicular thyroid neoplasm with papillary-like nuclear features (NIFTP) (25), reported data will need to be modified in the near future to use the updated 4th edition of the WHO thyroid tumor classification (please refer to Chapter 1). Indeed, thyroid carcinomas in the indeterminate category proved to be low-grade or early-stage lesions (58,59), and a significant number of borderline tumors (NIFTP) were also previously classified into the indeterminate category (60-62). The author of this chapter believes that the new thyroid tumor classification schema, including the borderline tumors, will help to determine the risk of malignancy for certain cytological categories and encourage a shift toward more conservative clinical management for patients with FT-UMP, WDT-UMP, capsular invasion-only FTC, papillary microcarcinoma, or encapsulated papillary carcinoma.

Prognosis of borderline thyroid tumors

Williams proposed two terminologies (FT-UMP and WDT-UMP) in 2000, although prognostic data were not included (20). No nodal or distant metastasis, tumor recurrence, or tumor-related deaths have been reported in the literature (44-48,63). Kakudo *et al*. proposed a new thyroid tumor classification characterized by the borderline tumor category, in which FT-UMP, WDT-UMP, capsular invasion-only FTC, papillary microcarcinoma, and encapsulated papillary carcinoma are included in the borderline tumor category because borderline (precursor) tumors are essential steps in the multi-step carcinogenesis theory. These are indolent tumors, and they are associated with significant interobserver variation in diagnoses (21-24). Nikiforov *et al*. proposed a name change from noninvasive encapsulated follicular variant PTC to NIFTP, without the use of cancer terminology, to prevent overtreatment and lessen the emotional burden on the patient (15,25). Their literature survey examined more than 300 published cases and identified an overall recurrence rate of less than 1% (25). They also collected an additional 210 cases (109 noninvasive cases and 101 invasive cases) and confirmed the absence of recurrence and metastasis in the noninvasive group after an average of 14 years of follow-up (25).

The recent reclassification of low-risk thyroid carcinomas in the borderline tumor category is currently under discussion, but this practice is becoming more widely accepted. The 4th edition of the WHO classification of endocrine organs incorporated hyalinizing trabecular adenoma/tumor (2-2), FT-UMP and WDT-UMP (2-2Ai), and NIFTP (2-2Aii) into either borderline (/1) or carcinoma in situ (/2) tumor categories in thyroid tumor classifications (please refer to Chapter 1).

The reasons for the differences between Western and Eastern practices:

The author of this chapter believes that there are cultural issues behind these different clinical approaches for patients with indeterminate thyroid nodules or low-risk thyroid carcinomas. Some of the issues have been solved with sufficient evidence, and some recommendations and clinical approaches will be shared in the future. However, there may be a few irreconcilable differences between the two practices. The following two examples were prepared to explain how our different cultural background affects our decision-making processes. The following two cases, different conclusions, and patients' reactions in Japan may not occur in Western societies, but they may be duplicated in other Asian societies.

Case 1:

A young woman visited Kuma Hospital for a second opinion consultation. The patient had been treated for Graves' hyperthyroidism with anti-thyroid medication at another hospital. She was found to be pregnant after low-dose RAI scintigraphy, and she was advised to undergo artificial abortion by her doctor. It was her first pregnancy, and she wished to have the baby. Her questions to us included what types of abnormalities the baby could experience and their probabilities of occurrence. Dr. Kuma, the president of Kuma Hospital, advised her to have the baby after a thorough explanation. The patient stopped crying and agreed with his advice. After she left our consultation room, I asked Dr. Kuma how sure about his advice he was. He told me, "At this moment, nobody knows whether her baby will have an abnormality or not (only God knows what will happen to the baby), and she needs someone who supports her choice to have her baby." Several years later, Dr. Kuma told me that the patient had a healthy baby. Dr. Kuma, as a Christian, thanked God that he could save a life. In Japan, many physicians would probably advise her to have an induced abortion, similar to the advice of her previous doctor, which is the only method to avoid possible abnormalities that might occur in the baby due to RAI radiation; however, she decided to have the baby. The author of this chapter believes that diagnostic surgery in all patients with indeterminate nodules to avoid missing the rare occurrence of malignancy is similar to a physician recommending an induced abortion to avoid the relatively rare chance of radiation-induced congenital anomalies in an unborn baby. As thyroid cancer is indolent and delayed surgery does not create any harm in the patient (32-34,64), the author of this chapter believes that the choice to opt for surgical intervention should not be rushed, and it should be applied only when high-risk clinical features are observed during active surveillance (watchful follow-up). This is largely because we cannot replace the resected thyroid lobe when the nodule is benign, and a significant number of patients with thyroid lobectomy develop hypothyroidism, which is harmful to patients (65-68).

Case 2:

A young woman visited a hospital for her thyroid nodule. Thyroid FNA cytology was performed, and it was interpreted as suspicious for PTC-type malignancy (Figure 1). The patient was advised to have surgery according to the clinical guidelines of the Japan Thyroid Association. She initially did not accept this advice, and she was followed up clinically at her hospital because she knew that many thyroid cancers were indolent and that active surveillance was an option. The doctor advised her three times to have surgery. She finally accepted his advice, and the histologic diagnosis of her thyroid nodule was a benign adenomatous goiter. The patient filed a lawsuit and asked for damages from the hospital and the cyopathologist. This was the first lawsuit in Japan involving a diagnosis of thyroid FNA cytology using the key words "thyroid" and "FNA cytology" and ("false positive" or "false negative" or "missing malignancy") in a database of judicial precedent in Japan. I was invited to provide a written expert opinion on cytologic diagnosis. Although the small probability of benign diseases had been explained to her before the surgery, she was not happy with the unnecessary alarm caused to her and the surgery. Her biggest concern was the suture wound on the anterior neck. Some Japanese people do not like to damage their bodies, which they believe were given to them by God/Buddha/Deities/Nature, and they consider it important to keep their bodies in as natural a state as possible. Cosmetic surgery and tattoos are not popular in Japan compared to other countries, which is related to this principle. There have been no lawsuits related to missed malignancies of thyroid FNA cytology in Japan. This author assumed that missed thyroid malignancy can usually be rectified by surgery when malignancy was clinically evidenced, and delayed surgery does not usually create any harm in patients with low-risk thyroid cancer (32-34,64), which is different from other organ systems in which many tumors are lethal and delayed surgery should be avoided.

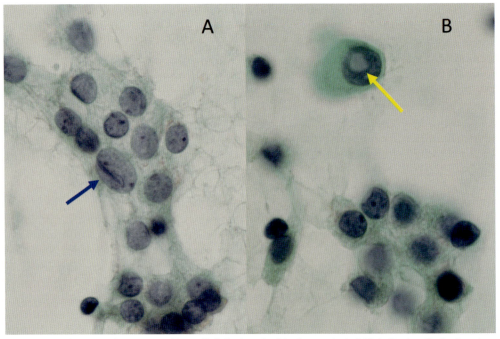

Figure 1. A: Nuclear enlargement with small distinct nucleoli is demonstrated. Note the longitudinal nuclear groove (blue arrow) in a large nucleus with powdery chromatin. B: A follicular cluster in the lower field and an isolated large cell in the upper field are present. An intranuclear cytoplasmic pseudoinclusion (yellow arrow) is noted in the isolated cell (conventional smear, Papanicolaou stain, ×1000).

Standardization of clinical management of patients with indeterminate nodules:

The 2015 revised ATA guidelines provide updated recommendations for the management of thyroid nodules (6). The concept of low-risk versus high-risk thyroid carcinomas and the increased role of conservative management through the application of molecular testing, clinicoradiologic risk stratification, and a multidisciplinary team approach are emphasized. The author of this chapter believes that thyroid FNA cytology, together with other clinical tests, plays a significant role in triaging patients for immediate surgery, active surveillance in lieu of surgery, periodic follow-up, or no further follow-up. As a result, the clinical management of patients with indeterminate nodules has been standardized in many areas of the world, and this change will build a bridge between Western and Eastern practices, creating better standards of care.

References

1. Haber RS Thyroid nodules and the detection of thyroid cancer. Mt Sinai J Med 1996; 63:10-15.
2. St Luis JD, Leight GS, Tyler DS Follicular neoplasms: the role for observation, fine-needle aspiration biopsy, thyroid suppression, and surgery. Semin Surg Oncol 1999; 16:5-11.
3. Cooper DS, Doherty GM, Haigen BR *et al*. Revised American Thyroid Association management guidelines for patients with thyroid nodules and differentiated thyroid cancer. Thyroid 2009; 19:1167-1214.
4. Gharib H, Papini E, Paschke R *et al*. American Association of Clinical Endocrinologists, Associazione Medici Endocrinologi, and European Thyroid Association Medical guidelines for clinical practice for diagnosis and management of thyroid nodules: executive summary of recommendations. Endocr Pract 2010; 16:468-475.
5. Guidelines Task Force of the Japanese Thyroid Association 2013. Treatments and follow-up of thyroid nodules. In: Guidelines for Clinical Practice for the Management of Thyroid Nodules in Japan [in Japanese], Nankodo, Tokyo, Japan. pp139-172.
6. Haugen BR, Alexander EK, Bible KC, *et al*. American Thyroid Association management guidelines for adult patients with thyroid nodules and differentiated thyroid cancer. Thyroid 2015; 26:1-134.
7. Shah JP, Loree TR, Dharker D *et al*. Lobectomy versus total thyroidectomy for differentiated carcinoma of the thyroid: a matched-pair analysis. Am J Surg 1993; 166:331-335.
8. Hay I, Hutchison ME, Gonzalez-Losada T *et al*: Papillary thyroid microcarcinoma: a study of 900 cases observed in a 60-year period. Surgery 2008; 144:980-987.
9. Matsuzu K, Sugino K, Masudo K *et al*. Thyroid lobectomy for papillary thyroid cancer: long-term follow-up study of 1,088 cases. World J Surg 2014; 38:68-79.
10. Takami H, Ito Y, Okamoto T, *et al*. Revisiting the guidelines by the Japanese Society of Thyroid Surgeons and Japan Association of Endocrine Surgeons: a gradual move towards consensus between Japanese and Western practice in the management of thyroid carcinoma. World J Surg 2014; 38:2002-2010.
11. Adam MA, Pura J, Gu L *et al*. Extent of surgery for papillary thyroid cancer is not associated with survival: An analysis of 61775 patients. Ann Surg 2014; 260:601-607.
12. Wang TS, Goffredo P, Sosa JA *et al* Papillary thyroid microcarcinoma: an over-treated malignancy? World J Surg 2014; 38:2297-2303.
13. Brito JP, Hay ID, Morris JC Low risk papillary thyroid cancer. BMJ 2014; 348: g3045:1-10.
14. Macedo FI and Mitta VK Total thyroidectomy versus lobectomy as initial operation for small unilateral papillary thyroid carcinoma: A meta-analysis. Surg Oncol 2015; 24:117-122.
15. Hodak S, Tuttle RM, Mayatal G *et al*. Changing the cancer diagnosis: the case of follicular variant of papillary thyroid cancer – prinum non nocere and NIFTP. Thyroid 2016; 26:869-871.
16. Kakudo K, Katoh R, Sakamoto A *et al*: Thyroid gland: international case conference. Endocrine Pathol, 2002; 13:131-134.
17. Hirokawa M, Carney JA, Goellner JR *et al*: Observer variation of encapsulated follicular lesions of the thyroid gland. Am J Surg Pathol 2002; 26:1508-1514.

18. Cipriani NA, Nagar S, Kaplan SP et al.: Follicular thyroid carcinoma: How have histologic diagnosis changed in the last half-century and what are the prognostic implications? Thyroid 2015; 25:1209-1216.
19. Carney JA, Ryan J, GoellnerJR Hyalinizing trabecular adenoma of the thyroid gland. Am J Surg Pathol 1987; 11:583-591.
20. Williams ED: Guest Editorial: Two proposals regarding the terminology of thyroid tumors. Int J Surg Pathol 2000; 8: 181-183.
21. Kakudo K, Bai Y, Katayama S et al. Classification of follicular cell tumors of the thyroid gland: analysis involving Japanese patients from one institute. Pathol Int 2009; 59:359-367.
22. Liu Z, Zhou G, Nakamura M et al: Encapsulated follicular thyroid tumor with equivocal nuclear changes, so-called well-differentiated tumor of uncertain malignant potential: a morphological, immunohistochemical, and molecular appraisal. Cancer Sci 2011; 102:288-294.
23. Kakudo K, Bai Y, Liu Z, et al. Classification of thyroid follicular cell tumors: with special reference to borderline lesions. Endocr J 2012; 59:1-12.
24. Kakudo K, Bai Y, Liu Z, et al. Encapsulated papillary thyroid carcinoma, follicular variant: A misnormer. Pathol Int 2012; 62:155-60.
25. Nikiforov YE, Seethala RR, Tallini G et al: Nomenclature revision for encapsulated follicular variant of papillary thyroid carcinoma: A paradigm shift to reduce overtreatment of indolent tumors. JAMA Oncol 2016 Apr 14. doi: 10.1001/jamaoncol.2016.0386. [Epub ahead of print]
26. Esserman LJ, Thompson IM, Reid P et al. Addressing overdiagnosis and overtreatment in cancer: a prescription for change. Lancet Oncol 2014; 15:e234-42.
27. Hay ID, Hutchinson ME, Gonzalez-Losada T et al. Papillary thyroid microcarcinoma: a study of 900 cases observed in a 60-year period. Surgery 2008; 144:980-987.
28. Ito Y, Hirokawa M, Uruno T et al. Biological behavior and prognosis of encapsulated papillary carcinoma of the thyroid: experience of a Japanese hospital for thyroid care. World J Surg 2008; 32:1789-1794.
29. Geffredo P, Cheung K, Roman SA et al: Can minimally invasive follicular thyroid cancer be approached as a benign lesion? Ann Surg Oncol 2013; 20:767-772.
30. Iyer NG, Morris LG, Tuttle RM et al. Rising incidence of second cancers in patients with low-risk (T1N0) thyroid cancer who receive radioactive iodine therapy. Cancer 2011; 117:4439-4446.
31. Hay ID Selective use of radioactive iodine in the postoperative management of patients with papillary and follicular thyroid carcinoma. J Surg Oncol 2006; 94:692-700.
32. Ito Y, Uruno T, Nakano K et al. An observation trial without surgical treatment in patients with papillary microcarcinoma of the thyroid. Thyroid 2003; 13:381-387.
33. Ito Y, Miyauchi A, Inoue H et al. An observational trial for papillary thyroid microcarcinoma in Japanese patients. World J Surg 2010; 34:28-35.
34. Sugitani I, Tada K, Yamada K et al. Three distinctly different kinds of papillary thyroid microcarcinoma should be recognized: our treatment strategies and outcomes. World J Surg 2010; 34:1222-1231.
35. Yoo WS, Choi HS, Cho SW et al. The role of ultrasound findings in the management of thyroid nodules with atypia or follicular lesions of undetermined significance. Clin Endocrinol (Oxf) 2014; 80:735-742.
36. Nikiforov YE, Carty SE, Chiosea ST et al. Highly accurate diagnosis of cancer in thyroid nodules with follicular neoplasm/suspicious for a follicular neoplasm cytology by ThyroSequ v2 next-generation sequencing assay. Cancer 2014; 120:3627-3634.
37. Hyeon J, Ahn S, Shin JH, et al. The prediction of malignant risk in the category 'atypia of undetermined significance/follicular lesion of undetermined significance' of the Bethesda System for Reporting Thyroid Cytopathology using subcategorization and BRAF mutation results. Cancer Cytopathol 2014; 122:368-376.
38. Ferris RL, Baloch Z, Bernet V et al. American Thyroid Association statement on surgical application of molecular profiling for thyroid nodules: Current impact on perioperative decision making. Thyroid 2015; 25:760-768.
39. Nikiforov YE, Carty SE, Chiosea ST et al. Impact of multi-gene ThyroSequ next-generation sequencing assay on cancer diagnosis in thyroid nodules with atypia of undetermined significance/follicular lesion of

undetermined significance cytology. Thyroid 2015; 25:1217-1223.

40. Kakudo K, Kameyama K, Miyauchi A, *et al*. Introducing the reporting system for thyroid fine-needle aspiration cytology according to the new guidelines of the Japan Thyroid Association. Endocr J 2014; 61:539-552.
41. Nakamura H, Hirokawa M, Ota H *et al*. Is an increase in thyroid nodule volume a risk factor for malignancy? Thyroid 2015; 25:804-811.
42. Zhu Yun, Dai J, Lin X *et al*.: Fine needle aspiration of thyroid nodules: experience in a Chinese population. J Basic & Clin Medicine 2015; 4:65-69.
43. Sugino K, Kameyama K, Ito K: Characteristics and outcome of thyroid cancer patients with indeterminate cytology. J Basic Clin Med 2015; 4:92-98.
44. VanHeerden JA, Hay ID, Goellner, JR *et al*: Follicular thyroid carcinoma with capsular invasion alone: a nonthreatening malignancy. Surgery1992; 112:1130-1138.
45. Liu J, Singh B, Tallini G *et al*: Follicular variant of papillary carcinoma. A clinicopathologic study of a problematic entity. Cancer 2006; 107:1255-1264.
46. Bai Y, Kakudo K, Li Y *et al*: Subclassification of non-solid type papillary carcinoma, identification of high-risk group in common type. Cancer Sci 2008; 99:1908-1915.
47. Piana S, Frasoldati A, Di Felice E *et al*: Encapsulated well-differentiated follicular-patterned thyroid carcinomas do not play a significant role in the fatality rates from thyroid carcinoma. Am J Surg Pathol 2010; 34:868-872.
48. Liu Z, Zhou G, Nakamura M *et al*: Encapsulated follicular thyroid tumor with equivocal nuclear changes, so-called well-differentiated tumor of uncertain malignant potential: a morphological, immunohistochemical, and molecular appraisal. Cancer Sci. 2011; 102:288-294.
49. Cibas ES, Ali SZ, NCI Thyroid FNA State of the Science Conference. The Bethesda system for reporting thyroid cytopathology. Am J Clin Pathol 2009; 132:658-665.
50. Ali SZ and Cibas ES (ed) 2010. The Bethesda system for reporting thyroid cytopathology. Definitions, criteria and explanatory notes. Springer, New York, USA: pp1-166.
51. Kuma K, Matsuzuka F, Yokozawa T *et al*. Fate of untreated benign thyroid nodules: results of long-term follow-up. World J Surg 1994; 18:495-498.
52. Lee A, Skelton TS, Zheng F *et al*. The biopsy proven benign thyroid nodule: Is long-term follow-up necessary? J Am Coll Surg 2013; 217:81-89.
53. Ajmal S, Rapoport S, Battle HR *et al*. The natural history of the benign thyroid nodule: What is the appropriate follow-up strategy? J Am Coll Surg 2015; 220:982-992.
54. Medici M, Liu X, Kwong N *et al*. Long- versus short-interval follow-up of cytologically benign thyroid nodules: a prospective cohort study. BMC Med 2016; Jan 27;14:11. doi: 10.1186/s12916-016-0554-1.
55. Nou E, Kwong N, Alexander LK *et al*. Determination of the optimal time interval for repeat evaluation after benign thyroid nodule aspiration. J Clin Endocrinol Metab 2014; 99:510-516.
56. Ohori NP, Schoedel KE. Variability in the atypia of undetermined significance/follicular lesion of undetermined significance diagnosis in the Bethesda system for reporting thyroid cytopathology: sources and recommendation. Acta Cytol 2011; 55:492-498.
57. Bongiovanni M, Crippa S, Baloch Z, *et al*. Comparison of 5-tired and 6-tired diagnostic systems for the reporting of thyroid cytopathology: a multi-institutional study. Cancer Cytopathol 2012; 120:117-125.
58. Rago T, Scutari M, Latrofa F *et al*. The large majority of 1520 patients with indeterminate thyroid nodule at cytology have a favorable outcome, and a clinical risk score has a high negative predictive value for a more cumbersome cancer disease. J Clin Endocrinol Metab 2014: 99:3700-3707.
59. Trimboli P, Bongiovanni M, Rossi F *et al*. Differentiated thyroid cancer patients with a previous indeterminate (Thy 3) cytology have a better prognosis than those with suspicious or malignant FNAC reports. Endocrine 2015: 49:191-195.
60. Strickland KC, Howitt BE, Marquesee E, *et al*. The impact of non-invasive follicular variant of papillary thyroid carcinoma on rates of malignancy for fine-needle aspiration diagnostic categories. Thyroid 2015; 25:987-992.
61. Faquin WC, Wong LQ, Afrogheh AH, *et al*. Impact of reclassifying noninvasive follicular variant of papillary

thyroid carcinoma on the risk of malignancy in the Bethesda system for reporting thyroid cytopathology. Cancer Cytopathol 2015 Oct 12. doi: 10.1002/cncy.21631. [Epub ahead of print]

62. Maletta F, Massa F, Torregrossa L et al. Cytological features of "noninvasive follicular thyroid neoplasm with papillary-like nuclear features" and their correlation with tumor histology. Hum Pathol 2016, doi: 10.1016/j.humpath.2016.03.014. [Epub ahead of print]

63. Sobrinho-Simoes M, Eloy C, Magalhaes J et al. Follicular thyroid carcinoma. Mod Pathol 2011; Suppliment 2:A10-18.

64. Amit M, Rudnick Y, Binenbaum Y et al. Defining the outcome of patients with delayed diagnosis of differentiated thyroid cancer. Larygoscope 2014; 124:2837-2840.

65. Stoll SJ, Pitt SC, Liu J et al. Thyroid hormone replacement after thyroid lobectomy. Surgery 2009; 146:554-558.

66. Farkas EA, King TA, Bolton JS et al. A comparison of total thyroidectomy and lobectomy in the treatment of dormant thyroid nodules. Am Surg 2002; 68:678-682.

67. Park HK, Kim DW, Ha TK et al. Factors associated with postoperative hypothyroidism after lobectomy in papillary thyroid microcarcinoma patients. Endocr Res 2015; 40:49-53.

68. Grossman A, Weiss A, Koren-Maraq N et al. Subclinical thyroid disease and mortality in the elderly: a retrospective cohort study. Am J Med 2016; 129:423-430.

Supplemental Chapter 3

Cyst Fluid Only (CFO)

Nami Takada

Case:

A case involved a 56-year-old woman. Ultrasound revealed a large cystic nodule in the left thyroid lobe measuring 59 mm × 23 mm × 27 mm. The nodule was irregular in shape, and the border was well defined. The cystic nodule contained a solid area. The ultrasound interpretation was nodular goiter with cystic degeneration or cystic papillary thyroid carcinoma. Aspiration cytology was performed for both the cystic and solid areas, and the diagnoses were cyst fluid only (CFO) and nondiagnostic (ND), respectively. Fourteen months later, she underwent repeat ultrasound. As the nodule had increased in size (Figure 1), and cystic papillary thyroid carcinoma was suspected by repeat aspiration cytology, she underwent total thyroidectomy with central lymph node dissection.

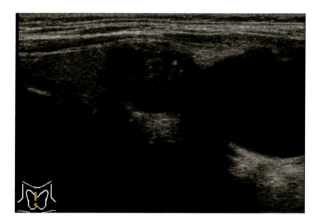

Figure 1. A gourd-shaped cystic lesion is noted in the thyroid. The border of the lesion is irregular and rough. A solid area is present in the cystic space (ultrasound B-mode image).

Figure 2. Foamy histiocytes are seen in the proteinaceous background. There are no follicular cells (Papanicolaou, ×40).

Figure 3. Atypical cells appear as cell clusters. Nuclear irregularity and grooving are noted (Papanicolaou, ×40).

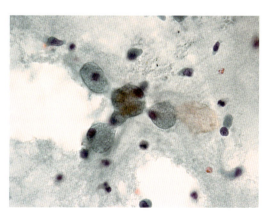
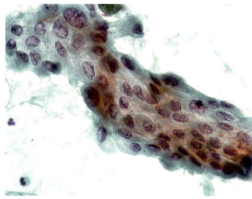

Cytologic findings

The first aspiration cytology from the cystic area revealed a large number of foamy histiocytes and degenerative red blood cells in the proteinaceous background (Figure 2). There were no follicular cells. The second aspiration cytology from both cystic and solid areas uncovered similar findings. In the proteinaceous background with foamy histiocytes, cell clusters composed of atypical cells were scattered (Figure 3). The clusters were three-dimensional or sheet-like. The nuclei of the atypical cells were slightly elongated, and they exhibited grooving. No intracytoplasmic inclusions were found.

The cytology report was suspicious for papillary thyroid carcinoma.

Pathologic findings

The tumor measured 46 mm × 25 mm, and it was composed of mixed multilocular cystic and solid areas (Figure 4). The former was predominant. Small papillary projections were focally observed on the inner surface of the cysts. The solid portion was whitish in color, and it invaded the surrounding thyroid tissue. Microscopically, the tumor was conventional papillary carcinoma (Figure 5). The cystic space contained foamy histiocytes, degenerative red blood cells, and proteinaceous materials (Figure 6). There were no metastatic lesions in dissected lymph nodes.

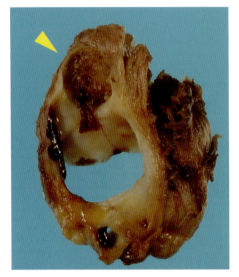

Figure 4. The tumor is predominantly composed of cystic lesions. Papillary growth (arrow) is observed on the inner surface of the cyst.

Figure 5. The carcinoma cells exhibit papillary growth into the cystic space (hematoxylin and elosin, ×2).

Figure 6. Foamy histiocytes, degenerative red blood cells, and proteinaceous materials are observed in the cystic space (hematoxylin and elosin, ×10).

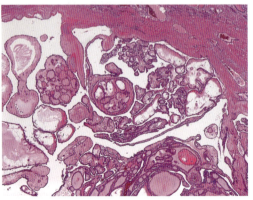
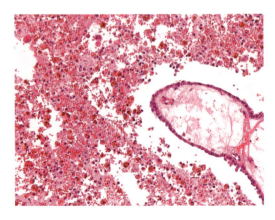

Discussion

The Bethesda System for Reporting Thyroid Cytopathology (TBSRTC) was developed to address terminology and other issues related to thyroid fine-needle aspiration (FNA) cytology.[1,2] According to the system, the recommended diagnostic categories are as follows: "ND," "benign," "atypia of undetermined significance," "follicular neoplasm," "suspicious for malignancy," and "malignant." ND applies to specimens that are unsatisfactory owing to the following: 1. Fewer than six groups of well-preserved, well-stained follicular cell groups with 10 cells each; 2. Poorly prepared, poorly stained, or obscured follicular cells; or 3. Cyst fluid, with or without histiocytes, and fewer than six groups of 10 benign follicular cells. Cystic papillary thyroid carcinoma cannot be excluded in the last "CFO" scenario, resulting in these cases being classified as ND.[1]

The cytologic interpretation of thyroid FNA cytology specimens consisting of cystic contents only, including only macrophages, remains controversial. CFO specimens were traditionally reported as benign.[3] At the National Cancer Institute Thyroid FNA State of the Science Conference in 2007,[4] because the possibility of cystic papillary thyroid carcinoma cannot be excluded in CFO cases, it was decided that such cases should be classified as a subset of ND. Subsequently, based on the conference proceedings, many laboratories adopted the reporting system. As a result, CFO cases accounted for more than half of those classified as ND, and 18–42% of aspiration cases became to be ND.[5-8] It is generally recommended that the incidence of ND specimens should ideally be <10% of thyroid FNAs, excluding CFO cases.[2] Therefore, we should calculate the incidences of both CFO and other-ND, but this is complicated given that CFO and other-ND exist in the same category.

The TBSRTC recommends that nodules with an initial ND result should be re-aspirated. However, follow-up strategies for CFO specimens from cystic nodules differ from those for solid nodules. When a nodule is determined to be a simple unilocular cyst on ultrasound, the specimen may be considered clinically adequate, even if it was reported as ND. Hence, the re-aspiration rate of CFO nodules should be lower than that of other-ND. We recommend that these two different cytologic findings, which necessitate different clinical management, should be classified into separate categories.

As ND cases are mostly benign and rarely require surgical resection, it is difficult to estimate the malignancy rates accurately. However, it has been reported that the rates range from 0 to 35%.[9] According to a report by MacDonald and Yazdi, the malignancy rates of CFO and other-ND nodules were 0 and 4.2%, respectively.[5] Renshaw reported no difference in the rates (3.9% in each group).[7] Garcia-Pascual et al. reported that the malignancy rate of CFO nodules was higher (14.3%) than that of other-ND nodules (6.7%), but this difference was not statistically significant.[8] In our experience, malignant rates in cases classified as CFO and other-ND nodules were 2.0% and 5.6%, respectively. That was significantly different. The former was similar to those (0–3%) of the benign category of the TBSRTC.[1] Therefore, we believe that the clinical management of CFO should conform to the benign category of the TBSRTC.

In conclusion, as CFO and other-ND nodules differ regarding clinical management and malignancy rates, they should be categorized separately. We propose that CFO should be a novel diagnostic category separately from ND. In terms of clinical management, we propose that only CFO cases with concerning sonographically worrisome features, such as suspected cystic PTC, should be re-aspirated. In Japan, the "cyst fluid" category was officially established as an independent diagnosis term in Japanese Society of Thyroid Surgery in 2015[11]. In UK Royal College of Pathologists Diagnostic category, CFO cases are included in nondiagnostic category (Thy1) and subclassified as nondiagnostic cystic thyroid lesions (Thy1c)[12]. Similarly, in Italy, ND is classified into TIR1 (inadequate) and TIR1C (cystic lesion)[12,13].

References

1. Ali SZ, Cibas, ES. The Bethesda System for Reporting Thyroid Cytology, Definitions, Criteria and Explanatory Notes. Springer, New York, 2010.
2. Cibas ES, Ali, SZ. The Bethesda System for Reporting Thyroid Cytopathology. Am J Clin Pathol. 2009;132:658–65.
3. Yang J, Schnadig V, Logrono R, Wasserman PG. Fine-needle aspiration of thyroid nodules: a study of 4703 patients with histologic and clinical correlations. Cancer. 2007;111:306–15.
4. Baloch ZW, Cibas ES, Clark DP, et al. The National Cancer Institute Thyroid fine needle aspiration state of the science conference: a summation. Cytojournal. 2008;5:6.
5. MacDonald L, Yazdi HM. Nondiagnostic fine needle aspiration biopsy of the thyroid gland: a diagnostic dilemma. Acta Cytol. 1996;40:423–8.
6. Yeoh GP, Chan KW. The diagnostic value of fine-needle aspiration cytology in the assessment of thyroid nodules: a retrospective 5-year analysis. Hong Kong Med J. 1999;5:140–4.
7. Renshaw AA. Accuracy of thyroid fine-needle aspiration using receiver operator characteristic curves. Am J Clin Pathol. 2001;116:477–82.
8. Jo VY, Stelow EB, Dustin SM, Hanley KZ. Malignancy risk for fine-needle aspiration of thyroid lesions according to the Bethesda System for Reporting Thyroid Cytopathology. Am J Clin Pathol. 2010;134:450–6.
9. Arul P, Akshatha C, Masilamani S. A study of malignancy rates in different diagnostic categories of the Bethesda system for reporting thyroid cytopathology: An institutional experience. Biomed J. 2015;38:517–22.
10. García-Pascual L, Barahona MJ, Balsells M, et al. Complex thyroid nodules with nondiagnostic fine needle aspiration cytology: histopathologic outcomes and comparison of the cytologic variants (cystic vs. acellular). Endocrine. 2011;39:33–40.
11. Japanese Society of Surgery. General Rules for the Description of Thyroid Cancer. Kanehara, Tokyo, 2015. [in Japanese]
12. Rossi ED et al. Thyroid FNA: International Perspectives from the European Congress of cytopathology –Can we cross the bridge of classifications?. Cancer cytopathology. 2015;123:207-11.
13. Fadda G and Rossi ED. Italian and national systems for thyroid cytology. JBCM 2015;4:46-51.

Supplemental Chapter 4

Thyroglossal Duct Cyst and Other Ectopic Thyroid Tissue in the Neck

Andrey Bychkov

Clinical History

A 49-year-old female presented with a 3-year history of a slowly growing asymptomatic mass along the neck midline. The patient complained that the swelling was slightly increasing in size since her last visit approximately a year ago. The patient had no significant past medical and surgical history. She denied any family history of thyroid disease or a history of head and neck irradiation. Physical examination revealed a 2 cm × 2 cm soft mass at the level of the hyoid bone, which was moving with both deglutition and tongue protrusion. There was no associated cervical lymphadenopathy. The rest of the physical examination was unremarkable. (Case courtesy of Prof. Pichet Sampatanukul, Department of Pathology, Faculty of Medicine, Chulalongkorn University, Bangkok, Thailand)

Ultrasound Findings

A 1.7 cm × 1.9 cm × 2.3 cm well-defined hypoechoic lesion was located at the level of the hyoid bone in the submental area (Figure 1). Color Doppler demonstrated no increased vascularity. The lesion was not related to the thyroid gland. There was an accompanying mass in lower pole of the left thyroid lobe. The thyroid nodule appeared as 2.2 cm × 1.1 cm × 1.6 cm well-defined mixed hyper-hypoechoic mass with a hypoechoic rim exhibiting internal microcalcification and increased vascularity. Both clinical data and sonography of the upper neck gave the impression of a thyroglossal duct (TGD) cyst.

Cytologic Findings

Three milliliters of watery, slightly hazy fluid were evacuated during ultrasound-guided fine-needle aspiration (FNA) of the cystic lesion. The aspirate was centrifuged, and

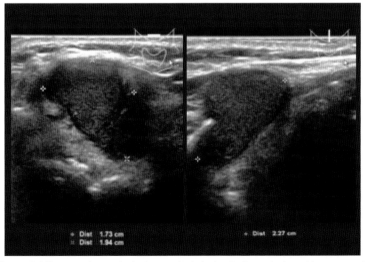

Figure 1. Ultrasound revealed a hypoechoic lesion in the anterior mid-upper neck.

sediment was further processed for cell block preparation. Review of the Papanicolaou-stained slides revealed a hypocellular aspirate with predominant inflammatory cells admixed with infrequent squames (Figure 2). Squamous cells were benign in appearance and rarely anucleated (Figure 3). No columnar or follicular epithelium was found. Numerous hemosiderin-laden macrophages were often arranged in small clusters. Abundant polymorphs and lymphocytes were scattered across most of the fields of view.

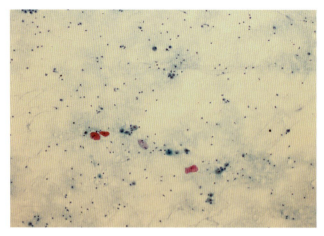

Figure 2. Low-power view shows sparsely cellular aspirate with inflammatory cells and infrequent squames (cell block, Papanicolaou stain, ×10).

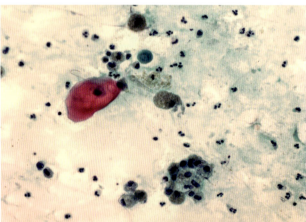

Figure 3. Benign squamous cell in an inflammatory background composed of histiocytes, lymphocytes, and scattered polymorphs (cell block, Papanicolaou stain, ×40).

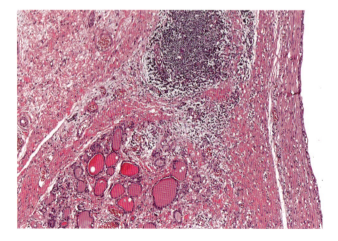

Figure 4. Cyst lined by cuboid epithelium contains thyroid follicles and lymphoid infiltrate (hematoxylin and eosin, ×10).

Histologic Findings

The surgical specimen consisted of the TGD with focal cystic dilation (2 cm × 2 cm sac with a smooth inner surface) submitted with part of the hyoid bone. Microscopically, the cyst lining was presented by nonkeratinizing squamous, and sometimes flattened to cuboid, epithelium (Figure 4). The underlying stroma was fibrotic with lymphocytic infiltrate, rarely arranged in aggregates, resembling lymphoid follicles. In some sections, the fibrotic cyst wall was partially denuded, and it contained granulation tissue. There were no evident signs of acute inflammation. Thyroid follicles were found lying in small groups under the lining epithelium. Thyroid follicular cells exhibited a benign appearance.

TGD Cyst

A TGD cyst is a midline neck developmental anomaly caused by persistent and cystic dilation of the TGD. TGD cysts are the most common congenital neck mass and the most common developmental anomaly of the thyroid gland. The main histologic components of the TGD are epithelial lined tubular structures and heterotopic thyroid tissue. Serial sections on autopsy identified latent TGD remnants in 7% of both pediatric and adult cohorts (1, 2). Scintigraphy after thyroid-stimulating hormone stimulation identified TGD remnants in more than 40% of thyroidectomized patients (3).

Similarly as thyroid lesions, FNA biopsy plays an important role in the diagnosis of neck masses. Most TGD cysts are located between the hyoid bone and thyroid cartilage, with only exceptional cases reported within the thyroid. However, the intimate developmental relationship between the TGD and thyroid gland *per se* gives us an opportunity to discuss this anatomically distinct lesion among other entities approached by thyroid FNA.

Most patients with TGD cysts are asymptomatic, with a slowly enlarging painless mass (1–4 cm) in the midline anterior neck, which moves upward on swallowing or protrusion of the tongue. Up to 30% of cases manifest with infected cysts, which may further progress to a draining sinus. Despite being a congenital anomaly, patients with TGD cysts exhibit a bimodal age distribution (first and fifth decades), and up to 25% of cases present after 50 years of age (4). Diagnosis is based on typical clinical manifestations supported by radiologic findings and confirmed by postoperative histopathology. Ultrasound is the preoperative investigation of choice, and it is aimed to evaluate the cyst location, echotexture (anechoic or pseudosolid appearance), and relation to the hyoid bone and thyroid gland (5). Complete surgical excision with removal of part of the hyoid bone (Sistrunk procedure) is routinely recommended for all patients with TGD cysts. As such, FNA of the cyst does not add much value to the preoperative triage of patients if the diagnosis is obvious. Histopathologic confirmation is a final step in the diagnostic workup of TGD cysts (Figure 5).

Microscopically, cystic or tubular structures are covered by epithelium. The type of epithelial lining varies by site, and combinations of several types can be noted in a single cyst (6). Ciliated pseudostratified columnar epithelium is regularly found in samples from the lower neck, probably due to the close proximity to the upper respiratory tract. Nonkeratinizing squamous epithelium is typical for the upper neck (near the tongue and foramen caecum), and it can be of metaplastic origin in the inflammatory setting. Stratified cuboidal epithelium is often found at the level of the hyoid bone. Often, the cyst is denuded of lining, at least focally, which reflects epithelial damage by inflammation. The cyst wall is fibrotic with foci of granulation tissue. Secondary inflammation is common, especially in the sinus tract, and it is denoted by intense lymphocytic infiltration (rarely arranged into lymphoid follicles) with admixture of neutrophils if the cyst is infected.

Ectopic thyroid follicles are found in 30–70% of cases, with higher yields on serial sections (routine number of blocks per case is three). Irregular groups of thyroid follicles with a mean size of 5 mm are noted in the cyst wall, being positioned under the lining epithelium or deeply situated and embedded by fibrosis (Figure 6). One study reported that ectopic thyroid tissue was more common in infra- *vs.* suprahyoid remnants (2). Thyroid epithelium is usually normal, but in exceptional cases, it can be hyperplastic or neoplastic. Thyroid tissue is often hidden by inflammation (7). However, the absence of thyroid follicles does not exclude the diagnosis of a TGD cyst. Occasional inclusions found in the cyst wall are skin adnexal structures, cholesterol granuloma, and mucous salivary-type glands. The latter are frequently reported in lingual and suprahyoid locations (8).

The histopathologic diagnosis of TGD cysts optimally requires evidence of respiratory or squamous epithelial lining and thyroid follicles, which sometimes can be difficult to locate due to inflammation and fibrosis; in these situations, a diagnosis of a developmental cyst with comment (favor TGD cyst or branchial cleft cyst) may be an option.

Preoperative FNA for routine cases is not advised because it is only moderately sensitive with many false negatives (4, 9). In a recently reported large series of TGD cysts, preoperative FNA was performed only in 13–21% of all cases submitted for surgery (4, 9, 10). Furthermore, the series reported by Thompson *et al.*, which had the highest rate of preoperative cytology, obtained unsatisfactory results in 85% of cases according to The Bethesda System for Reporting Thyroid Cytopathology (4). FNA of TGD cysts is warranted for the evaluation of suspicious cysts, for example those that appear as firm fixed lesions or exhibit a solid component on sonography. These findings may raise the possibility of malignancy (Please refer to Chapter 7). It is known that less than 1% of TGDs develop a cancer, usually papillary thyroid carcinoma. Ultrasound guidance is highly recommended as an aid for FNA, especially in children. Cell block preparation or liquid-based cytology of cystic fluid, along with sampling of residual mass after fluid evacuation, may substantially increase the FNA yield.

FNA smears of TGD cysts are of low cellularity, with predominant inflammatory cells, which outnumber epithelial cells, a picture similar to that for branchial cleft cysts. The most common cell populations are macrophages, either foamy or hemosiderin-laden, as well as mature lymphocytes and neutrophils. The latter are especially abundant in infected cysts. Squamous or ciliated columnar epithelium is not a frequent finding, being reported in less than half of cases (Please refer to Chapter 32: Mini-test case 8). Anucleated squames or parakeratotic cells can be noticed. Benign follicular epithelium is found rarely (2–10% of aspirates), most likely due to deep embedding in the cyst wall. A colloid or mucoid background is common, ranging from thick and fragmented to thin and watery. Admixtures of cholesterol crystals may be noted.

The differential diagnosis of TGD cysts is potentially large due to the anatomy of the thyroglossal tract, which spans from the foramen caecum to the thyroid. Most of the cases are resolved easily because of the typical clinical manifestation with a mobile painless mass in the midline neck. Nevertheless, diagnostic challenges can be posed during presentation, sonography, and evaluation of aspirated or resected specimens. We grouped all potential lesions from the differential diagnosis list into solid and cystic (Table 1). The main difficulty for pathologists is when ectopic thyroid tissue is not found in the cyst wall. In this scenario, a wide array of cystic lesions may be considered, especially in children (Figure 7).

It is believed that accurate review of the surgical samples may finally yield the presence of ectopic thyroid remnants, which, by definition, is the only pathognomonic sign of TGD cysts. The Sistrunk procedure is a relatively extensive surgery with cosmetic consequences, which is not advocated for other neck cysts, such as common dermoid or epidermal inclusion cysts. Hence, a surgeon can only consider pathologic diagnoses other than TGD cysts after the Sistrunk procedure. Careful examination of slides, recut of blocks, and the use of descriptive terminology (e.g., "consistent with TGD cysts" or "favor TGD

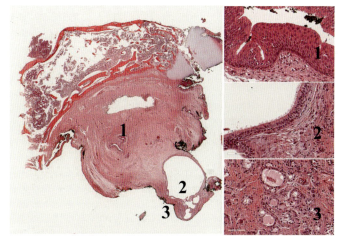

Figure 5. Diagnostic appearance of thyroglossal duct cysts. Perihyoid tubular and cystic structures, fibrotically embedded and covered with variable epithelial lining (Hematoxylin and eosin [HE], panoramic).
Insets: stratified squamous epithelium (upper), ciliated epithelium (middle), thyroid follicles (lower). Numbers show corresponding areas on the panoramic microphoto (HE, ×40).

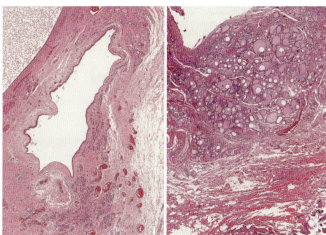

Figure 6. Appearance of ectopic thyroid tissue in the cyst wall. Irregular small follicles located under cyst epithelium (left); well arranged normofollicular "nodule" deeply embedded in the cyst wall (right) (hematoxylin and eosin, ×4).

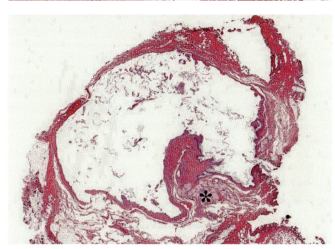

Figure 7. Specimen submitted as "thyroglossal duct cyst" displays the typical histologic appearance of a dermoid cyst lined by keratinized epithelium and contains sebaceous glands in the wall (asterisk) (hematoxylin and eosin, panoramic).

cyst") may assist in some cases involving a lack of thyroid tissue. It should be noted in this regard that thyroid remnants are often found in the vicinity of the hyoid bone, which is an essential part of the submitted surgical specimen. Bone tissue processing takes additional time, and a preliminary diagnosis based on microscopy of soft tissue specimens of TGD cysts can sometimes be corrected after the delivery of decalcified samples.

Table 1. Differential diagnosis of thyroglossal duct cysts

SOLID LESIONS	
Lingual thyroid	resolved by clinical and radiological modalities, orthotopic thyroid is often absent
Pyramidal lobe of thyroid gland	histologically large fragment of thyroid parenchyma enclosed by thin capsule
Lymph node with reactive hyperplasia	microscopic appearance of lymph node, no epithelium
Squamous cell carcinoma	atypical cells
Lipoma	adipose tissue
CYSTIC LESIONS	
Dermoid cyst	upper neck; filled with sebaceous material, lined by keratinizing epithelium, and having skin appendages in the wall, rarely inflamed; aspirate enriched with anucleated squames
Epidermoid cyst (epidermal inclusion cyst)	superficial location; histology similar to dermoid cyst, but without skin adnexa
Branchial cleft cyst	lateral location, lymphoid follicles in the wall; aspirate is more cellular with abundant squamous epithelium
Delphian lymph node metastasis of papillary thyroid carcinoma with cystic degeneration	typical papillary carcinoma; lymph node architecture, including lymphoid stroma and subcapsular sinus; lack of TGD epithelium and thyroid parenchyma
Cystic degeneration of colloid nodule	background of benign thyroid parenchyma
Rare developmental cysts:	
– lymphangioma	lymphatic channels, absence of epithelial lining
– lymphoepithelial cyst	wall contains lymphoid tissue with germinal centers
– thymic cyst (suprasternal)	contains Hassall's corpuscles or other thymic tissue
– cervical bronchogenic cyst	cyst wall with smooth muscle, mucoserous glands, and often cartilaginous tissue
– midline cervical cleft	linear cleft extending from hyoid bone to the suprasternal notch, always present at birth
– teratoma	presence of three germ cell layers in a surgical sample
Rare non-developmental cysts:	
– ranula (upper neck)	submental origin; pools of mucus surrounded by fibrous tissue, absence of epithelial lining
– laryngocele	intimate relation to larynx; clinical presentation and radiology

The most unusual sites at which TGD cysts have been described are suprasternal, mediastinal, and intrathyroidal locations. An intrathyroidal location may account for up to 1.5% of all TGD cysts (4). These lesions present difficulties for both histologic and cytologic interpretation. The histoarchitecture of intrathyroidal TGD cysts is similar to that of another rare thyroid lesion, known as lymphoepithelial or branchial cleft-like cysts. Most authors link the origin of thyroid lymphoepithelial cysts to solid cell nests, which undergo squamous metaplasia and cystic degeneration in the setting of chronic thyroiditis. Despite the common features with TGD cysts such as a squamous epithelial lining and chronic inflammation, lymphoepithelial cysts are located laterally in the lobes, they lack respiratory epithelium, and they often contain lymphoid follicles with germinal centers in the wall. Smears of intrathyroidal TGD cysts can be confused with primary thyroid carcinoma due to the presence of unusual epithelium (squamous or ciliated); however, no signs of atypia are observed.

TGD Carcinoma

The most serious consequence of TGD cysts is neoplastic transformation of the epithelium. Carcinoma is found in approximately 1% of TGD cysts (up to 5–7% in large referral centers); however, the risk of carcinoma over time is probably underestimated due to the routine removal of TGD cysts in childhood (11). There are two theories of the origin of TGD carcinoma, namely *de novo* and metastatic; however, a precise mechanism has not been resolved, probably due to the lack of molecular studies. The vast majority of cases are represented by papillary thyroid carcinoma (90%), mainly the classic variant, but follicular and tall cell variants have also been reported (12). Contrary to early reports, nodal involvement was found to be common, approaching a rate of 70% of cases in series with neck dissections (13). Rarely, TGD cancer can be squamous cell carcinoma derived from the actual cyst lining (5%) or follicular thyroid carcinoma (2–3%). Exceptional cases or unusual cancers (anaplastic, mucoepidermoid, adenosquamous) and combinations were also documented. To summarize, over 250 cases of TGD carcinoma have been reported to date (14).

The mean age of the patients is approximately 40 years old. A preoperative diagnosis of carcinoma in a patient presenting with a TGD cyst is unusual. Most TGD cancers are asymptomatic, and they are discovered by the pathologist on routine histological evaluation. Clinically, no clear distinction between a benign cyst and malignancy can be made. In some cases, cancer can be suspected on the basis of sudden growth of a preexisting cyst or enlargement of cervical lymph nodes. Routine workup is similar to that for TGD cysts, essentially including neck ultrasound, which can be complemented by computed tomography, magnetic resonance imaging, and FNA. Suspicious ultrasound findings include calcification, complex cysts with internal echoes, and solid vascularized vegetations. Most TGD carcinomas are managed initially by the Sistrunk procedure. Further steps may include total thyroidectomy, neck dissection, and radioiodine ablation.

Histopathology reveals typical thyroid carcinoma, mainly papillary (nuclear features and microarchitecture compatible with a specific histotype) in the context of a TGD cyst with an epithelial lining. Invasion of the hyoid bone and adjacent soft tissue is common. The criteria for diagnosis include histopathological confirmation of thyroglossal remnants in a specimen with carcinoma coupled with clinical or histologic evidence of a normal thyroid gland (to exclude a metastasis from a primary thyroid cancer). Recent studies found that coincident cancer in orthotopic thyroid glands, mainly papillary microcarcinoma, occurred in 30–60% of patients with TGD carcinoma when thyroidectomy was performed (15).

FNA biopsy of TGD cysts may be helpful in confirming the clinical suspicion, being most efficient in adults. FNA findings range from a nonspecific cystic lesion to features characteristic of papillary or squamous cell carcinoma (16). However, FNA cytology has relatively low sensitivity, similarly as observed in cases of benign TGD cysts. Some authors recommend intraoperative frozen section as a more robust diagnostic modality (17).

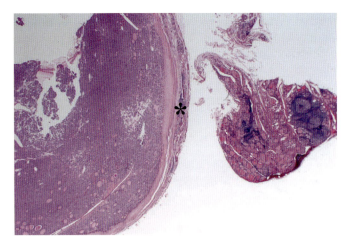

Figure 8. Excised nodule above thyroid cartilage was suspected to be follicular carcinoma (capsular invasion found in other fragments) developed from thyroglossal duct remnants. The presence of a pericapsular rim of well-developed thyroid tissue (asterisk) and separated piece with signs of Hashimoto's thyroiditis favor a diagnosis of follicular thyroid carcinoma of the pyramidal lobe (hematoxylin and eosin, ×2).

The first line of differential diagnosis should consider TGD carcinoma to be metastasis from primary thyroid cancer whether occult or evident. Such an assumption needs to be ruled out during the thyroid diagnostic workup with imaging and FNA. In addition to clinical relevance (extent of surgery), this may add missing knowledge to the scarce field of theories of the origin of TGD cancer. TGD-associated carcinoma also should be distinguished from either primary pyramidal thyroid lobe cancer or Delphian (prelaryngeal) lymph node metastasis, both of which appear at a similar anatomic location. This differential diagnosis is critically important for staging and treatment. Primary cancer of the pyramidal lobe presents as carcinoma surrounded by a background of benign thyroid parenchyma with the absence of TGD epithelium (respiratory or squamous) and lymph node structures (Figure 8). It should be noted that isolated cancer of the pyramidal lobe is extremely rare, and most "pyramidal cancers" are seeded from the index tumor elsewhere within thyroid lobes, which can be disclosed by ultrasound. Delphian node metastasis is distinguished on the basis of lymph node architecture, including lymphoid stroma and subcapsular sinus, a lack of TGD epithelium and thyroid parenchyma, and the presence of occult or evident cancer in the thyroidectomy specimen. Recently, a new term, upper neck papillary thyroid carcinoma, was proposed to combine TGD cyst cancer, pyramidal lobe cancer, and Delphian lymph node metastasis, which are often difficult to distinguish (14).

Ectopic Thyroid Inclusions in the Lower Neck

It has been well illustrated by the case of thyroid carcinoma arisen in the pyramidal lobe (Figure 8) that an accidental finding of normal or abnormal thyroid tissue in unusual sites poses a serious diagnostic challenge. This holds especially true for FNA when the tissue context and histologic relationships visible in surgical samples are not evident. Perhaps a level of confusion is the best described by the surgical term "**lateral aberrant thyroid**". An aberrant thyroid is a mass of tissue having the structure of a normal or pathological thyroid gland but being situated at some definite distance from the normal thyroid (more strictly, lateral to the jugular vein), with which it has no connection. A trick is that this collective term is imprecise, and it is actually represented by various conditions both benign and malignant in nature. We recommend avoiding such outdated terminology, at least in pathology practice.

All lesions formerly called "lateral aberrant thyroid" can be divided into malignant and benign. Nodal metastasis of papillary thyroid carcinoma accounts for most malignant cases. In addition, soft tissue implants of thyroid cancer or exceptional cases of branchial cleft with thyroid carcinoma can be considered. The benign group includes thyroid parasitic nodules and displaced thyroid tissue after surgery or trauma. A true ectopic thyroid with a lateral location is extremely rare compared to a midline location. In summary, lateral aberrant thyroid is largely represented by metastatic carcinoma or benign parasitic nodules.

The classic presentation and pitfalls in the diagnosis of lymph node metastasis of papillary thyroid carcinoma are well described in detail in the major head-neck and thyroid pathology books. In this text, we would like to address the more enigmatic issue of ectopic thyroid tissue in cervical lymph nodes. **Benign thyroid inclusion** is a tiny fragment of thyroid tissue incidentally discovered in cervical nodes during histologic examination of neck dissections performed for non-thyroidal disease, e.g., head and neck cancer. For several decades, it was suggested that all thyroid tissue within lymph nodes is metastatic thyroid cancer; however, the possibility of benign inclusions is widely accepted today (18). The incidence of unsuspected benign thyroid tissue in lymph nodes of patients with head and neck carcinoma treated with neck dissection is 0.6–1.5% (19, 20). Meticulous study of cervical lymph nodes identified benign thyroid inclusions in up to 5% of unselected autopsies (21).

Benign thyroid inclusions involve medial inferior neck lymph nodes, whereas any thyroid tissue found lateral to large neck vessels (carotid artery or jugular vein) should be considered metastatic tumors rather than benign ectopia (22). However, occasional cases of benign inclusions in lateral (up to level II) lymph nodes have been described (18). It is believed that aberrations during migration of the embryonic thyroid may result in entrapment of structures that terminally differentiate into thyroid follicles and remain quiescent in lymph nodes (heterotopia). Another theory speculates that tiny fragments of ruptured thyroid tissue float into sentinel lymph nodes ("benign metastasis"), similar to the proposed mechanism for endometriosis. Benign nodal thyroid inclusions are not unique, as similar benign foci of the parathyroid, salivary gland tissue and nevus cells were described in cervical lymph nodes. A diagnosis of benign nodal thyroid inclusions is possible only after excluding primary thyroid carcinoma on an extensive workup including imaging and possibly surgery. Unequivocally benign inclusions confirmed by morphology and negative thyroid imaging may require no further action, but clinical correlation and follow-up are advised.

Inclusions are 0.1–2.3 mm in size, and they contain up to 100 (average 30) normal-appearing thyroid follicles usually arranged in a wedge-shaped focus with the base adjacent to the nodal capsule and the apex directed toward the cortex (18). Benign inclusion should be located within the nodal capsule or in the marginal sinus (subcapsular) and present in no more than two cervical lymph nodes. The probability of obtaining tiny benign thyroid inclusions during FNA of cervical lymph nodes is extremely low, with only one case reported (23). Thus, the presence of thyroid follicles in cervical lymph node aspirate should be considered metastatic thyroid carcinoma or a technical error, for instance, if an orthotopic or heterotopic thyroid nodule is sampled instead of the lymph node. Key points for the differential diagnosis between benign and malignant thyroid inclusions in cervical nodes are presented in Table 2.

A parasitic nodule is a more rare condition that is believed to represent a substantial number of benign cases of lateral aberrant thyroid. It is a peripheral nodule of goiter that is anatomically separate from the main thyroid gland (8). This lesion is also known as sequestered goiter or an accessory thyroid nodule. Spontaneous detachment of thyroid tissue may occur in nodular goiter and Hashimoto's thyroiditis and less commonly in Grave's disease. A portion of nodular thyroid may be separated by the mechanical action of neck muscles and subsequently implanted in the lateral neck.

Table 2. Differential diagnosis of thyroid inclusions in cervical lymph nodes

	Benign inclusions	Metastatic carcinoma
Primary tumor	• No evidence	• Thyroid carcinoma (mainly papillary), often occult and ipsilateral • Extremely rare can be extrathyroidal primary
Cervical node location	• Only medial to jugular vein (basically midline)	• Any, mainly inferior • All thyroid inclusions in nodes lateral to jugular vein/carotid artery irrespective of benign appearance should be considered metastatic
Extent	• Single focus of few follicles, located within node capsule or in marginal sinus (subcapsular) • One, rarely two nodes	• From few follicles to total (and cystic) replacement of lymph node • Often multiple nodes involved
Microscopy	• Normal appearing thyroid follicles • No features of PTC	• Features of PTC: – cellular (nuclear enlargement, clearing, etc.; tall eosinophilic cells) – architectural (papillary formations) – secondary (psammoma bodies, stromal reaction)
Ancillary tests	• IHC: TTF1+, Tg+; CK19-, Galectin-3-, HBME1- • Molecular: no aberrations • Clonality assay: polyclonal	• IHC: CK19+, Gal-3+, HBME1+ (immunophenotype of thyroid cancer) • Molecular: BRAF+, or RET/PTC+, or RAS+ • Clonality assay: monoclonal

A parasitic nodule can be located in the lateral neck anywhere from the submandibular to the mediastinal area, including the retroclavicular area and the sternocleidomastoid and sternohyoid muscles (24). However, most nodules are found in the perithyroidal area near the gland (<1 cm). Parasitic nodules imitate enlarged cervical lymph nodes clinically, and they are usually removed to rule out metastasis. Hence, the diagnosis is essentially made on histopathology after excluding metastatic cancer. The following criteria should be satisfied to consider a lesion to be a parasitic nodule: it should be in the same fascial plane as the thyroid gland and exhibit a similar histologic appearance as the main gland without evidence of lymph node structures. Grossly, these are 0.5–6.5-cm nodules that are separate from the thyroid gland, and they are singular in more than 80% of cases. The histology of the nodule is similar to that of benign-appearing thyroid tissue with colloid-filled or hyperplastic follicles, sometimes including the signs of Hashimoto's thyroiditis. Similar features are found in the orthotopic gland. Scarce cytologic reports described unremarkable findings of benign follicular cells (25).

Parasitic nodules should be differentiated from nodal metastasis of papillary thyroid carcinoma. The cytologic and architectural features of carcinoma are the crucial signs aiding the diagnosis. Primary tumor in the main thyroid favors a diagnosis of a metastatic lesion; however, it may be occult. Diagnostic difficulty appears when Hashimoto's thyroiditis in parasitic nodules simulates lymph node tissue. In this situation, careful assessment of lymph node structures helps to render a diagnosis; for example, subcapsular sinuses can be highlighted by reticulin stain. Ancillary studies, including immunohistochemistry with markers of thyroid carcinoma (CK19, galectin-3, HBME-1) and molecular analysis (BRAF and RAS mutations), can potentially assist in challenging cases.

The core part of this chapter is devoted to TGD-related lesions, which by definition are examples of **ectopic thyroid**. This term covers a range of developmental abnormalities characterized by the presence of thyroid tissue in any location other than its normal anatomic position. The target area for thyroid ectopia lies along the track of medial anlage descent between the base of the tongue and normal thyroid location. The most common and clinically important types of ectopic thyroid are lingual thyroid and thyroid remnants within TGD cysts. Rare sites of thyroid ectopia are mainly distributed in the neck area, including midline (larynx and trachea) and non-midline structures (retropharyngeal space, salivary glands, and branchial cleft cysts). It should be noted that benign thyroid follicles are commonly found in perithyroid soft tissue and muscles. These microscopic inclusions located in the immediate vicinity of the gland (often around the isthmus) are silent and harmless (26). One other condition may provide a reasonable explanation of the accidental finding of thyroid follicles in the cervical region. This is so-called displacement or seeding of thyroid tissue due to prior surgery or trauma (27). Seeded nodules are often multiple and superficial, i.e., subcutaneous. Microscopically identified suture material and talc crystals accompanied by reactive fibrosis may give a clue for the differential diagnosis with other ectopic thyroid inclusions.

Take Home Message

The path taken by the developing thyroid during embryogenesis encompasses a wide area in the anterior neck, which may harbor ectopic thyroid remnants. The most common entity, which requires attention of the pathologist, is the TGD cyst. This midline neck developmental lesion is diagnosed by the presence of an epithelial lining and thyroid follicles. Rarely, follicular epithelium in the TGD cyst wall of may undergo malignant transformation, giving rise to papillary thyroid carcinoma. FNA findings in TGD are well described; however, the utility of cytologic examination in controversial due to its low sensitivity. The major indication for FNA is the evaluation of suspicious TGD cysts, for which cytology may yield atypical cells with characteristic features of papillary carcinoma. Various types of microscopic thyroid inclusions accidentally found in the cervical region are important in the context of the differential diagnosis with metastatic thyroid cancer. A meticulous search for the primary thyroid tumor is a rule of thumb in such a challenging situation.

References

1. Ellis PD, van Nostrand AW. The applied anatomy of thyroglossal tract remnants. Laryngoscope 1977; 87:765-70.
2. Sprinzl GM, Koebke J, Wimmers-Klick J, et al. Morphology of the human thyroglossal tract: A histologic and macroscopic study in infants and children. Ann Otol Rhinol Laryngol 2000; 109:1135-9.
3. Lee M, Lee YK, Jeon TJ, et al. Frequent visualization of thyroglossal duct remnant on post-ablation 131I-SPECT/CT and its clinical implications. Clin Radiol 2015; 70:638-43.
4. Thompson LD, Herrera HB, Lau SK. A clinicopathologic series of 685 thyroglossal duct remnant cysts. Head Neck Pathol 2016.
5. Zander DA, Smoker WR. Imaging of ectopic thyroid tissue and thyroglossal duct cysts. Radiographics 2014; 34:37-50.
6. Ali AA, Al-Jandan B, Suresh CS, et al. The relationship between the location of thyroglossal duct cysts and the

epithelial lining. Head Neck Pathol 2013; 7:50-3.
7. Chandra RK, Maddalozzo J, Kovarik P. Histological characterization of the thyroglossal tract: implications for surgical management. Laryngoscope 2001; 111:1002-5.
8. Assi A, Sironi M, Di Bella C, et al. Parasitic nodule of the right carotid triangle. Arch Otolaryngol Head Neck Surg 1996; 122:1409-11.
9. Shahin A, Burroughs FH, Kirby JP, et al. Thyroglossal duct cyst: a cytopathologic study of 26 cases. Diagn Cytopathol 2005; 33:365-9.
10. Wei S, LiVolsi VA, Baloch ZW. Pathology of thyroglossal duct: an institutional experience. Endocr Pathol 2015; 26:75-9.
11. Foley DS, Fallat ME. Thyroglossal duct and other congenital midline cervical anomalies. Semin Pediatr Surg 2006; 15:70-5.
12. Klubo-Gwiezdzinska J, Manes RP, Chia SH, et al. Ectopic cervical thyroid carcinoma - Review of the literature with illustrative case series. J Clin Endocrinol Metab 2011; 96:2684-91.
13. Choi YM, Kim TY, Song DE, et al. Papillary thyroid carcinoma arising from a thyroglossal duct cyst: a single institution experience. Endocr J 2013; 60:665-70.
14. Zizic M, Faquin W, Stephen AE, et al. Upper neck papillary thyroid cancer (UPTC): A new proposed term for the composite of thyroglossal duct cyst-associated papillary thyroid cancer, pyramidal lobe papillary thyroid cancer, and Delphian node papillary thyroid cancer metastasis. Laryngoscope 2016; 126:1709-14.
15. Pellegriti G, Lumera G, Malandrino P, et al. Thyroid cancer in thyroglossal duct cysts requires a specific approach due to its unpredictable extension. J Clin Endocrinol Metab 2013; 98:458-65.
16. Bardales RH, Suhrland MJ, Korourian S, et al. Cytologic findings in thyroglossal duct carcinoma. Am J Clin Pathol 1996; 106:615-9.
17. Danilovic DL, Marui S, Lima EU, et al. Papillary carcinoma in thyroglossal duct cyst: role of fine needle aspiration and frozen section biopsy to guide surgical approach. Endocrine 2014; 46:160-3.
18. Triantafyllou A, Williams MD, Angelos P, et al. Incidental findings of thyroid tissue in cervical lymph nodes: old controversy not yet resolved? Eur Arch Otorhinolaryngol 2015.
19. Gerard-Marchant R, Caillou B. Thyroid inclusions in cervical lymph nodes. Clin Endocrinol Metab 1981; 10:337-49.
20. Leon X, Sancho FJ, Garcia J, et al. Incidence and significance of clinically unsuspected thyroid tissue in lymph nodes found during neck dissection in head and neck carcinoma patients. Laryngoscope 2005; 115:470-4.
21. Meyer JS, Steinberg LS. Microscopically benign thyroid follicles in cervical lymph nodes. Serial section study of lymph node inclusions and entire thyroid gland in 5 cases. Cancer 1969; 24:302-11.
22. Wenig BM. Atlas of head and neck pathology. 3 ed. USA: Elsevier; 2015. 1600 p.
23. Lee YJ, Kim DW, Park HK, et al. Benign intranodal thyroid tissue mimicking nodal metastasis in a patient with papillary thyroid carcinoma: A case report. Head Neck 2015; 37:E106-8.
24. Rodriguez J, Rosai J. Parasitic nodules of the thyroid. A metastasis simulator. A study of 76 cases. Lab Invest 2006; 86:96A.
25. Nasrallah MP, Pramick MR, Baloch ZW. Images in endocrine pathology: Parasitic nodule of thyroid in neck of patient with family history of papillary thyroid carcinoma. Endocr Pathol 2015; 26:273-5.
26. Komorowski RA, Hanson GA. Occult thyroid pathology in the young adult: An autopsy study of 138 patients without clinical thyroid disease. Hum Pathol 1988; 19:689-96.
27. Harach HR, Cabrera JA, Williams ED. Thyroid implants after surgery and blunt trauma. Ann Diagn Pathol 2004; 8:61-8.

Supplemental Chapter 5

Diagnostic Clues for Thyroid Fine Needle Aspiration Cytology

Aki Ito and Ayana Suzuki

Smear Background

Watery Colloid

Colloid is the semifluid material that occupies the lumen of thyroid follicles, and it mainly contains thyroglobulin. The character of colloid plays a central role in thyroid fine-needle aspiration (FNA) cytology. In general, colloid aspirated from active follicles is paler and thinner, and that from inactive glands or neoplastic lesions is denser. Grossly, a colloid-predominant aspirate often resembles honey. Colloid may be lost from the glass slide during processing (1).

Watery colloid spreads as a thin, acellular, homogeneous film on the glass slide. In Giemsa staining, it has a tendency to crack or represent uneven spread on the slide glass, resulting in a

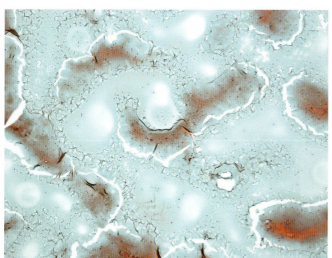

Figure 1. Watery colloid in nodular goiter (Papanicolaou, ×4).

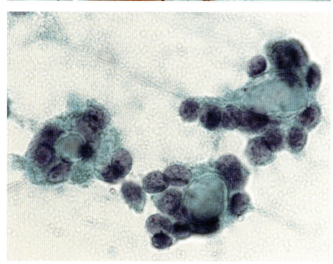

Figure 2. Dense colloid in follicular neoplasm (Papanicolaou, ×100).

geometric pattern, stained glass appearance, spider web-like appearance, or chicken wire pattern. In Papanicolaou staining, it is cyanophilic to eosinophilic, and thin to thick. It may resemble plastic wrap or parched earth with cracks (Figure 1). Abundant watery colloid indicates a benign condition. Note that watery colloid tends to be lost in liquid-based cytology (LBC) specimens (2,3).

Dense colloid

Dense inspissated colloid usually resembles irregular or rounded chips of translucent, homogeneous materials. It stains blue, green, pink, or orange (please refer to Figures 3–4 of Chapter 20) in Papanicolaou staining and deep purple in Giemsa or Diff-Quik staining (please refer to Figure 8 of Chapter 24). The size and shape of dense colloid reflects those of the follicles. Large, small, and clubbed forms of colloid indicate macrofollicular, microfollicular (Figure 2), and trabecular growth, respectively. Occasionally, especially in elderly patients and those with chronic marantic disease, dense colloid may be granular. In LBC specimens, dense colloid resembles small droplets, saber, or feathers (please refer to Figure 6A of Chapter 19 and Figure 4 of Chapter 27).

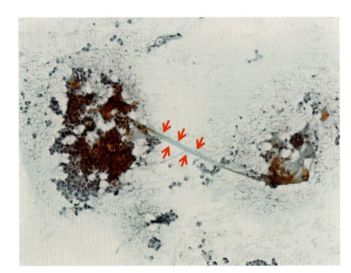

Figure 3. Ropy colloid in papillary thyroid carcinoma (arrows) (Papanicolaou, ×10).

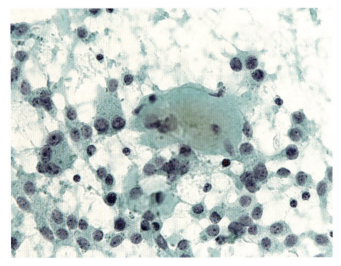

Figure 4. Amyloid in medullary thyroid carcinoma (Papanicolaou, ×40).

Ropy colloid

Densely staining strands of colloid, termed "ropy colloid," is characteristic of papillary thyroid carcinoma (PTC) (4). Ropy colloid is known by various other names such as bubble gum colloid, ropy strand, viscous colloid, sticky colloid, cord-like colloid, and chewing gum colloid. It is pink-purple or blue-green in Papanicolaou staining (Figure 3). It appears in up to 25% of PTCs (5). The shape is not a smearing artifact. Ropy colloid could be present in situ, and its formation is related to inspissated colloid and a papillary structure.

Amyloid

Amyloid is characteristic of medullary thyroid carcinoma (MTC). It is derived from either a prohormone of calcitonin or calcitonin itself (6). Amyloid is histologically present in >80% of cases of MTC (7), but it is cytologically identified in only 40–80% of cases (8). It may appear in other thyroid diseases, including mucosa-associated lymphoid tissue (MALT) lymphoma associated with plasma cell differentiation (9) and amyloid goiter. Amyloid is a Light Green-positive, flocculent or dense, acellular material in Papanicolaou staining (Figure 4) (please also refer to Figure 16 of Chapter 16). It occasionally resembles dense colloid. Special stains can be used for identification. Amyloid stains "brick red" with Congo red stain, exhibiting characteristic apple green birefringence under polarized microscopy.

Inflammatory cells

Lymphocytes are usually observed in conditions of chronic inflammatory conditions, such as Hashimoto's thyroiditis. Regarding neoplastic disease, PTC, but not follicular neoplasm, is frequently associated with lymphocytes in the background. The presence of numerous plasma cells may indicate IgG4-related thyroiditis or MALT lymphoma associated with plasma cell differentiation. Neutrophils are characteristic of acute suppurative thyroiditis. Anaplastic carcinoma may reveal a large number of neutrophils that outnumber carcinoma cells. Therefore, it is important not to overlook a few anaplastic carcinoma cells in abscess-like materials (please refer to Figures 1–3 of Case 2 in Chapter 32). Multinucleated giant cells associated with lymphocytes and epithelioid cells suggest subacute thyroiditis (please refer to Chapter 11). Multinucleated foreign body type giant cells that are bizarre in shape are present in half of cases of PTC (Figure 5A) (please also refer to Figures 5 and 8 of Chapter 4). The cytoplasm is dense and not dirty. The nuclei may resemble those of PTC cells, but they are histiocytic in origin (please also refer to Figures 2–3 of

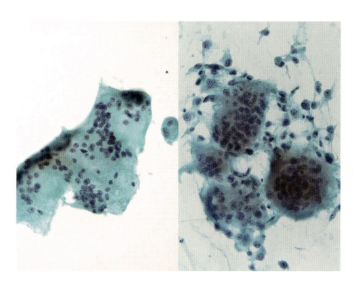

Figure 5. A (right): Bizarre foreign body-type multinucleated giant cells in papillary thyroid carcinoma (Papanicolaou, ×40), B (left): Osteoclast-type multinucleated giant cells in anaplastic carcinoma (Papanicolaou, ×20)

Chapter 11). Anaplastic carcinoma may be associated with osteoclast-type multinucleated giant cells (Figure 5B).

Psammoma bodies

Psammoma bodies are calcified, concentrically laminated, spherical bodies. They stain hematoxyphilic on hematoxylin and eosin (HE) in staining, but they are lavender, golden brown, or amphophilic in Papanicolaou staining (Figure 6) (please refer to Figure 9D in Chapter 7). They may be starburst and refractile. They are 5–100 μm in diameter. They are surrounded by tumor cells, or they appear as naked structures in the background. Although not pathognomonic, psammoma bodies in the thyroid FNA strongly indicate PTC. The incidence of psammoma bodies is <25% of PTCs in cytology (10). The pathogenesis is still debated. Theories include dystrophic calcification around infarcted tips of papillae (11,12), individual necrotic tumor cells (13), or intracytoplasmic substances (14). Hyalinizing trabecular tumors and the oxyphilic cell variant of follicular neoplasm may display psammoma bodies that are formed from inspissated colloid.

Lymphoglandular bodies (LGBs)

LGBs are cytoplasmic fragments of lymphoid cells (Figure 7). They are round, pale,

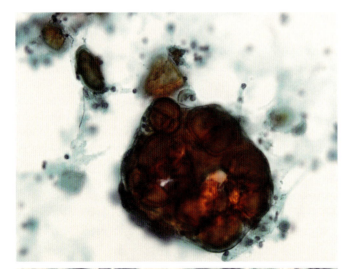

Figure 6. Psammoma bodies in papillary carcinoma (Papanicolaou, ×20).

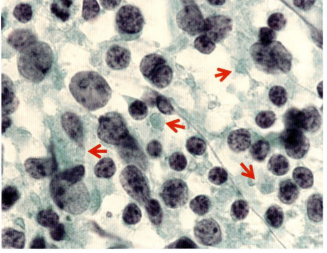

Figure 7. Lymphoglandular bodies in diffuse large B cell lymphoma (arrows) (Papanicolaou, ×100).

basophilic fragments in Giemsa-stained specimens. Their size varies between 2 and 7 μm in diameter. The presence of lymphoid cells with numerous LGBs supports a diagnosis of malignant lymphoma.

Necrotic materials

Anaplastic carcinoma is frequently associated with necrotic cells and/or materials. When only necrotic materials are aspirated, we should consider a possibility of anaplastic carcinoma. The oxyphilic cell variant of follicular neoplasm and PTC with infarction feature necrotic tumor cells (Figure 8) (please refer to Chapter 25).

Cellular Arrangements

Microfollicles

It has been proposed that the "microfollicle" designation must be limited to crowded, flat groups of less than 15 follicular cells arranged in a circle that is at least two-thirds complete (Figure 9) (15). The follicles may or may not be associated with a small amount of central colloid. Microfollicular arrangements are more likely to be neoplastic. Crowded, three-dimensional syncytial-like aggregates of microfollicles are particularly characteristic of follicular neoplasms

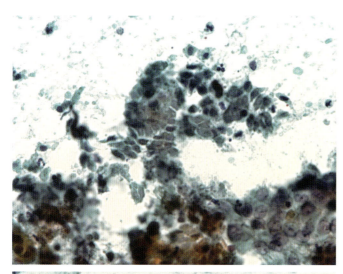

Figure 8. Necrotic materials caused by the infarction of papillary thyroid carcinoma (Papanicolaou, ×40).

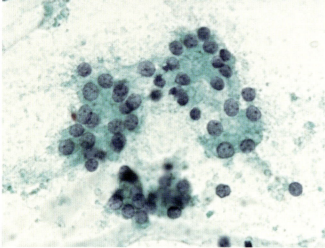

Figure 9. Microfollicles in follicular neoplasm (Papanicolaou, ×40).

(1). Aggregation of microfollicles should be differentiated from multiple microfollicles within a large solid nest. The latter is observed in insular carcinoma with cribriform patterns (please refer to Figure 11 of Chapter 20).

Papillary tissue fragment

Three-dimensional branching papillae with fibrovascular cores are highly characteristic of PTC (Figure 10). A duct-like structure or trabecular pattern containing spindle-shaped nuclei representing endothelial cells or fibroblasts within the clusters indicates non-branching papillary tissue fragments. Adenomatous goiter may exhibit a papillary arrangement (please refer to Figure 6 of Chapter 4).

Crinkled (bended) monolayered sheets

Large monolayered sheets of bland tumor cells are common and characteristic findings of PTC with papillary growth. The sheets are partially crinkled or bended (Figure 11). The nuclei are linearly arranged, and they display palisading at the folded portion.

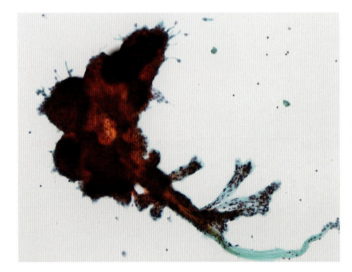

Figure 10. Papillary tissue fragment in papillary thyroid carcinoma (Papanicolaou, liquid-based cytology, ×20).

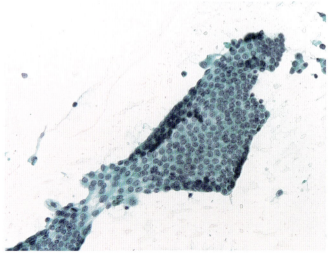

Figure 11. Crinkled monolayered sheet in papillary thyroid carcinoma (Papanicolaou, ×20).

Caps

Three-dimensional dome-shaped structures composed of epithelial cells are called caps (Figure 12). The structure represents the tips of papillae without a stromal component and indicates PTC.

Cellular swirls

Cellular swirls are defined as concentrically organized aggregates of tumor cells (Figure 13). The structures are relatively flat and two-dimensional, and they do not contain any colloid. The most peripherally situated cells have ovoid nuclei that are oriented perpendicularly to the radius of the swirl. The structures represent a finding that is highly specific to PTC and is easily visible upon screening magnification (16).

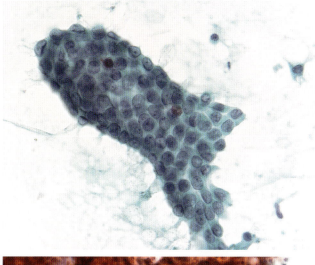

Figure 12. Cap in papillary thyroid carcinoma (Papanicolaou, ×40).

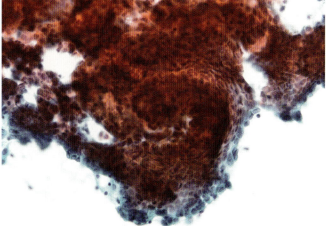

Figure 13. Cellular swirl in papillary thyroid carcinoma (Papanicolaou, ×20).

Hobnail pattern

A hobnail pattern denotes apically placed nuclei and surface bulging. The hobnail variant of PTC is an aggressive variant, and it requires that at least 30% of the tumor cells have hobnail features. The variant is identified as isolated single cells exhibiting eccentric nuclei with teardrop or tapering cytoplasm, so-called comet-like cells (Figure 14). Micropapillary fragments displaying a hobnail appearance can be also observed. The hobnail pattern more often appears in LBC specimens than in conventional specimens (17), and it can be also observed in cystic PTC and the diffuse sclerosing variant of PTC.

Ball-like clusters

Ball-like clusters are composed of spherical stromal components entirely surrounded by epithelial cells. The clusters represent a type of papillary structure, and they usually appear in fluid, such as pleural effusion and ascites. In thyroid FNA cytology, ball-like clusters can be present in cystic PTC and the diffuse sclerosing variant of PTC. They are floating in the cystic spaces of the former or dilated lymphatic vessels of the latter. The clusters may be hollow because the stroma is extremely edematous (Figure 15). The stroma present in diffuse sclerosing variants frequently contains lymphocytes or psammoma bodies.

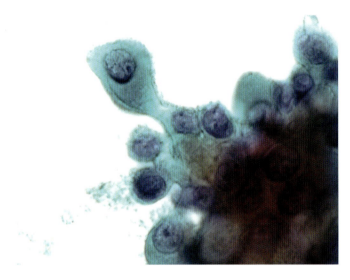

Figure 14. Hobnail pattern in papillary thyroid carcinoma (Papanicolaou, ×100).

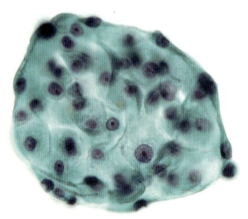

Figure 15. Ball-like cluster in papillary thyroid carcinoma (Papanicolaou, ×40).

Cell Shapes

Tall cells

Tall cells are defined as cells with a height more than three times larger than the width. Thyroid carcinomas with tall cells include the cribriform, tall cell, and columnar cell variants of PTC (Please refer to chapters 8, 9, and 10) and metastatic colonic adenocarcinoma. The latter three are clinically aggressive, but the cribriform variant of PTC has a better prognosis. It is not easy to recognize tall cells in conventional specimens. Parallelly arranged, tail-like cytoplasmic elongation toward the outside of cell clusters may be a clue indicating tall cells (Figure 16). Tall cell features are more easily recognized in LBC specimens.

Spindle cells

Spindle cells can appear in a variety of thyroid conditions. Differential diagnoses of monotonous neoplastic spindle cells include MTC (Figure 17), solitary fibrous tumor, spindle epithelial tumor with thymus-like differentiation, anaplastic carcinoma, and sarcoma. The former three exhibit bland tumor cells. By contrast, the latter two feature strikingly atypical tumor cells. Nodular goiter, follicular neoplasm, and PTC rarely contain spindle cell components. When the tall

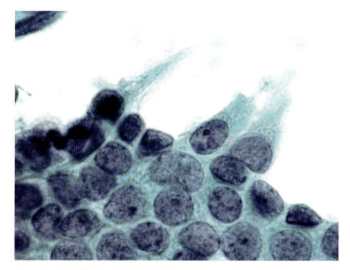

Figure 16. Tall cells in the cribriform variant of papillary thyroid carcinoma (Papanicolaou, ×100).

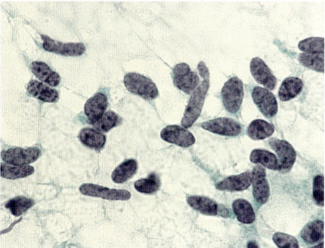

Figure 17. Spindle cells in medullary thyroid carcinoma (Papanicolaou, ×100).

cell variant of PTC is isolated, they may resemble spindle cells. Schwannoma is rarely aspirated as a thyroid tumor.

Tail-like cytoplasmic elongation

MTC cells have tail-like cytoplasmic elongation. As the cytoplasm is faintly stained and the cell border is indistinct, the findings are frequently obscure in Papanicolaou staining. Immunocytochemical staining using calcitonin or carcinoembryonic antigen can highlight the tail-like extension (Figure 18). The tall cell and cribriform variants of PTC also display cytoplasmic elongation toward the outside of cell clusters.

Cytoplasm

Oxyphilic cells

Oxyphilic cells (Hürthle cells, oncocytes) are polygonal cells with abundant, fine granular, acidophilic cytoplasm, and a distinct cell border, and they contain a vast number of mitochondria. They are found throughout the body, including the kidneys, salivary gland, and parathyroid, as well as the thyroid gland. Oxyphilic cells can appear in a variety of thyroid conditions, such as

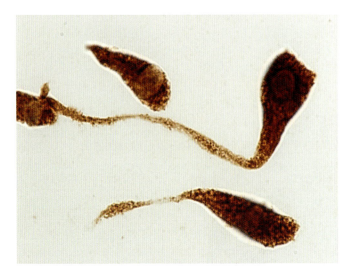

Figure 18. Tail-like cytoplasmic elongation in medullary thyroid carcinoma (calcitonin immunostaining, liquid-based cytology, ×100).

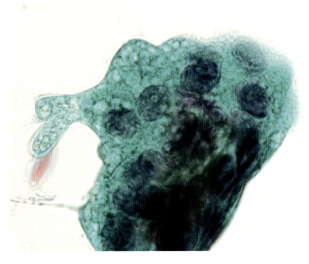

Figure 19. Septate intracytoplasmic vacuoles in papillary thyroid carcinoma (Papanicolaou, ×100).

Hashimoto's thyroiditis (please refer to Chapter 13), nodular goiter, Warthin tumor-like PTC, the oxyphilic cell variant of follicular neoplasm, and MTC (please refer to Chapter 15). Hashimoto's thyroiditis and Warthin tumor-like PTC are associated with lymphocytes in the background

Septate intracytoplasmic vacuoles (SIVs)

SIVs, which represent one of the characteristic findings of PTC, are small, uniform, well-defined vacuoles separated by defined strands of cytoplasm, resembling tiny champagne bubbles (Figure 19). SIVs are present in some cells in approximately 50% cases of PTC, whereas they are rarely observed in other thyroid diseases (18). Histologically, PTC cells with SIVs are limited to the hobnail-shaped cells located at papillary configurations or floating tumor cells within the papillary lumen (19).

Intracytoplasmic lumina (ICLs)

ICLs are distinct, intracytoplasmic spherical structures (Hector's hole) enclosed by the cell membrane. ICLs are 5–10 μm in diameter, and they sometimes contain inspissated secreted material (magenta body). They have been observed in adenocarcinomas, particularly of the

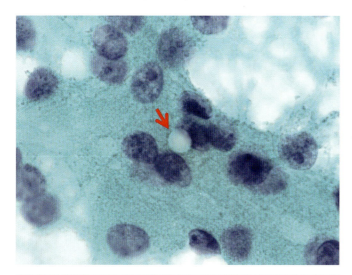

Figure 20. Intracytoplasmic lumina in the oxyphilic cell variant of follicular neoplasm (arrow) (Papanicolaou, ×100).

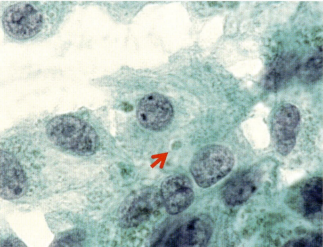

Figure 21. Yellow body in hyalinizing trabecular tumor (arrow) (Papanicolaou, ×100).

breast. In general, their presence is a cytological clue indicating adenocarcinoma. However, in the thyroid, they have not always indicated malignancy. ICLs have been observed in both benign and malignant thyroid lesions, including nonneoplastic oxyphilic cell lesions, oxyphilic cell adenomas/carcinomas (Figure 20), and medullary carcinomas (20). We should be aware that ICLs may appear in nonmalignant thyroid lesions.

Yellow bodies

Yellow bodies are highly characteristic of hyalinizing trabecular tumors. The bodies are usually round (spherical), but they may be irregular or vacuolated. They can measure up to 5 μm in diameter, and they are surrounded by a clear space (Figure 21). They are slightly refractile and yellow in HE staining and pale blue-green in Papanicolaou staining (please refer to Figures 9 and 13 in Chapter 12). They probably represent giant lysosomes (1).

Paravacuolar granules

Paravacuolar granules are tiny granules of lipofuscin or hemosiderin in small, clear

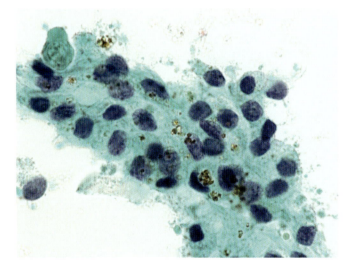

Figure 22. Paravacuolar granules in nodular goiter (Papanicolaou, ×100).

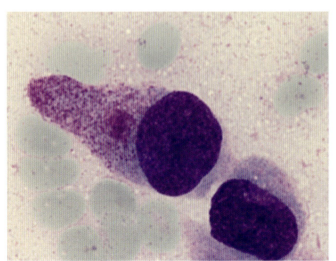

Figure 23. Metachromatic granules in medullary thyroid carcinoma (Giemsa, ×100).

cytoplasmic vacuoles (Figure 22). The findings are common in nodular goiter with degenerative changes (1), as highlighted by Giemsa staining. As paravacuolar granules do not appear in follicular neoplasms and PTC, their presence is a hallmark of nonneoplastic lesions.

Metachromatic granules

Metachromasia describes the appearance of a color different from that of the dye used for staining (please refer to Chapter 31). Cytoplasmic granules in the cytoplasm of neuroendocrine tumors are metachromatic, and they stain red-purple in Giemsa staining. MTC cells with abundant cytoplasm may represent metachromatic granules (Figure 23) (21). The finding is useful for distinguishing MTC from oxyphilic cell tumors that have granular cytoplasm.

Emperipolesis

Emperipolesis is the presence of an intact cell within the cytoplasm of another cell. The phenomenon is not phagocytosis, in which the engulfed cells are killed by the lysosomal enzymes of macrophages. Emperipolesis is due to the active penetration of one cell into another cell. Its etiopathogenesis is uncertain. We frequently encounter megakaryocytes containing neutrophils in normal bone marrow or myeloproliferative disorders. The hallmark of Rosai-Dorfman disease is emperipolesis, in which there are lymphocytes within the cytoplasm of histiocytes. In the thyroid, anaplastic carcinoma cells may contain neutrophils (Figure 24) (22). Rosai-Dorfman disease may involve the thyroid.

Nuclei

Ground-glass nuclei

The chromatin of PTC is usually pale and finely granular, producing a powdery, dusty chromatin, or ground-glass appearance (Figure 25). The heterochromatin is scant and pushed to the edge of the nuclei. As the clear appearance resembles the empty eyes of a popular comic character called Orphan Annie, the nuclei are also called "orphan Annie eye nuclei." The chromatin pattern is highly specific for PTC, but the chromatin in some PTCs can be coarse and dark (23). In LBC specimens, ground-glass nuclei are not recognized (17).

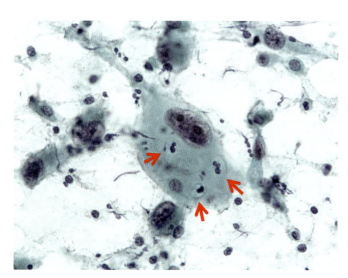

Figure 24. Emperipolesis (arrows) in anaplastic carcinoma (Papanicolaou, ×100).

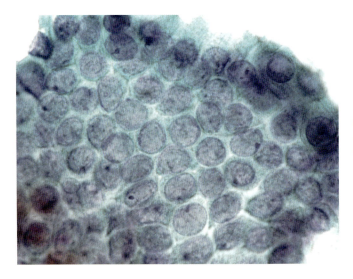

Figure 25. Ground glass nuclei in papillary thyroid carcinoma (Papanicolaou, ×100).

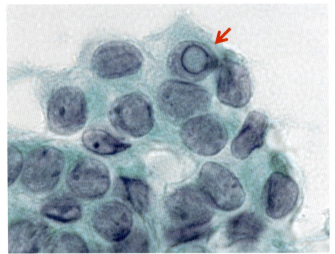

Figure 26. Intranuclear cytoplasmic inclusion in papillary thyroid carcinoma (arrow) (Papanicolaou, ×100).

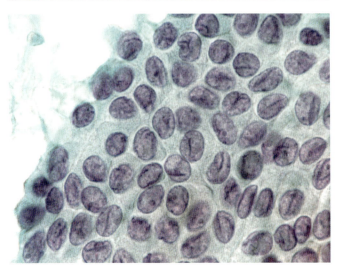

Figure 27. Nuclear grooves in papillary thyroid carcinoma (Papanicolaou, ×100).

Intranuclear cytoplasmic inclusions

Nuclear (intranuclear) cytoplasmic inclusions (NCIs) are cytoplasmic components enclosed by the nuclear membrane within nuclei (24,25). They are formed by invagination of the nuclear membrane by cytoplasmic components. Therefore, NCIs are called pseudoinclusions. NCIs are round, sharply demarcated, and similar to cytoplasmic staining in color (Figure 26). It is important to identify chromatin clumping at the outer edge of the nuclear membrane enclosing the inclusion. On careful search of adequate cytologic specimens, NCIs can be found in the vast majority of PTCs (>90%) (26,27). NCIs are not specific for PTC, and they can occur in other thyroid tumors, such as hyalinizing trabecular tumor, MTC, anaplastic carcinoma, and metastatic renal cell carcinoma. Hyalinizing trabecular tumors contain NCIs more frequently than PTC. Multiple intranuclear pseudoinclusions ("soap bubbles") in the nucleus may strongly suggest PTC.

Nuclear grooves

Nuclear grooves are longitudinal folds along the long axis of nuclei (Figure 27). They are usually present in PTC, but they may be sparse in 25% of cases (28) and absent in up to 10% of cases (29). Nuclear grooves are not specific for PTC, and they can be present in the other thyroid diseases, both benign and malignant (30). In our experience, the presence of prominent nuclear grooves or more than two folds in one nuclear is highly suggestive of PTC.

Nuclear overlapping

Nuclear overlapping is one of the nuclear findings characteristic of PTC. It reflects an extremely high nuclear/cytoplasmic ratio, and it is typified by haphazardly arranged nuclei with enlargement. The aggregates of such nuclei are called an "egg-basket" on histologic sectioning. In cytologic specimens, nuclear overlapping is observed as a thickened nuclear membrane at the point of contact of two nuclei (Figure 28) (31). In LBC specimens, nuclear overlapping is rarely observed because of the shrinkage of the nuclei and cytoplasm (17).

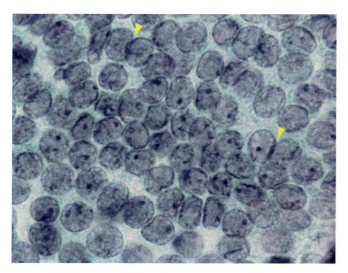

Figure 28. Nuclear overlapping in papillary thyroid carcinoma (arrowheads) (Papanicolaou, ×100).

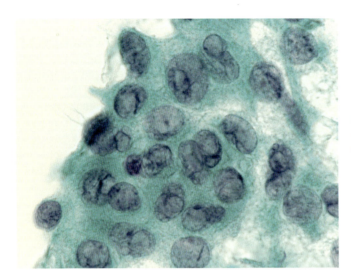

Figure 29. Polylobated nuclei in papillary thyroid carcinoma (Papanicolaou, ×100).

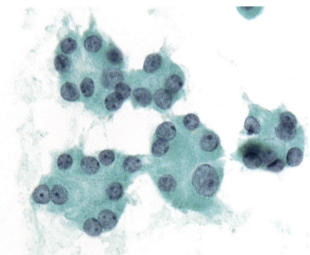

Figure 30. Binucleated cells in the oxyphilic cell variant of follicular neoplasm (Papanicolaou, ×100).

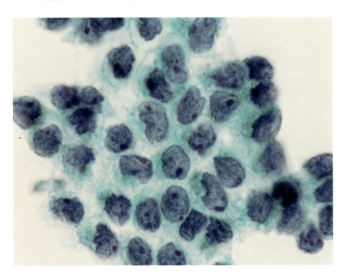

Figure 31. Convoluted nuclei in papillary thyroid carcinoma (Papanicolaou, liquid-based cytology, ×100)

Polylobulated nuclei

The nuclei of PTC frequently exhibit nuclear indentation. When the indentation is marked and multiple, the nuclei become be polylobulated (Figure 29). The appearance resembles that of the convoluted nuclei of T-cell lymphoma. Polylobulated nuclei can be present in poorly differentiated carcinoma.

Binucleated cells

Binucleated cells may be found in neoplastic cells. Concerning FNA cytology of the thyroid, the oxyphilic cell variant of follicular neoplasm (Figure 30) and MTC frequently exhibit binucleated cells (please refer to Chapter 15) (32).

Convoluted nuclei

Convoluted nuclei denote a zigzag irregularity occupying more than half of the nuclear membrane, and they are characteristic of PTC in LBC specimens (Figure 31). They are observed in 40% of LBC specimens in cases of PTC, but they are rarely detected in conventional specimens (17). The findings are rarely observed in nodular goiter and never observed in follicular neoplasms.

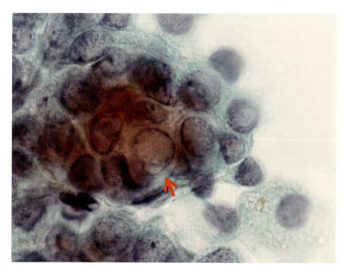

Figure 32. Peculiar nuclear clearing in the cribriform variant of papillary thyroid carcinoma (arrow) (Papanicolaou, ×100).

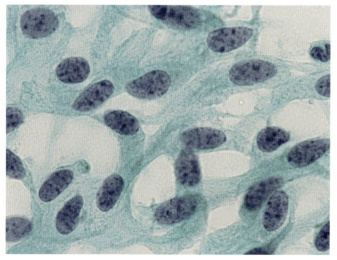

Figure 33. Salt-and-pepper chromatin in medullary thyroid carcinoma (Papanicolaou, ×100).

Peculiar nuclear clearing (PNC)

PNC is a pale-staining area occupying most of the nuclei (Figure 32). Condensed chromatin may be observed at the periphery of the nuclei. PNC is a true inclusion that is rich in biotin. PNC is characteristically observed in the cribriform variant of PTC (CV-PTC), and the presence has not been reported in any other thyroid conditions (please refer to Chapter 9). On FNA cytology, the incidence of PNC is 63% in CV-PTCs (33). PNC may resemble NCIs. Whereas NCIs exhibit similar staining as the cytoplasm and they are surrounded by the nuclear membrane, PNC is clear, and it does not display cytoplasmic staining (33). In addition, the border is obscure.

Salt-and-pepper chromatin

Salt-and-pepper chromatin (stippled chromatin) denotes a coarse granular, stippled chromatin pattern. It is characteristic of neuroendocrine tumors, such as MTC (Figure 33) (please refer to Chapters 15–16) (1), parathyroid tumor (please refer to Figure 12 in Chapter 18), pheochromocytoma, pituitary adenoma, and other neuroendocrine tumors/carcinomas. The nuclei of oxyphilic cell tumor may exhibit a similar chromatin pattern. We should know that parathyroid adenoma with salt-and-pepper chromatin can occur in the thyroid.

Reference

1. DeMay RM. Thyroid. In: The art and science of cytopathology. 2nd edit. Volume 2, Superficial Aspiration cytology, Chicago: ASCP Press; 2012: p.860-924.
2. Afify AM, Liu J, Al-Khafaji BM. Cytologic artifacts and pitfalls of thyroid fine-needle aspiration using ThinPrep: a comparative retrospective review. *Cancer* 2001;93:179-186.
3. Fadda G, Rossi ED, Raffaelli M, et al. Fine-Needle aspiration biopsy of thyroid lesions processed by thin-layer cytology: one-year institutional experience with histologic correlation. *Thyroid* 2006;16:975-981.
4. Löwhagen T, Granberg PO, Lundell G, et al. Aspiration biopsy cytology (ABC) in nodules of the thyroid gland suspected to be malignant. *Surg Clin North Am* 1979;9:3-18.
5. Basu D, Jayaram G: A logistic model for thyroid lesions. *Diagn Cytopathol* 1992;8:23-27.
6. Khurana R, Agarwal A, Bajpai VK, et al. Unraveling the amyloid associated with human medullary thyroid carcinoma. *Endocrinology* 2004;145:5465-5470.
7. Albores-Saavedra J, LiVolsi VA, Williams ED. Medullary carcinoma. *Semin Diagn Pathol* 1985;2:137-146.
8. Bose S, Kapila K, Verma K. Medullary carcinoma of the thyroid: a cytological, immunocytochemical and ultrastructural study. *Diagn Cytopathol* 1992;8:28-32.
9. Nobuoka Y, Hirokawa M, Kuma S, et al. Cytological findings and differential diagnoses of primary thyroid MALT lymphoma with striking plasma cell differentiation and amyloid deposition. *Diagn Cytopathol* 2014;42:73-77.
10. Das DK, Mallik MK, HajiBE,et al. Psammoma body and itsprecursors in papillary thyroid carcinoma: a study by fine-needle aspiration cytology. *Diagn Cytopathol* 2004;31:380-386.
11. Johannessen JV, Sobrinho-Simões M. The originand significance of thyroid psammoma bodies. *Lab Invest* 1980;43:287-296.
12. Klinck GH, WinshipT. Psammomabodiesand thyroid cancer. *Cancer* 1959;12:656-662.
13. Rosai J. Papillary carcinoma. *Monogr Pathol* 1993;35:138-165.
14. Das DK, Sheikh ZA, George SS, et al. Papillary thyroid carcinoma: evidence for intracytoplasmic formation of precursor substance for calcification and its release from well-preserved neoplastic cells. *Diagn Cytopathol* 2008;36:809-812.
15. Ali SZ, Cibas ES. The Bethesda system for reporting thyroid cytopathology: Definitions, criteria and explanatory notes. New York: Springer; 2010. p15-51.
16. Szporn AH, Yuan S, Wu M, et al. Cellular swirls in fine needle aspirates of papillary thyroid carcinoma: a new diagnostic criterion. *Mod Pathol* 2006;19: 1470–1473.

17. Suzuki A, Hirokawa M, Higuchi M, et al. Cytological characteristics of papillary thyroid carcinoma on LBC specimens, compared with conventional specimens. *Diagn Cytopathol* 2015;43:108-113.
18. Miller TR, Bottles K, Holly E, et al. A stepwise logistic regression analysis of papillary carcinoma of the thyroid. *Acta Cytol* 1986;30:285-293.
19. Hirokawa M, Kanahara T, Habara T, et al. Dilated rough endoplasmic reticulum corresponding to septate cytoplasmic vacuoles in papillary thyroid carcinoma. *Diagn Cytopathol* 2000;23:351-353.
20. Suzuki A, Hirokawa M, Takada N, et al. Thyroid follicular adenoma with numerous intracytoplasmic lumina mimicking yellow bodies: a case report. *Cytopathol* 2016 [Epub ahead of print].
21. Kini SR. Color atlas of differential diagnosis in exfoliative and aspiration cytopathology. Philadelphia: Lippincott Williams & Wilkins; 1999. p. 271.
22. Kini SR. Color atlas of differential diagnosis in exfoliative and aspiration cytopathology. Philadelphia: Lippincott Williams & Wilkins; 1999. p. 251.
23. Albores-Saavedra J, Wu J. The many faces and mimics of papillary thyroid carcinoma. *Endocr Pathol* 2006;17:1-18.
24. Kaneko C, Shamoto M, Niimi H, et al. Studies on intranuclear inclusions and nuclear grooves in papillary thyroid cancer by light, scanning electron and transmission electron microscopy. *Acta Cytol* 1996;40:417-422.
25. Serra S, Asa SL. Controversies in thyroid pathology: the diagnosis of follicular neoplasms. *Endocr Pathol* 2008;19:156-165.
26. Christ ML, Haja J. Intranuclear cytoplasmic inclusions (invaginations) in thyroid aspirations. Frequency and specificity. *Acta Cytol* 1979;23:327-331.
27. Das DK. Intranuclear cytoplasmic inclusions in fine-needle aspiration smears of papillary thyroid carcinoma: a study of its morphological forms, association with nuclear grooves, and mode of formation. *Diagn Cytopathol* 2005;32:264-268.
28. Harach HR, Soto MS, Zusman SB, et al. Parenchymatous thyroid nodules: a histocytological study of 31 cases from a goitrous area. *J Clin Pathol* 1992;45:25-29.
29. Bhambhani S, Kashyap V, Das DK. Nuclear grooves: Valuable diagnostic feature in May-Grünwald-Giemsa-stained fine needle aspirates of papillary carcinoma of the thyroid. *Acta Cytol* 1990;34:809-812.
30. Carney JA, Ryan J, Goellner JR. Hyalinizing trabecular adenoma of the thyroid gland. *Am J Surg Pathol* 1987;11:583-591.
31. Hirokawa M, Odawara Y, Kanahara T. Cytologlcal findings corresponding to overlapping nuclei seen in histological sections. *J Jpn Soc Clin Cytol* 1998;37:10-12 [in Japanese].
32. Kini SR. Color atlas of differential diagnosis in exfoliative and aspiration cytopathology. Philadelphia: Lippincott Williams & Wilkins; 1999. p. 280.
33. Hirokawa M, Maekawa M, Kuma S, et al. Cribriform-morular variant of papillary thyroid carcinoma--cytological and immunocytochemical findings of 18 cases. *Diagn Cytopathol* 2010;38:890-896.

Subject Index

A

Active surveillance *4, 283, 284, 286, 287, 288, 289*

Adenomatous nodule *53, 64, 142, 257, 259*

American system (see also Bethesda system and TBSRTC) *14, 17, 18, 23, 24, 26, 177, 278*

American Thyroid Association *12, 14, 21, 27, 29, 57, 58, 174, 241, 289, 290*

Amyloid *130, 131, 132, 133, 135, 139, 142, 146, 148, 150, 214, 252, 271, 273, 310, 311, 326*

Anaplastic thyroid carcinoma (see also Undifferentiated carcinoma) *12, 13*

Architectural atypia *34, 51, 52, 59, 275, 278*

Artifact *17, 45, 47, 51, 52, 54, 57, 171, 196, 231, 251, 279, 311, 326*

Atypia of Undetermined Significance *12, 21, 29, 42, 47, 53, 58, 59, 60, 192, 241, 250, 277, 278, 281, 290, 291, 295*

Atypical adenoma *67, 144, 163*

B

Beta-catenin *86, 87, 90, 91, 187*

Bethesda system *9, 10, 13, 21, 22, 28, 29, 33, 38, 41, 42, 46, 49, 50, 52, 58, 59, 60, 62, 64, 67, 77, 174, 183, 231, 241, 281, 282, 283, 290, 291, 292, 295, 296, 300, 326*

Borderline tumor *8, 24, 42, 180, 283, 286, 287*

BRAF *12, 21, 26, 29, 59, 60, 67, 92, 93, 98, 237, 239, 241, 242, 306, 307*

British system *23, 24, 27, 49, 56, 62, 64, 123, 177, 278*

C

Calcification *39, 43, 47, 61, 69, 70, 146, 148, 201, 213, 214, 225, 228, 244, 245, 246, 260, 269, 270, 271, 303, 312, 326*

Calcitonin *12, 111, 133, 134, 138, 139, 141, 144, 145, 146, 147, 148, 198, 200, 206, 232, 234, 243, 271, 273, 311, 318*

Carcinoembryonic antigen *12, 138, 150, 234, 318*

Carcinoma showing thymus-like differentiation *12, 16, 151, 156, 157, 185, 191, 232*

C cell *3, 12, 18, 51, 64, 132, 134, 142, 144, 145, 146, 147, 149, 150, 155, 162, 163,*

187, 200, 202, 203, 232, 255, 261, 263, 266, 271

CD5 *154, 155, 156, 157, 232, 234*

CD10 *192, 194, 195, 196, 197, 232, 234*

Cellular follicular adenoma *178, 179, 182, 183*

Chromogranin A *148, 163, 166, 232, 234*

Clear cell *142, 196, 197*

Columnar cell *2, 80, 81, 82, 89, 93, 95, 96, 97, 98, 272, 317*

Complications *4, 11, 216, 217, 220, 221, 223, 224, 243, 246, 283*

Core needle biopsy *12, 130, 221, 223, 244*

Cribriform *2, 12, 81, 82, 83, 84, 86, 89, 90, 91, 92, 187, 188, 232, 314, 317, 318, 325, 326, 327*

Cyst *2, 4, 12, 30, 33, 34, 38, 51, 52, 53, 57, 58, 69, 70, 71, 74, 75, 77, 167, 210, 256, 259, 262, 269, 272, 278, 293, 294, 295, 297, 298, 299, 300, 301, 302, 303, 304, 307, 308*

Cytokeratin *43, 111, 113, 114, 127, 129, 154, 157, 187, 234*

D

Differentiated carcinoma *3, 11, 185, 190, 289*

E

Ectopic thyroid *4, 297, 299, 300, 304, 305, 307*

Endocrine atypia *163*

F

False negative *219, 285, 288, 300*

False positive *67, 172, 288*

Follicular lesion of undetermined significance *12, 21, 29, 47, 53, 58, 59, 60, 192, 241, 255, 258, 290, 291*

Follicular neoplasm *3, 12, 23, 26, 28, 31, 34, 42, 47, 49, 50, 51, 57, 62, 64, 89, 107, 111, 132, 144, 162, 163, 164, 168, 170, 171, 172, 177, 183, 184, 186, 192, 194, 196, 197, 221, 223, 229, 258, 260, 261, 263, 265, 268, 270, 277, 278, 279, 283, 289, 290, 295, 309, 311, 312, 313, 317, 319, 321, 324, 325, 327*

Follicular thyroid carcinoma *12, 15, 17, 22, 64, 182, 184, 189, 214, 238, 242, 284, 290, 291, 292, 303, 304*

Follicular tumor of uncertain malignant potential *8, 12, 15, 182*

Follicular variant *8, 9, 12, 15, 16, 17, 22, 24, 26, 28, 29, 34, 42, 46, 47, 49, 50, 54, 59, 62, 64, 66, 67, 68, 120, 124, 177, 180, 184, 196, 257, 267, 275, 279, 282, 286, 289, 290, 291*

G

GATA-3 *163, 164, 167, 234*

Giant cell *33, 39, 41, 43, 44, 45, 47, 99, 100, 101, 102, 103, 105, 106, 113, 115, 116, 117, 118, 132, 133, 141, 142, 144, 146, 148, 149, 150, 207, 211, 214, 216, 226, 268, 273, 274, 311, 312*

Ground glass *19, 44, 45, 52, 64, 80, 81, 84,*

85, 86, 89, 90, 228, 229, 267, 321, 322

H

Hashimoto's thyroiditis *3, 12, 33, 115, 117, 118, 119, 120, 122, 123, 124, 131, 138, 140, 141, 208, 212, 219, 264, 304, 306, 311, 319*

HBME-1 *43, 187, 279, 282, 307*

Hurthle cell *12, 16, 31, 32, 33, 34, 35, 52, 56, 57, 255, 264, 274, 275, 279, 280*

Hyalinizing trabecular *3, 8, 9, 11, 16, 41, 42, 64, 89, 107, 111, 113, 114, 232, 287, 290, 312, 319, 320, 323, 327*

I

Immunohistochemical *9, 12, 22, 29, 46, 68, 86, 92, 100, 102, 103, 109, 111, 127, 148, 154, 155, 167, 184, 187, 194, 197, 233, 234, 246, 275, 279, 290, 291*

Inadequate *17, 18, 23, 47, 50, 54, 55, 56, 57, 201, 228, 231, 246, 247, 250, 256, 259, 278, 295*

Indeterminate *2, 4, 9, 14, 16, 17, 18, 19, 21, 23, 24, 26, 27, 28, 29, 41, 42, 46, 47, 49, 50, 51, 53, 55, 56, 57, 58, 59, 62, 64, 67, 68, 115, 116, 123, 132, 144, 162, 170, 171, 172, 173, 174, 177, 178, 179, 180, 181, 182, 183, 184, 186, 194, 237, 241, 255, 256, 257, 258, 259, 260, 261, 263, 267, 268, 270, 271, 276, 277, 278, 279, 280, 281, 282, 283, 284, 286, 287, 289, 291*

Insular *89, 144, 155, 182, 189, 190, 191, 265,*
268, 314

Isolated cells *20, 61, 63, 70, 143, 144, 148, 175, 214, 229, 230*

Italian system *19, 23, 24, 26, 27, 49, 62, 64, 123, 177, 278*

K

Ki-67 (see also MIB-1) *80, 109, 111, 112, 113, 148, 154, 187, 194, 221, 228, 232, 233, 234*

L

Liquid-based cytology *11, 12, 70, 82, 164, 171, 192, 225, 228, 231, 247, 250, 279, 282*

Lobectomy *4, 26, 67, 68, 83, 88, 100, 102, 179, 182, 192, 203, 217, 283, 284, 287, 289, 292*

Lymphocytic thyroiditis *12, 38, 124, 208, 211, 212*

Lymphoepithelial lesion *127, 128, 130*

Lymphoglandular bodies *125, 130, 312*

Lymphoma *3, 12, 16, 18, 52, 125, 129, 130, 131, 252, 256, 260, 270, 285, 311, 312, 313, 325, 326*

M

Malignant lymphoma *12, 18, 52, 125, 256, 260, 270, 285*

Medullary *3, 12, 16, 18, 33, 46, 64, 89, 132, 133, 134, 135, 136, 137, 138, 139, 141, 142, 144, 146, 147, 148, 150, 155, 162, 163, 187, 200, 202, 203, 206, 232, 252,*

255, 261, 265, 271, 310, 311, 317, 318, 320, 325, 326

Metastatic *3, 33, 44, 81, 96, 97, 98, 142, 144, 145, 146, 151, 155, 162, 185, 187, 190, 192, 194, 195, 196, 197, 198, 199, 201, 202, 206, 214, 216, 232, 239, 255, 258, 264, 267, 268, 294, 303, 305, 306, 307, 317, 323*

MIB-1 (see also Ki67) *109, 111, 112, 113, 114, 146, 154, 187, 194, 232, 233, 234, 235, 236*

Microfollicle *17, 20, 27, 40, 47, 52, 56, 57, 171, 176, 180, 182, 185, 190, 268, 276, 279, 313, 314*

Mitosis *130, 142, 148, 178*

Morule *81, 84, 86, 89, 90, 92*

Mucoepidermoid carcinoma *16*

Multiple endocrine neoplasia *138*

N

Necrosis *39, 43, 46, 47, 62, 129, 142, 144, 148, 153, 154, 175, 177, 178, 211, 213, 214, 216, 217, 218, 219, 248, 256, 265, 266, 268, 271*

Neuroendocrine *17, 144, 148, 149, 155, 163, 252, 265, 321, 326*

Non-diagnostic *23, 250, 277, 278, 293, 295*

Non-Invasive Follicular Thyroid Neoplasm with Papillary-like Nuclear Features *2, 8, 11, 12, 15, 24, 41, 54, 61, 64, 120*

Nuclear atypia *17, 21, 24, 26, 51, 52, 60, 89, 117, 119, 122, 170, 177, 180, 181, 182, 216, 220, 271, 278*

Nuclear clearing *81, 84, 85, 86, 87, 89, 90, 92, 325, 326*

Nuclear crowding *17, 20, 33, 39, 48, 49, 51, 52, 53, 54, 61, 63, 168, 170, 171, 172, 176, 177, 178, 181, 182, 214*

Nuclear cytoplasmic inclusions *12, 39, 40, 47, 50, 175, 251, 265, 268*

Nuclear grooves *19, 33, 34, 38, 39, 40, 42, 43, 44, 45, 47, 49, 50, 51, 52, 62, 67, 78, 81, 82, 84, 89, 93, 96, 97*

Nuclear irregularity *19, 54, 130, 187, 195, 214, 229, 293*

Nuclear overlapping *26, 61, 168, 171, 172, 175, 180, 181, 323*

O

Observer variation *16, 17, 22, 28, 29, 64, 66, 67, 120, 184, 239, 283, 286, 289*

Overtreatment *9, 22, 26, 27, 29, 67, 68, 124, 275, 282, 283, 286, 290*

Oxyphilic *3, 42, 49, 64, 81, 107, 122, 132, 137, 138, 142, 164, 190, 255, 265, 312, 313, 318, 319, 320, 321, 324, 325, 326*

P

Pain *100, 104, 207, 213, 217, 219, 222*

Papillary cluster *42, 45, 70, 71, 73, 74, 78, 83, 225, 226, 227*

Papillary microcarcinoma *12, 14, 17, 49, 241, 284, 286, 290, 303*

Papillary thyroid carcinoma *2, 3, 8, 9, 11, 12, 15, 19, 20, 22, 28, 29, 30, 31, 38, 39, 42, 43, 46, 47, 54, 59, 62, 67, 68, 78, 82,*

83, 90, 91, 92, 93, 98, 99, 107, 112, 113, 114, 115, 120, 124, 132, 141, 151, 170, 175, 184, 191, 196, 198, 200, 214, 219, 223, 225, 231, 233, 242, 246, 248, 264, 265, 267, 269, 270, 271, 275, 279, 282, 284, 289, 290, 291, 293, 294, 295, 300, 302, 303, 304, 305, 306, 307, 308, 310, 311, 313, 314, 315, 316, 317, 318, 322, 323, 324, 325, 326, 327

Papillary thyroid carcinoma type nuclear features *2, 12, 20, 39, 265, 267, 271*

Papillary thyroid microcarcinoma *12, 93, 100, 117, 238, 289, 290, 292*

Parathyroid *3, 6, 7, 11, 12, 46, 158, 159, 160, 161, 162, 163, 164, 165, 166, 167, 170, 198, 203, 204, 205, 206, 220, 221, 234, 263, 273, 274, 305, 318, 326*

Piriform sinus *210, 262, 272*

Poorly differentiated carcinoma *3, 11, 12, 15, 16, 17, 51, 98, 144, 146, 151, 155, 162, 163, 177, 178, 179, 185, 187, 190, 191, 194, 214, 216, 255, 258, 263, 265, 266, 268, 273, 274, 325*

Powdery chromatin *33, 34, 39, 45, 52, 61, 64, 70, 73, 78, 81, 82, 113, 115, 123, 216, 275, 288, 321*

Precursor tumor *15, 16, 24, 67, 183*

Primary hyperparathyroidism *12, 158, 198, 206*

Psammoma bodies *33, 39, 42, 43, 47, 62, 73, 78, 81, 82, 86, 90, 111, 138, 252, 270, 306, 312, 316, 326*

R

Radioactive iodine *13, 51, 52, 67, 182, 207, 284, 287, 290*

Rapid on-site evaluation *4, 13, 251, 252, 254, 264*

Rapid stain *4, 251, 252*

RAS *29, 67, 237, 306, 307*

Renal cell carcinoma *3, 192, 197, 232, 323*

Repeat FNA cytology *14, 49, 51, 54, 57*

RET *26, 237, 241, 306*

Risk of malignancy *9, 10, 14, 22, 24, 26, 54, 55, 58, 59, 67, 178, 179, 183, 250, 277, 279, 280, 286, 292*

Risk stratification *2, 14, 27, 39, 42, 68, 179, 181, 283, 289*

Romanowsky *135, 148, 251, 252, 254*

S

Salt and pepper *18, 135, 139, 146, 148, 149, 163, 164, 165, 265, 271, 273, 325, 326*

Solid *14, 23, 39, 47, 61, 65, 69, 78, 86, 89, 90, 99, 109, 110, 129, 132, 142, 144, 146, 151, 152, 153, 154, 155, 157, 161, 162, 168, 175, 177, 185, 187, 189, 190, 191, 192, 193, 194, 196, 197, 202, 205, 213, 228, 250, 265, 269, 271, 291, 293, 294, 295, 299, 300, 302, 303, 314*

Specimen adequacy *17, 21, 243, 246, 252, 253*

Spindle cell *34, 81, 89, 149, 317, 318*

Squamous cell *16, 74, 145, 155, 156, 157, 167, 214, 216, 252, 272, 298, 302, 303*

Subacute thyroiditis *3, 51, 99, 100, 103, 104,*

105, 106, 195, 211, 212, 214, 219, 266, 311

Suspicious for malignancy *13, 16, 17, 18, 42, 47, 49, 50, 51, 53, 54, 55, 57, 64, 83, 123, 170, 177, 181, 263, 277, 295*

T

Tall cell *2, 78, 81, 82, 89, 96, 97, 98, 229, 231, 303, 317, 318*

TBSRTC (see also American system and Bethesda system) *13, 33, 50, 54, 55, 58, 277, 279, 283, 295*

Thymoma *3, 12, 16, 151, 155, 156, 157, 232*

Thyroglobulin *13, 43, 69, 78, 86, 88, 90, 111, 125, 133, 134, 139, 146, 148, 151, 154, 155, 164, 185, 187, 192, 196, 197, 198, 206, 207, 221, 232, 234, 283, 309*

Thyroglossal duct cyst *4, 210, 272, 297, 299, 307, 308*

Thyroidectomy *34, 69, 78, 88, 93, 96, 104, 107, 119, 123, 125, 133, 134, 135, 137, 146, 151, 158, 161, 177, 182, 185, 196, 201, 220, 221, 223, 225, 270, 275, 283, 284, 285, 289, 292, 293, 303, 304*

Thyroiditis *3, 12, 31, 33, 34, 38, 41, 42, 47, 49, 50, 51, 52, 56, 57, 62, 64, 99, 100, 103, 104, 105, 106, 115, 117, 118, 119, 120, 122, 123, 124, 125, 127, 129, 130, 131, 138, 140, 141, 151, 195, 207, 208, 210, 211, 212, 214, 216, 219, 224, 256, 260, 261, 262, 264, 266, 270, 272, 275, 303, 304, 305, 306, 311, 319*

Trabecular *3, 8, 9, 11, 16, 17, 20, 41, 42, 61,* *63, 64, 78, 79, 80, 81, 82, 89, 90, 107, 109, 110, 111, 113, 114, 144, 155, 159, 160, 163, 164, 165, 172, 178, 182, 187, 188, 189, 190, 194, 196, 197, 214, 229, 232, 265, 280, 287, 290, 310, 312, 314, 319, 320, 323, 327*

TTF1 *13, 148, 234, 306*

U

Ultrasound *7, 30, 39, 47, 48, 61, 69, 83, 93, 103, 107, 115, 120, 125, 132, 142, 151, 158, 168, 192, 199, 200, 201, 202, 204, 207, 211, 213, 225, 249, 250, 260, 272, 273, 293, 297, 300*

Undifferentiated carcinoma (see also Anaplastic carcinoma) *12, 13, 16, 100, 144, 145, 146, 149, 214, 216, 256, 263, 266, 271, 273*

W

Warthin *81, 319*

Well Differentiated Tumor of Uncertain Behavior *13*

Well differentiated tumor of uncertain malignant potential *8, 13, 42, 64, 267*

World Health Organization *13, 189, 219*

Worrisome histologic alterations following fine needle aspiration of the thyroid *13, 220, 223*

Y

Yellow bodies *108, 109, 110, 111, 112, 113, 320, 327*

How to order this book (print edition). Please enter your order through BookWay Global at http://bookway-global.com
The eBook version (reduced size version) is also available from the S&S Publications and distributed by Smashwords. (https://www.smashwords.com/books/view/655745) at $39.99.

Thyroid FNA Cytology
Differential Diagnoses & Pitfalls

Copyright ©2016 by Kakudo Medical Education
All rights reserved.
Printed by Onokousoku Insatsu Co., LTD.
Distributed by BookWay GLOBAL (https://bookway-global.com/)
 For Japanese customers, please visit at BookWay
(http://www.ohp.co.jp/webcontents/bookway.html).

No part of this publication may be reproduced, stored in a retrieval system, or transmitted in any form or by any means, electronic, mechanical, photocopying, recording, or otherwise, without the prior permission of the publisher.

Published in Japan.　　　　　　　　　　　　ISBN978-4-86584-182-4

For information contact : BookWay
ONO KOUSOKU INSATSU CO.,LTD.
62, HIRANO-MACHI, HIMEJI-CITY, HYOGO 670-0933 JAPAN
(Phone) 079-222-5372 (Fax) 079-223-3523